METHODS IN CANCER RESEARCH

Volume XIX

TUMOR MARKERS

Contributors to This Volume

V. P. BHAVANANDAN

REBECCA BLACKSTOCK

HARRIS BUSCH

ROSE K. BUSCH

SUBHAS CHAKRABARTY

PUI-KWONG CHAN

BYUNG-KIL CHOE

T. M. CHU

E. A. DAVIDSON

SHELDON DRAY

HAROLD A. HOPKINS

G. BENNETT HUMPHREY

DAVID KELSEY

M. KURIYAMA

K. W. LO

WILLIAM B. LOONEY

R. M. LOOR

MARGALIT B. MOKYR

G. P. MURPHY

L. D. PAPSIDERO

NOEL R. ROSE

KEI TAKAHASHI

CHARLES W. TAYLOR

K. C. TSOU

L. A. VALENZUELA

M. C. WANG

LYNN C. YEOMAN

METHODS IN CANCER RESEARCH
Volume XIX
TUMOR MARKERS

Edited by

HARRIS BUSCH

DEPARTMENT OF PHARMACOLOGY
BAYLOR COLLEGE OF MEDICINE
HOUSTON, TEXAS

and

LYNN C. YEOMAN

DEPARTMENT OF PHARMACOLOGY
BAYLOR COLLEGE OF MEDICINE
HOUSTON, TEXAS

ACADEMIC PRESS 1982

A Subsidiary of Harcourt Brace Jovanovich, Publishers

New York   London
Paris   San Diego   San Francisco   São Paulo
Sydney   Tokyo   Toronto

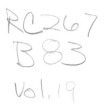

ACADEMIC PRESS, INC.
111 Fifth Avenue, New York, New York 10003

United Kingdom Edition published by
ACADEMIC PRESS, INC. (LONDON) LTD.
24/28 Oval Road, London NW1 7DX

LIBRARY OF CONGRESS CATALOG CARD NUMBER: 66–29495

ISBN 0–12–147679–0

PRINTED IN THE UNITED STATES OF AMERICA

82 83 84 85   9 8 7 6 5 4 3 2 1

Contents

CELL SURFACE MARKERS FOR NEOPLASIA

CHAPTER I.　**Surface Markers in the Characterization of Leukemias**

Rebecca Blackstock and G. Bennett Humphrey

CHAPTER II.　**Cell Surface Glycoprotein Markers for Neoplasia**

V. P. Bhavanandan and E. A. Davidson

ANTIGEN MARKERS OF TUMOR CELLS AND NUCLEI

CHAPTER III.   **Nucleolar Antigens of Human Tumors**

Harris Busch, Rose K. Busch, Pui-Kwong Chan, David Kelsey, and Kei Takahashi

CHAPTER IV.   **Prostate Antigen of Human Cancer Patients**

M. C. Wang, M. Kuriyama, L. D. Papsidero, R. M. Loor, L. A. Valenzuela, G. P. Murphy, and T. M. Chu

CHAPTER V.   **Prostatic Acid Phosphatase: A Marker for Human Prostatic Adenocarcinoma**

Byung-Kil Choe and Noel R. Rose

CHAPTER VI.   **Human Colon Tumor Antigens**

Lynn C. Yeoman, Charles W. Taylor, and Subhas Chakrabarty

CHAPTER VII.   **5′-Nucleotide Phosphodiesterase and Liver Cancer**

K. C. Tsou and K. W. Lo

MODELS AND METHODS FOR DIAGNOSIS AND THERAPY

CHAPTER VIII.   **Solid Tumors as a Model for the Development of Antineoplastic Therapy**

William B. Looney and Harold A. Hopkins

CHAPTER IX.   *In Vitro* **Immunization as a Method for Generating Cytotoxic Cells Potentially Useful in Adoptive Immunotherapy**

Margalit B. Mokyr and Sheldon Dray

List of Contributors

Numbers in parentheses indicate the pages on which the authors' contributions begin.

V. P. BHAVANANDAN (53), Department of Biological Chemistry, The Milton S. Hershey Medical Center, Pennsylvania State University, Hershey, Pennsylvania 17033

REBECCA BLACKSTOCK (3), Department of Pediatrics, University of Oklahoma Health Sciences Center, Oklahoma City, Oklahoma 73190

HARRIS BUSCH (109), Department of Pharmacology, Baylor College of Medicine, Houston, Texas 77030

ROSE K. BUSCH (109), Department of Pharmacology, Baylor College of Medicine, Houston, Texas 77030

SUBHAS CHAKRABARTY (233), Nuclear Protein Laboratory, Department of Pharmacology, Baylor College of Medicine, Houston, Texas 77030

PUI-KWONG CHAN (109), Department of Pharmacology, Baylor College of Medicine, Houston, Texas 77030

BYUNG-KIL CHOE (199), Department of Immunology and Microbiology, Wayne State University School of Medicine, Detroit, Michigan 48201

T. M. CHU (179), Department of Diagnostic Immunology Research and Biochemistry, Roswell Park Memorial Institute, Buffalo, New York 14263

E. A. DAVIDSON (53), Department of Biological Chemistry, The Milton S. Hershey Medical Center, Pennsylvania State University, Hershey, Pennsylvania 17033

SHELDON DRAY (385), Department of Microbiology and Immunology, University of Illinois at the Medical Center, Chicago, Illinois 60612

HAROLD A. HOPKINS (303), Division of Radiobiology and Biophysics, University of Virginia School of Medicine, Charlottesville, Virginia 22908

G. BENNETT HUMPHREY (3), Department of Hematology/Oncology, Oklahoma Children's Memorial Hospital, Oklahoma City, Oklahoma 73126

DAVID KELSEY (109), Department of Pharmacology, Baylor College of Medicine, Houston, Texas 77030

M. KURIYAMA (179), Department of Diagnostic Immunology Research and Biochemistry, Roswell Park Memorial Institute, Buffalo, New York 14263

K. W. LO (273), Westvaco Research Center, 11101 Johns Hopkins Road, Laurel, Maryland 20810

ix

WILLIAM B. LOONEY (303), Division of Radiobiology and Biophysics, University of Virginia School of Medicine, Charlottesville, Virginia 22908

R. M. LOOR (179), Department of Diagnostic Immunology Research and Biochemistry, Roswell Park Memorial Institute, Buffalo, New York 14263

MARGALIT B. MOKYR (385), Department of Microbiology and Immunology, University of Illinois at the Medical Center, Chicago, Illinois 60612

G. P. MURPHY (179), National Prostatic Cancer Project, Roswell Park Memorial Institute, Buffalo, New York 14263

L. D. PAPSIDERO (179), Department of Diagnostic Immunology Research and Biochemistry, Roswell Park Memorial Institute, Buffalo, New York 14263

NOEL R. ROSE (199), Department of Immunology and Microbiology, Wayne State University School of Medicine, Detroit, Michigan 48201

KEI TAKAHASHI (109), Department of Pharmacology, Baylor College of Medicine, Houston, Texas 77030

CHARLES W. TAYLOR (233), Nuclear Protein Laboratory, Department of Pharmacology, Baylor College of Medicine, Houston, Texas 77030

K. C. TSOU (273), Harrison/Surgical Research, University of Pennsylvania, Philadelphia, Pennsylvania 19104

L. A. VALENZUELA (179), Department of Diagnostic Immunology Research and Biochemistry, Roswell Park Memorial Institute, Buffalo, New York 14263

M. C. WANG (179), Department of Diagnostic Immunology Research and Biochemistry, Roswell Park Memorial Institute, Buffalo, New York 14263

LYNN C. YEOMAN (233), Nuclear Protein Laboratory, Department of Pharmacology, Baylor College of Medicine, Houston, Texas 77030

Preface

The subject of "tumor markers" is becoming of great interest to oncologists. A number of opportunities exist in this area, particularly for diagnosis of cancer and assessment of body burden either by direct interactions between antigens of cancer cells and specific antibodies or by the products produced in cancer cells that may exhibit sufficiently distinctive features for clinical utility.

Beginning with Volume II, this treatise has dealt with immunology and special products of cancer cells. Volumes XIX and XX are specifically related to newer information on tumor markers. In Volume XIX, cell surface markers for leukemias and other neoplasms are dealt with in the first section. The second section deals with nucleolar antigens, colon tumor antigens, and prostate antigens, as well as with acid phosphatase and phosphodiesterase as specific markers. It also deals with specific models and methods for diagnosis and therapy.

Not much is understood about the mechanisms involved in the production of tumor markers at the level of either gene control, activation of fetal genes, or quantitative variations in phenotypic differentiation.

It is a pleasure to welcome Dr. Lynn Yeoman as coeditor of these two volumes, and I am grateful for his willingness to participate. It is our hope that the topics presented are timely and useful to investigators in these and related fields.

HARRIS BUSCH

Contents of Other Volumes

VOLUME V

VOLUME VI

VOLUME XIV

VOLUME XV

CELL SURFACE MARKERS FOR NEOPLASIA

CHAPTER I

CELL SURFACE MARKERS IN THE CHARACTERIZATION OF LEUKEMIAS

REBECCA BLACKSTOCK AND G. BENNETT HUMPHREY

I. Introduction

The decade of the 1970s saw a redefinition of acute lymphoblastic leukemia (ALL) by the use of immunological markers. Three major groups having prognostic significance and therapeutic implications have already been defined within ALL. Immunological markers have also illustrated the remarkable heterogeneity within this malignancy.

There is now intensive research activity relating to the use of immunological markers in ALL. Various aspects of this application of markers to leukemia have recently been reviewed: management (Bowman and Mauer, 1981), anatomy (Kay *et al.*, 1979), enumeration of subpopulations (Ross, 1979), T lymphoblastic malignancies (Nadler *et al.*, 1980a), histopathologic and histochemical correlations in lymphomas (Collins *et al.*,

3

1979), interrelationships between leukemia and lymphoma in children (Kersey *et al.*, 1979), morphological correlations (Palutke and Tabaczka, 1980), cytochemical correlations (Huhn, 1980), cellular interactions of subgroups (Miller, 1979), subpopulations in immunodeficiency and lymphoproliferative disorders (Gupta and Good, 1980), and lymphoma and acute and chronic leukemias (Aisenberg, 1981; Callihan and Berard, 1980). The reader is referred to these review articles for additional information.

It has been necessary to limit the scope of this present chapter in several ways. Methods used to identify receptors or antigens on lymphoid cells and lymphoblasts freshly isolated from human subjects will be emphasized. The recent clinical application (publications of the last 2 to 3 years) of immunological markers will be limited to ALL although it should be noted that the principles described apply as well to their use with the myeloid leukemias, the chronic leukemias, and immunodeficiency diseases. ALL was chosen because it affects both children and adults and because of the large number of cases which have been under study for a number of years. Results of the analysis of human lymphoblastic cell lines will not be included because of the possible selection of subtypes in the culturing process even though much can be learned from the study of them (Minowada *et al.*, 1980, 1981a,b).

TABLE I

RESEARCH STUDIES BEING UNDERTAKEN TO BETTER DEFINE ALL

Host	Lymphoblast
Genetics	Morphology
Acton and Barger (1981)	Bennett *et al.* (1981)
Immune status	Hormone receptors
Kersey *et al.* (1979)	Mastrangelo *et al.* (1980)
Clinical status	Enzymes
Boyd *et al.* (1979)	Blatt *et al.* (1980)
Race	Cytochemistry
Olisa *et al.* (1975)	Raney *et al.* (1979)
Response to therapy	Cytogenetics
Leimert *et al.* (1980)	Kaneko and Rowley (1981a)
Nutritional status	Immunological markers
van Eys (1977)	Gupta and Good (1980)
Age	Cytokinetics
Leimert *et al.* (1980)	Park (1980)
Carcinogenetic exposure (ecogenetics)	Metabolism
Harris *et al.* (1980)	Nishida *et al.* (1980)
Epidemiology (ecosocial)	Virology
Alderson (1980)	Stass *et al.* (1980)

It is important to remember that immunological markers are only one area of research currently being undertaken to better define ALL. Table I lists examples of studies which focus on either an analysis of the patient population with ALL (host) or evaluation of malignant lymphoblasts isolated from these patients. All of these host factors and tumor characteristics suggest heterogeneity and some are currently influencing clinical trials. The results should aid in determining the relative importance of many of the subclasses which are currently being proposed, whether they have been identified by immunological markers or by other research approaches.

II. Methods

Observations made in immune-deficient patients and in animal models led to the division of the immune system into two major arms (Miller, 1961; Miller *et al.*, 1963; Glick *et al.*, 1956; Good and Bach, 1974). Cells which differentiated in the bursa of Fabricius of avian species (or the bursa-equivalent of mammals) were identified as B-lymphocytes. These cells mature as antibody-secreting plasma cells and are responsible for humoral immunity. The thymus was found to be the site of differentiation for the other major component of the immune response, the T-cell system. T cells exhibit a variety of functions which have been described under the general heading of cell-mediated immunity.

Initial observations which indicated a greater heterogeneity of the two major subsets occurred when *in vitro* assays for the function of lymphocytes were developed. Among these advances were the ability to generate a primary humoral immune response *in vitro* (Mishell and Dutton, 1966) and various assays for cell-mediated immunity including cytotoxicity (Cerottini and Brunner, 1971), suppressor cell (Rich and Rich, 1975), and lymphokine assays (David and David, 1971). Through examination of the results of functional assays, it became apparent that subpopulations of T and B cells existed. Further delineation of lymphocytic subsets occurred after it was discovered that lymphoid subsets could be identified and separated on the basis of their differing membrane structures (Chess and Schlossman, 1977). These membrane characteristics have been called "markers." A variety of markers for T cells, B cells, and their subpopulations have been described, and they will be explained below. This discussion will emphasize the populations of normal lymphocytes which express the markers and, when possible, the functional correlate of the expression of the marker. In addition, we will mention if these markers have been detected in the leukemias. In a later section, we will describe the clinical significance of the detection of the various lymphocyte markers in the acute leukemias.

A. E-Rosettes

The first important commonly used marker for human T-lymphocytes was first described in the early 1970s (Brian *et al.*, 1979; Lay *et al.*, 1970; Jondal *et al.*, 1972). The test was performed by mixing sheep erythrocytes and lymphocytes together. Most, but not all, T-lymphocytes had SRBC attached to their membranes resulting in the formation of a "rosette." The incubation was a two-step procedure. The initial short incubation was at room temperature or 37°C (Lay *et al.*, 1971; Mendes *et al.*, 1973). After a brief centrifugation step, the pellet was incubated at 4°C from 1 to 24 hours. After careful resuspension of the cells, the rosettes could be seen by microscopic examination of the wet mount preparations. Stains were sometimes added to the cell suspension. Mahowald and co-workers (1977) reported that fluorescein staining of the lymphocytes increased the percentage of rosette-forming cells detected due to better enumeration of lymphocytes in morulas.

Many technical variations in the rosette procedure have been described, from those performed in test tubes (Jondal *et al.*, 1972) to a microrosette assay carried out in tissue typing microplates (Tilz, 1978). The presence of fetal calf serum (Mahowald *et al.*, 1977; Hepburn and Ritts, 1974) or fetuin (Gupta *et al.*, 1976a) in the buffer was reported to enhance the formation of rosettes. Rosette formation was also enhanced by increased incubation from 4 to 18 hours (Mahowald *et al.*, 1977). Other authors (Whitehead *et al.*, 1978) reported that the greatest difference between numbers of rosette-forming cells detected in patients with cancer and healthy, age-matched controls was detected when the incubation time was limited to 1.5 hours at 4°C. Various modifications of the procedure for enumeration have been reported such as direct counts on wet preparations (Jondal *et al.*, 1972; Mahowald *et al.*, 1977), differential counts on stained smears (Hepburn and Ritts, 1974; Campbell and Watter, 1979), and by automated quantitation of E-rosettes on a particle size analyzer (Brown *et al.*, 1979).

Several different treatments of the sheep erythrocytes prior to their use in the rosette assay may also result in detection of a higher percentage of T cells. Neuraminidase treatment of SRBCs or treatment of SRBCs with the sulfhydryl reagent AET enhanced the stability of the rosette and caused an increase in the number of rosettes detected (Gilbertsen and Metzgar, 1976; Kaplan and Clark, 1974; Pellegrino *et al.*, 1975a; Moore and Zusman, 1978). Since these two treatments also stabilized the rosettes from mechanical disruption, they were useful in experiments where lymphocyte subpopulations were isolated by centrifugation of rosetted cells through a Ficoll–Hypaque barrier (Wahl *et al.*, 1976). Gelfand and colleagues (1979) warned against exclusive use of AET or neuraminidase-treated sheep erythrocytes when T cells were determined as a part of an immunologic evaluation. They found that such erythrocytes prevent detection of differences in T-cell subpopulations which may exist between normal individuals and patients who had diseases which affected the T-cell system.

A modification of the E-rosette assay commonly used for determination of the total number of T-lymphocytes was developed by Wybran and his colleagues (1972, 1973). The assay depended upon the interaction of SRBC with lymphocytes which had been preincubated for 1 hour at 37°C. A lower RBC-to-lymphocyte ratio was used in this assay; lymphocytes and red blood cells were combined in a tube, which was centrifuged for 5 minutes at 200 *g* and read immediately. This assay was termed the "active" E-rosette test (Wybran *et al.*, 1976). Twenty-eight percent of peripheral blood lymphocytes formed "active" E-rosettes (Wybran and Fudenberg, 1973). It was believed that the assay detected an immunocompetent subpopulation of T-lymphocytes and therefore might be valuable in assessing the immunocompetence of cancer patients and of patients with certain immunodeficiency diseases (Wybran and Fudenberg, 1973; Wybran *et al.*, 1973, 1976; Nekam *et al.*, 1977; Horowitz *et al.*, 1975; Kerman *et al.*, 1976). Traycoff and co-workers (1979) published evidence that active rosette-forming cells behave like activated T cells. Some authors have found that the active E-rosette assay was a reliable *in vitro* correlate to the delayed hypersensitivity reaction (Felsburg and Edelman, 1977). Kerman and co-workers (1976) refuted the usefulness of the active E-rosette assay in the evaluation of cancer patients, however, they did not follow the active E-erosette methodology as originally described.

Mature T cells isolated from the peripheral blood were reported to form rosettes at 4°C, however, the rosettes were unstable and dissociated upon incubation at 37°C (Sen *et al.*, 1976). On the other hand, T cells activated by mitogens (Katoh and Charoensiri, 1978; Richie and Patchen, 1978; Sen *et al.*, 1976; Schlesinger and Kertes, 1979) or in mixed lymphocyte cultures (Galili and Schlesinger, 1976; Wybran and Govaerts, 1978) formed rosettes which were stable at 37°C.

The sensitivity of E-rosette formation to the presence of theophylline was used to divide T-lymphocytes into subgroups by Limatibul and co-workers (1978). Those T cells which did not rosette following theophylline treatment were called suppressor T-lymphocytes (Shore *et al.*, 1978).

Other adrenergic drugs also inhibited E-rosette formation while cholenergic drugs stimulated E-rosette formation (Ferreira *et al.*, 1976).

A subgroup of patients with ALL has been defined based on the ability of the leukemic blasts to rosette with sheep erythrocytes (Borella and Sen, 1974; Kersey *et al.*, 1975; Sen and Borella, 1975; Brouet *et al.*, 1976; Tsukimoto *et al.*, 1976; Humphrey *et al.*, 1978a; Thiel *et al.*, 1980; Pullen *et al.*, 1981; and Melvin, 1979). The rosettes formed by T-cell leukemias are usually stable at 37°C (Melvin, 1979; Borella and Sen, 1974; Sen and Borella, 1975), however, some investigators have reported that a small percentage of T-cell leukemias will rosette at 4 but not at 37°C (Humphrey *et al.*, 1978b, 1979; Koziner *et al.*, 1978). The T-cell leukemias have exhibited a poorer response to therapy than null ALL (to be reviewed in a later section), and therefore determination of the presence or absence of this marker has become clinically significant for the management of this disease.

B. ROSETTES WITH MOUSE ERYTHROCYTES

Stathopoulos and Elliott (1974) reported that lymphocytes from patients with chronic lymphocytic leukemia formed rosettes when mixed with mouse erythrocytes. Subsequently, Catovsky *et al.* (1975) made a similar observation using lymphocytes from hairy-cell leukemia patients. These authors also reported that 5 to 10% of normal peripheral blood lymphocytes would rosette with mouse red blood cells. This observation was confirmed by Forbes and Zalewski (1977), Gupta and Grieco (1975), and Bertoglio *et al.* (1977) who reported that normal M-rosette-forming cells were a subclass of B-lymphocyte. Double labeling experiments showed that most of the B-lymphocytes which rosetted with mouse red blood cells (MRBC) had IgM, IgD, or both on their surface (Gupta *et al.*, 1976b). Although earlier work suggested that the receptor for MRBC might be a part of the immunoglobulin molecule (Forbes and Zalewski, 1977), later investigations indicated that this receptor was different from surface Ig, C_3, or Fc receptors (Gupta *et al.*, 1976b,c).

The MRBC rosette method has been used to separate T-lymphocytes from B-lymphocytes. Papain treatment of the mouse red blood cells gave sufficient stability to the rosettes to allow subsequent separation by centrifugation through Ficoll (Zola, 1977). Others (Forbes and Zalewski, 1977) reported increased binding by prior treatment of the MRBC with neuraminidase or trypsin.

The expression of the M-rosette receptor was reported in both CLL (Stathopoulos and Elliott, 1974; Gupta *et al.*, 1976d) and in hairy-cell leukemia (Catovsky *et al.*, 1975). Others reported that hairy cell leukemia cases were negative for rosette formation with MRBC (Rosenszajn *et al.*, 1976; Catovsky *et al.*, 1975). Burns and Cawley (1980) found 8 to 15% cases of hairy cell leukemia to rosette with MRBC. They found that a higher percentage of splenic hairy cells rosetted than did hairy cells taken from the peripheral blood. Cells which expressed multiple heavy chain isotypes, including IgD, rosetted, while those that expressed sIgG only (i.e., more mature B cells) did not form rosettes. Based on these data, it appeared that the M-rosette receptor may be expressed early in B-cell differentiation and that expression on individual cells depends on the stage of development of the cell.

C. HUMAN AUTOLOGOUS ROSETTES

Human thymocytes and T cells from tonsils and peripheral blood were found to rosette with autologous erythrocytes (Baxley *et al.*, 1973). The T-cell nature of such rosette-forming cells was confirmed in several different laboratories (Kaplan, 1975; Gluckman and Montambault, 1975; Sandilands *et al.*, 1975; Caraux *et al.*, 1979). The percentage of human lymphocytes which rosetted with autologous RBC varied from 0.3% (Charreire and Bach, 1974) to 28% (Yu, 1975). The variation in reported results may be attributed to differences in the techniques used in the performance of the rosette test (Charreire and Bach, 1974; Gluckman and Legrain, 1975; Gluckman and Montambault, 1975; Yu, 1975; Lambermont *et al.*, 1977). Serum or albumin enhanced rosette formation, however, enhancement varied from one lot of serum to the next (Lambermont *et al.*, 1977; Yu, 1975). Caraux and co-workers (1979) used autologous serum in the rosette assay and they obtained $26.2 \pm 5.9\%$ rosette-forming cells among 60 normal individuals. Enhanced rosette formation occurred when lymphocytes were preincubated in autologous serum at 4°C for 30 minutes. Additionally, an 8 hour incubation of the RBC–lymphocyte mixture was required for maximal rosette-forming cells (RFC) to be detected. The ratio of RBC to lymphocyte in the assay was also important to maximize rosette formation. A 30:1 ratio was optimal. Lower ratios may be responsible for the low percentage of autologous RFC reported by others (Gluckman and Montambault, 1975). Gallinger and co-workers (1980) substituted human albumin for autologous serum and detected an increase of rosette formation. They confirmed the necessity of long, cold incubation and for counting rosettes while still cold. They reported that both $T\mu$ and $T\gamma$ T cells could rosette with H-RBC.

Initially, H-rosette-forming cells (RFC) were thought to be involved in RBC destruction (Baxley *et al.*, 1973), and autoimmunity (Charreire and Bach, 1974) or to be immature T cells (Fournier and Charreire, 1977).

These hypotheses were based on the detection of only small numbers of RFC by the investigators. These theories now seem implausible because of the high percentages of H-RFC which have since been detected by others.

D. Rosettes with Other Erythrocytes

Erythrocytes from several other species were reported to form spontaneous rosettes with human lymphocytes. Rhesus monkey red blood cells rosette primarily with T-lymphocytes (Lohrman and Novikovs, 1974) but also with "null" or "third population" lymphocytes (Chiao et al., 1978). Erythrocytes of the Macaca speciosa monkey were shown by Pellegrino and co-workers (1975a) to rosette with B-lymphocytes and perhaps some third-population lymphocytes. Pandolfi et al. (1978) described the binding of goat erythrocytes to human T-lymphocytes. Inhibitor data indicated that the receptor on the lymphocyte which binds goat RBC was the same as that responsible for binding sheep erythrocytes (Indiveri et al., 1979).

E. Surface and Cytoplasmic Immunoglobulin

B-lymphocytes carry immunoglobulin molecules on their membrane. These structures serve as the antigen recognition unit of the lymphocyte and are an integral membrane component, as opposed to immunoglobulins which are absorbed to the cell via an Fc receptor. This structure has therefore been called surface immunoglobulin (sIg). Twenty percent of peripheral blood lymphocytes in man are B-lymphocytes as determined by sIg determinations. Most B-lymphocytes express IgM alone or IgM and IgD together. A much smaller proportion of B-lymphocytes express either IgG or IgA. Abo and Kumagai (1978) reported that the total number of B cells exhibited a circadian as well as seasonal variation.

The most common method used to detect sIg is by incubation of lymphocytes with fluorescein-conjugated antiimmunoglobulin reagents. Certain precautions should be maintained to ensure the detection of sIg and not Ig absorbed to lymphocytes or monocytes via Fc or C receptors. Preincubation of lymphocytes at 37°C for at least 1 hour has been used to elute immunoglobulins bound to receptors from such cells. Some investigators have trypsinized cells and then incubated them under tissue culture conditions to allow resynthesis of sIg molecules. Additionally, many investigators use antiglobulin reagents which have had their Fc portion removed by enzymatic digestion. Reagents with high FP ratios (4 or greater) and microscopes utilizing epifluorescence have been found to be useful in the detection of B-lymphocytes (Dyer, 1976). Another detection system for sIg utilizes rosetting with polyacrylamide beads precoated with anti-globulin reagents (Chao and Yokoyama, 1977; Ammann *et al.*, 1977). Gordon and co-workers (1977) described a two-stage antiglobulin procedure in which polymeric microspheres were coated with the second antibody. Labeled cells were visualized in Giemsa-stained preparations allowing the preparation of permanent slides and evaluation of morphological detail. Rosettes formed between lymphocytes and antiimmunoglobulin-coated RBC were the basis of the mixed antiglobulin rosette assay for B-lymphocytes described by Haegert (1978). Immunoperoxidase methods (Lees, 1977; Laurent *et al.*, 1980) used to detect sIg on B-lymphocytes have the advantage of allowing permanent slides to be made. A quantitative immunoperoxidase method was described by Dighiero and co-workers (1980). The procedure allowed quantitation of surface Ig density. The authors reported that the density of sIg on chronic lymphocytic leukemia cells was less than that of normal B-lymphocytes and that the density varied less from cell to cell when malignant cells were evaluated. On the other hand, sIg was more dense on lymphocytes of prolymphocytic leukemia and densities were more heterogeneous from cell to cell than that observed with CLL cells. Recent evidence has shown that about 2% of cases of acute lymphoblastic leukemia can be classified as B-cell leukemia on the basis of their expression of surface immunoglobulin (Brouet *et al.*, 1975; Kawashima *et al.*, 1978).

In animals and in man, during the ontogeny of the lymphoreticular system, a pre-B cell develops in the fetal liver before the appearance of sIg-bearing lymphocytes (Raff *et al.*, 1976; Gathings *et al.*, 1977). The pre-B cell has IgM in its cytoplasm but lacks detectable surface immunoglobulin. Pre-B cells are found normally in adult bone marrow and it is for this reason that the adult bone marrow is thought to be analogous to the avian Bursa of Fabricius (Pearl *et al.*, 1978).

Recently, it was realized that a subgroup of patients with ALL could be classified as having leukemia of the pre-B type (Vogler *et al.*, 1978; Brouet *et al.*, 1979). Prior to testing for cytoplasmic Ig, these patients would have been classified as non-T, non-B leukemia or "null" ALL. Kaneko and co-workers (1980) described an ALL patient with the pre-B phenotype who also had an 8:14 (14q +) chromosome translocation. This chromosome abnormality is often found in cells of B-cell leukemia and Burkitt's lymphoma in which it carries a poor prognosis (Berger *et al.*, 1979; Zech *et al.*, 1976). As yet, a large series of pre-B leukemias have not been examined by karyotyping, and therefore the prognostic significance of the 14q + chromosome in pre-B leukemia has not been determined.

The J chain of an IgM or IgA polymeric molecule is synthesized within the B-lymphocyte (Kaji and Parkhouse, 1974). J-chain is also present in circulating immunoblasts which synthesize cytoplasmic immunoglobulins (Mestecky *et al.*, 1980; Brandzaeg, 1976). The report by Isaacson (1979) indicates that J chain is present in lymphomas which produce monotypic light chains and may, therefore, be a useful marker for B-cell lymphomas.

F. Fc Receptors

Most hematopoietic cells, including polymorphonuclear leukocytes, mononuclear leukocytes, eosinophils, and "third-population" lymphocytes possess Fc receptors. Both T- and B-lymphocytes have been shown to express Fc receptors for different immunoglobulin classes including IgG, IgM, IgA, and IgE (Romagnani *et al.*, 1978, 1979; Pichler and Broder, 1978; Gonzales-Molina and Spiegelber, 1977; Gupta *et al.*, 1979a; Dickler *et al.*, 1974; Lum *et al.*, 1979; Moretta *et al.*, 1975, 1976; Yodoi and Ishizaka, 1979; Golightly and Golub, 1980).

A variety of methods have been described for the detection of receptors for the Fc portion of immunoglobulin molecules. Those most commonly employed include the EA rosette assay (Zighelboim *et al.*, 1974), the Ripley rosette assay (Froland *et al.*, 1974), and binding of heat-aggregated human immunoglobulin (Arbeit *et al.*, 1976). The EA rosette assay measures binding of an EA complex to the cell surface. The complex is prepared by incubating a subagglutinating dose of antierythrocyte antibody (A) with erythrocytes (E). After washing, the EA complex is incubated with the cellular population under study. Incubations are usually at a temperature of 25 or 37°C. Ripley rosettes are determined by a type of EA assay in which the erythrocyte–antibody complex consists of "Ripley" anti-CD antiserum (Waller and Lawler, 1962) and human type O Rh-positive red blood cells (Froland and Wisloff, 1976). Ripley antibody-coated erythrocytes do not bind to all Fc receptor-bearing lymphocytes but rather to a subpopulation of lymphocytes which is responsible for antibody-dependent cell-mediated cytotoxicity (ADCC) (Eremin *et al.*, 1977). Ripley rosettes are also formed with monocytes and with neutrophils (Shaw *et al.*, 1979b), although the avidity of binding to each of these different cell types varies. Arbeit and co-workers (1976) described procedures for detection of Fc receptors by binding heat-aggregated immunoglobulin or antigen–antibody complexes. Similar assays have been developed which allow quantitative information to be obtained regarding the density of Fc receptors on the cell. These assays determine the amount of aggregated immunoglobulin bound to the cell by spectrofluorometric analysis (Schreiber *et al.*, 1978) or by use of ^{125}I-labeled aggregated HGG (Segal and Horowitz, 1977).

In studies which have directly compared several of the different methods for detection of Fc receptors (Clements and Levy, 1978; Winchester *et al.*, 1979), it was apparent that these assays might be detecting different lymphocyte subpopulations. So, the Fc receptors of cells are described as heterogeneous, differing in avidity, sensitivity to proteolytic enzymes, the subclass of immunoglobulin bound, the relationship with other membrane structures, and functional activity (Arbeit *et al.*, 1977; Clements and Levy, 1978; Winchester *et al.*, 1979; Gormus *et al.*, 1978a,b; Horowitz *et al.*, 1979; and Fanger and Lydyard, 1979). The function of Fc receptors on the third-population of lymphocytes is to allow the cell to participate in ADCC, whereas sIg-positive Fc receptor-bearing lymphocytes (B cells) do not exhibit ADCC activity (Eremin *et al.*, 1977). Pape *et al.* (1979) determined that Fc receptor expression was necessary for ADCC activity but was not necessary for natural killer activity, another function which Fc receptor-positive lymphocytes also possess.

LaVia and LaVia (1978) reported that the attachment of aggregated immunoglobulin to Fc receptors on B cells suppressed antibody production, suggesting that these receptors play an important role in immunoregulation. Recently, the presence of Fc receptors for IgG or IgM on T-lymphocytes has been correlated with their functional activity. Cells which rosetted with ox erythrocytes coated with IgM ($T\mu$) provided help for B-cell differentiation into plasma cells (Moretta *et al.*, 1977; Heijnen *et al.*, 1979). $T\gamma$ cells, those forming rosettes with ox erythrocyte–IgG complexes, were shown to function as suppressors of B-cell differentiation and of T-cell proliferation (Moretta *et al.*, 1977). $T\gamma$ cells were shown by Moretta and co-workers (1977) to express suppressor activity only after activation with antigen–antibody complexes. Hayward and colleagues (1978) induced $T\gamma$ cells to become suppressors following activation with Con A. These observations were confirmed by Cooke *et al.* (1979).

$T\mu$ cells produce the lymphokine, LMIF, in response to PHA (Moretta *et al.*, 1977). Lydyard and Fanger (1979) found that PHA induced modulation of the $T\mu$ receptor, and it was suggested that similar modulatory events may function as a regulatory response to antigens. $T\mu$ cells were reported by Shaw and co-workers (1979a) to contain the precursor of the cell responsible for cell-mediated lysis (CML); $T\gamma$ cells contained effectors for ADCC, natural killers, and mitogen-induced cellular cytotoxicity (MICC), while $T\mu$ contained only MICC activity (Pichler *et al.*, 1979; Shen *et al.*, 1979; Lum *et al.*, 1979). $T\mu$ and $T\gamma$ differ in their electrophoretic mobility (Platsoucas *et al.*, 1979), and morphology (Grossi *et al.*, 1977). $T\gamma$ cells have Ia antigens and histamine receptors; $T\mu$ cells do not (Gupta and Good, 1980). Incubation of peripheral blood lymphocytes with thymosin caused an increase in the percentage of $T\gamma$ cells with no change in $T\mu$ (Gupta and Good, 1977). Cells in the $T\gamma$ subclass were reported to be sensitive to radiation and to steroids (Gupta and Good, 1977). T-lymphocytes which possess Fc receptors for IgA and IgE have also been described (Gupta et al., 1979a,b; Yodoi and Ishizaka, 1979). However, to this date the function of these T-cell subsets has not been determined.

Gupta and Good (1978) reported the normal distribution of Tμ and Tγ cells in various lymphoid organs. Peripheral blood, tonsils, and bone marrow had comparable proportions of each subset, with 40–50% of the T cells present being Tμ and 8–10% Tγ. Tγ cells were present in higher proportions in cord blood and were not found in neonatal lymph nodes. With age, Tμ cells were found to decrease (Cobleigh et al., 1980). This decrease occurred mainly in males. The lowered number of Tμ cells found in older individuals could not be correlated with decreases in their PHA responsiveness.

Fc receptors have been detected on many different types of malignant lymphoid cells, including ALL (Huber et al., 1978; Rudders et al., 1980; Spiegelberg and Dainer, 1979), CLL (Rudders et al., 1980; Spiegelberg and Dainer, 1979), Sezery syndrome (Spiegelberg and Dainer, 1979), and myeloid leukemia (Ridway et al., 1979). Leukemic cells were sometimes shown to express Fc receptors for more than one immunoglobulin class simultaneously (Reaman et al., 1979; Spiegelberg and Dainer, 1979; Beck et al., 1981). In one case of T-ALL, Saxon and co-workers (1979) found some blasts which expressed Fcμ receptors while others expressed Fcγ receptors, an observation indicating that differentiation must have occurred after malignant transformation or that two different malignant lines were present. When tested in vitro the leukemic cells were able to provide helper and suppressor functions.

G. COMPLEMENT RECEPTORS

Two types of receptors for complement are found on the surface of lymphoid cells (Ross, 1979). They are distinct molecules and have been given the designations CR$_1$ and CR$_2$. A third complement receptor, CR$_3$, can be found on granulocytes and mononuclear phagocytes. The third component of complement, C3, can bind to CR$_1$ or CR$_2$ (Ross and Polley, 1975). However, it binds to these receptors via different regions on the C3 molecule. C4 binds to CR$_2$ sites after it has been activated to become C4b (Ross, 1979).

A number of assays have been described for the detection of complement receptors. The EAC rosette assay (Shannon and Hastings, 1977) was one of the first methods utilized for such analysis. Erythrocytes (E) coated with IgM antierythrocyte antibody (A) and complement (C) resulted in the formation of EAC complex. This complex, when incubated with lymphocytes at 37°C, bound to complement receptors and formed an EAC rosette. Other types of rosettes have been described which utilize other complement binding particles. Zymozan (Mendes *et al.*, 1974), baker's yeast (Rivero *et al.*, 1979), and certain bacteria (Gormus *et al.*, 1980) were shown to activate and bind complement when incubated in fresh serum. These particles were mixed with cells and attached to complement receptors on the cell. Alternatively, immunofluorescence was used to detect binding of fluid phase complement components to the cell membrane (Cossman *et al.*, 1978). Difficulties in distinguishing mononuclear phagocytes from lymphocytes in complement receptor assays were overcome by allowing mononuclear cells to ingest latex particles (Rothbarton *et al.*, 1978) or by a procedure which detected the cytoplasmic esterase of monocytes (Mullink *et al.*, 1979).

The complement receptors are functionally related to the phagocytic process in mononuclear cells (Mantovani *et al.*, 1972; Scribner and Fahrney, 1976). Feldman and Pepys (1974) suggested that complement receptors might play an important role in the presentation of thymus-independent antigens to B-lymphocytes.

The percentage of peripheral blood mononuclear cells which bind complement has been reported in the 10 to 19% range (Aiuti *et al.*, 1975; Slease *et al.*, 1980). Methods which allow distinction of the density of complement receptors have shown that malignant lymphocytes may express a different density of receptors or a different avidity for complement receptors as compared to normal lymphoid cells (Slease *et al.*, 1980).

H. LYMPHOCYTE DIFFERENTIATION ANTIGENS

Over the past decade there have been a number of reports in the literature on the development of antibody reagents which were specific to human T- or B-lymphocytes and mononuclear cells (Gross and Bron, 1978; Anderson and Metzgar, 1979; Braathen *et al.*, 1979; Stevens and Saxon, 1978; Stratton and Byfield, 1977; Espinouse *et al.*, 1978; Balch *et al.*, 1978; Stuart *et al.*, 1976). Many of these antibody reagents were developed by injecting nonhuman primates or xenogeneic species with human thymocytes, lymphoid cell lines, or brain tissue. The antisera developed required extensive absorption to assure specificity. Using similar approaches, some investigators were able to detect antigens on T-lymphocytes which defined subpopulations of the T-cell lineage (Boumsell *et al.*, 1979; Brouet and Chevalier, 1979; Pandolfi *et al.*, 1981; Evans *et al.*, 1978; Reinherz and Schlossman, 1979). One of the best characterized of the antigens on T-cell subsets defined by heteroantisera was the anti-TH$_2$ described by Evans and co-workers (1977). This antiserum was shown to react with 90% of thymocytes but only a portion of T cells in the peripheral blood (Evans *et al.*, 1977). The T-cell subset defined by the anti-TH$_2$ antiserum was found to contain that cellular subpopulation responsible for cell-mediated lympholysis. Cells lacking the TH$_2$ marker were those cells responsive in an MLC and in lymphocyte transformation assays to soluble antigens *in vitro*. TH$_2$(−) cells were amplifiers of the cytotoxic TH$_2$ subset (Evans *et al.*, 1978). The TH + subset was found to be the Con A-induced suppressor of an MLC reaction (Reinherz and Schlossman, 1979).

Strelkauskas and colleagues (1978a,b) reported that juvenile rheumatoid arthritis patients had an autoantibody in their serum which reacted with a subset of T-lymphocytes but not with B-lymphocytes. The population of cells defined by the JRA serum (JRA + cells) responded to Con A but not PHA, and was a poor responder in mixed lymphocyte cultures. JRA(−) T-cells provided helper function for immunoglobulin synthesis by B-lymphocytes, were stimulated by PHA but not Con A, and exhibited a strong reaction in MLR. The presence of the antibody in the serum of JRA patients could be correlated with loss of regulatory mechanisms for immunoglobulin synthesis *in vivo* (Strelkauskas *et al.*, 1978b). Although there was some apparent overlap in the JRA + and TH$_2$+ subsets, Reinherz *et al.* (1979a) presented evidence to show these are two distinct subsets.

The development of the monoclonal antibody technique has led to the development of a variety of very specific antibodies which react with various cellular subpopulations (Reinherz and Schlossman, 1981; Reinherz *et al.*, 1979b, 1980a,b; Kung *et al.*, 1979a; LeBien and Kersey, 1980; Trucco *et al.*, 1978; Taetle and Royston, 1980; Abramson *et al.*, 1981; Royston *et al.*, 1981). The best defined series of monoclonal antibodies has been given the designation OKT followed by a number designation. One of the antibodies reacted with thymocytes and peripheral T-lymphocytes, OKT11 (Kung *et al.*, 1979b). Others would only bind to thymocytes, OKT6 (Reinherz *et al.*, 1980a), or were restricted in reactivity with peripheral T cells only, OKT1 and OKT3 (Kung *et al.*, 1979a; Reinherz and Schlossman, 1980; Reinherz *et al.*, 1979b). A subset of T-lymphocytes were defined by the OKT4 antibody which reacted with T cells exhibiting helper activity (Reinherz *et al.*, 1979c,d, 1980a).

Suppressor/cytotoxic T-lymphocytes carry antigens defined by the OKT5 and OKT8 monoclonal antibodies (Reinherz *et al.*, 1979c, 1980a; Kung *et al.*, 1979b). Reinherz and co-workers (1980b) compared the T-cell subpopulations defined by Fc receptors (Tμ and Tγ) with those defined by monoclonal antibodies. The Tμ cells contained both OKT4 + (helper) and

OKT5 + (suppressor/cytotoxic) lymphocytes. The Tγ subset was found to contain very few T-lymphocytes (OKT3 +) and consisted mainly of cells which reacted with a monocyte-specific monoclonal antibody (OKM1).

Janossy and colleagues (1980) evaluated the tissue distribution of the T-cell subsets defined by the OKT series of monoclonal antibodies. Cells of the helper (or inducer) subset which are OKT4 + were found to predominate in the medulla of the thymus, the blood, the paracortex of the tonsils, and the lamina propria of the intestine. The T cells in the bone marrow and in the gut epithelium were mainly OKT8 +, suppressor T-lymphocytes. In addition, a microanatomical relationship between OKT4 + lymphocytes and Ia + macrophages was described.

Antisera prepared against T cells, B cells, and T-cell subsets have been used to classify lymphoid malignancies (Carrel et al., 1979; Netzel et al., 1979; Hsu and Morgan, 1978; Melvin, 1979; Tsubota et al., 1980; Boumsell et al., 1980; Thiel et al., 1980; Sallen et al., 1980; Nadler et al., 1980a, 1981; Turesson et al., 1979; Hattori et al., 1980; Espinouse et al., 1980). Further classification of lymphoid malignancies has been the result of combining the data from studies such as these with an analysis with marker assays such as E-rosettes and sIg determinations. The subclassification of ALL has been expanded into several subgroups. Null leukemia has also now been subcategorized. Reactions with anti-T- and B-cell reagents have subdivided this group (Melvin, 1979; Thiel et al., 1980; Sallen et al., 1980). Nadler and co-workers (1980b) found that cells from most patients with lymphoblastic lymphoma expressed the TH_2 antigen while lymphoblasts of T-cell ALL did not. These data have shown that these two T-cell diseases are probably different rather than a single disease process.

Antigens known as "Ia" antigens are readily detected on the surface of B cells (Metzgar and Mohanakumar, 1978). These antigens have received the "Ia" designation due to their similarity to Ia antigens of mice which are products of the I-region of the major histocompatibility complex (MHC). In humans Ia antigens are linked to the D-locus of the MHC. Although Ia antigens were originally thought to be expressed exclusively on B-lymphocytes, recent evidence has shown Ia antigen expression of T-lymphocytes (Kaszubowski et al., 1980a; De Wolf et al., 1979; Ko et al., 1979; Reinherz et al., 1979c; Yu et al., 1981).

Different authors have either been unable to detect Ia antigens on resting T cells or have detected them on only a small percentage (2–5%) of such cells (Reinherz et al., 1979c; Yu et al., 1981; Fu et al., 1978; De Wolf et al., 1979; Kaszubowski et al., 1980a). Activation of T-lymphocytes by mitogens, antigens, or in mixed lymphocyte cultures increased the percentage of T cells which expressed Ia (Ko et al., 1979; De Wolf et al.,

1979; Reinherz *et al.*, 1979c; Kaszubowski *et al.*, 1980a). Reinherz and co-workers (1979c) reported that Ia antigen expression increased in both the OKT4(+) subset and the OKT4(−) subset when the cells were activated with PHA, Con A, or allogeneic cells. Activation with tetanus toxoid increased Ia expression in the inducer (OKT4+) subset. Thus, Ia antigen expression after activation depends upon the agent used to activate the cell and the T-cell population which is responsive to the stimulant.

Macrophages, immature myeloid cells, and bone marrow cells of patients with megaloblastic anemia and patients with myeloid hyperplasia also express Ia antigens (Greaves and Janossy, 1978; Janossy *et al.*, 1978). Ia antigens were found on human myeloid and erythroid progenitors but were not detected on the pluripotential stem cell (Moore *et al.*, 1980). Ia antigens have been found in CML in blast crises, AML, non-T, non-B ALL, and ANLL (Balch *et al.*, 1978; Greaves *et al.*, 1978; Wernet *et al.*, 1977; Janossy *et al.*, 1980; Hiraoka *et al.*, 1980). The detection of Ia antigens in combination with other marker and biochemical analysis has been useful in the subclassification of these diseases (Billing *et al.*, 1981).

Numerous reports of detection of leukemia-specific antigens have appeared in the literature over the past several years. This literature has been reviewed by Metzgar and Mohanakumar (1978). Most of the antigens described were not extensively characterized, and it was not clear whether they were truly leukemia specific or if they represented fetal or differentiation antigens reexpressed on the surface of the leukemic blast.

One antigen found on the "common" form of ALL (or null ALL) has been extensively studied. It has a molecular weight of about 100,000 (Metzgar and Mohanakumar, 1977; Kabisch *et al.*, 1979; Sutherland *et al.*, 1978). The antigen has been designated as the cALL antigen. It is present, not only on "common" ALL, but also on AUL and CML in blast crisis (Brown *et al.*, 1975; Roberts *et al.*, 1978; Pesando *et al.*, 1980). The antigen can be found in the serum of ALL patients (Kabisch *et al.*, 1979). It is present on fetal bone marrow cells and on cells in regenerating bone marrow, but it cannot be detected on normal, mature lymphocytes (Janossy *et al.*, 1978). It has been proposed that the antigen is a normal differentiation antigen of bone marrow progenitors (Greaves and Janossy, 1978).

Pesando and co-workers (1980) isolated the cALL antigen in a highly purified form. They prepared an antiserum to the purified antigen and found that it reacted with cALL negative B- and T-cell lines. These authors proposed that the cALL-specific sera must detect a unique specificity present on a similar molecule which is found on other malignant and normal cells. Alternatively, the cALL antigen may be "hidden" on these other cell lines.

A monoclonal antibody (J5) was prepared which exhibited the same reactivity as anti-cALL produced by conventional procedures (Ritz *et al.*, 1980a). The J-5 antibody reacted with 80% of non-T ALL and some cases of CLL in blast crisis. J-5 monoclonal antibody was used for specific immunotherapy in one patient with the result of reducing by 90% the number of circulating blasts within 1 hour of infusion (Ritz *et al.*, 1981). After 3 days of therapy, the number of blasts returned to pretreatment levels. Examination of the markers present on lymphoblasts during the course of serotherapy indicated that the cALL antigen was modulated from the surface of the leukemic blast. This finding correlated with *in vitro* data of Ritz *et al.* (1980b) showing that the J-5 antibody modulated the cALL antigen from the surface of lymphoblasts without concomitant loss of other markers. Ritz and co-workers (1980b) also found that other cell surface markers could not be modulated from the surface of lymphoblasts following treatment with monoclonal antibodies directed toward them. It was apparent, therefore, that the ability to be modulated may be different from one cell surface component to another.

Kersey and co-workers (1981) described a monoclonal antibody (BA-2) produced against an ALL cell line of the pre-B phenotype. The monoclonal antibody detected a 24,000-dalton polypeptide present on most "common" ALL and on lymphohemopoietic bone marrow stem cells. Based on its molecular weight, the antigen detected by BA-2 is different from the cALL antigen.

I. Glucocorticoid Receptors

It has been known for a long time that glucocorticoids exert a suppressive effect on lymphoid cells of animals and man. Lymphocytes were shown to possess cytoplasmic receptors for glucocorticoids (Schmidt and Thompson, 1978). The hormone produced its effect by binding to the receptor followed by a series of steps which included nuclear transfer and culminated in inhibition of a number of biosynthetic and transport functions (Schmidt and Thompson, 1978).

A number of investigators have quantitatively examined the receptors present in the cytoplasm of normal lymphocytes, and it was found that cells stimulated by mitogens or antigens expressed more receptors than unstimulated cells (Smith *et al.*, 1977; Crabtree *et al.*, 1980a,b). Crabtree and colleagues (1980b) reported an increase in receptors occurred in cells in the S phase of the cell cycle, and therefore they believed that increased numbers of receptors only reflected that the cells examined were in S phase.

Initially, it was believed that sensitivity to glucocorticoids varied with the state of maturation or activation of the lymphocyte (Claman, 1972; Duval *et al.*, 1976). However, later information indicated that inhibition of macromolecular synthesis was not directly correlated with the level of receptors in the cell (Smith *et al.*, 1977). This finding was in contrast to the results of Galili and co-workers (1980) who reported that T cells activated in a mixed lymphocyte culture developed sensitivity to glucocorticoids. Activation per se apparently does not produce the sensitivity because Con A and PHA stimulated cells did not develop a similar sensitivity to the hormone.

Quantitation of the number of glucocorticoid receptors in the cytoplasm of leukemic blasts was compared to certain cell surface markers by Yarbro *et al.* (1977). These workers found that T-ALL had fewer receptors than null ALL. When the null group was subcategorized based upon the ability of the leukemic blast to act as a stimulator in mixed lymphocyte cultures (MLC+), it was found that MLC+ cells had an intermediate number of receptors between MLC(−), null ALL cells, and T-lymphoblasts. The evaluation of the quantity of glucocorticoid receptors in leukemic blasts has proven to be important because it was correlated with the sensitivity of the cell to glucocorticoids both *in vitro* and *in vivo*. It was determined that the presence of these receptors may serve as a prognostic indicator (Lippman *et al.*, 1978). Other authors (Iacobelli *et al.*, 1978; Kontula *et al.*, 1980) questioned that a correlation with clinical response and the quantity of steroid receptors can be made. Their criticisms relate to the fact that patients are on multidrug regimens, and, therefore, the correlation between the density of receptors and the effect of one among several drugs is difficult to determine. The data of Kontula and co-workers (1980) have led them to believe that the presence of glucocorticoid receptors cannot be used as a criterion for steroid sensitivity. It is important to note that very few of the patients in their study had ALL, and there was no attempt to subclassify the ALL patients examined. Studies with cell lines have failed to find a correlation between glucocorticoid receptor content and either immune phenotype or growth inhibition by glucocorticoids (Paavonen *et al.*, 1981).

J. Peanut Agglutinin Receptors

Observations made in the murine species showed that peanut agglutinin (PNA) would bind to immature T-lymphocytes such as those found in the hydrocortisone-sensitive subset of the thymus (Reisner *et al.*, 1976, 1978). Reisner and co-workers (1979) extended their observations to include humans and determined that 60 to 80% of human thymocytes carried the PNA receptor. A differential response of PNA + and PNA thymocytes to phytohemagglutinin led the authors to speculate that the PNA + subset was functionally more immature. PNA receptors were found on the surface of most cases of acute lymphocytic leukemia but could not be demonstrated in cases of chronic lymphocytic leukemia. PNA receptors were reported to occur on the surface of acute myeloid leukemia (Reisner *et al.*, 1979) but were not found on the surface of blasts from chronic myeloid leukemia (Taub *et al.*, 1980). Thus, the PNA receptor may define many lineages of hematopoietic cells which are in relatively early stages of differentiation.

A correlation between the PNA receptor and other markers in acute leukemia showed that the PNA receptor was found on some but not all cases of T cell, null cell, and B cell ALL. Preliminary evidence in a small series of patients indicated that the presence of the PNA receptors carried a poor prognosis (Levin *et al.*, 1980; Russell *et al.*, 1981).

K. Histamine Receptors

Kedar and Bonavida (1974) described a rosette assay which detected cells carrying receptors for histamine on their surface. This assay detected such receptors on B cells (about one-third of those in the peripheral blood), macrophages, and 10% of peripheral blood T-lymphocytes (Saxon *et al.*, 1977). Other techniques for the detection of histamine receptors have been described including affinity chromatography (Tartakovsky *et al.*, 1979) and flow cytometry (Osband *et al.*, 1980). When analyzed by flow cytometric analysis, 45% of T cells in the blood exhibited histamine receptors (Tartakovsky *et al.*, 1979). Using a guinea pig model, Rocklin (1976) reported that histamine would block the production of the lymphokine, macrophage inhibitor factor (MIF), *in vitro*. This block was later found to be the result of the production of histamine suppressor factors (HSF) which had a molecular weight of 23,000 to 40,000 (Rocklin, 1977). Rocklin and co-workers (1979) found that although HSF was produced by nonsensitized lymphoid cells, 2 weeks after immunization, increased HSF production occurred when MIF assays to the sensitizing antigen were evaluated. The HSF-producing cell was a T-lymphocyte which had histamine receptors on its surface. Histamine receptor antagonists of both the H_1 and H_2 types were able to induce HSF, however, H_2 antagonists were effective at concentrations 100 times less than H_1 antagonists. Rigal *et al.* (1979) reported similar observations to those of Rocklin in humans. They found inhibition of LIF production by histamine-stimulated T cells. At least one report in the literature has shown that humans receiving H_2 antagonist for the treatment of peptic ulcers exhibit an enhanced skin test reaction after several weeks of drug treatment (Avella et al., 1978).

Histamine receptors on the surface of cytotoxic lymphocytes functioned to inhibit cytotoxicity (Plaut et al., 1973, 1975). Shearer and co-workers (1972) reported that lymphoid cells possessing histamine receptors served to regulate the humoral immune response. Anderson and colleagues (1977) found that neutrophil random mobility was stimulated by histamine and true chemotaxis was inhibited. Histamine antagonists of the H_2 type were able to block the inhibition of chemotaxis. Histamine produced a respiratory burst in alveolar macrophages and the effect was found to depend upon H_1 receptors (Diaz et al., 1979).

L. MISCELLANEOUS MARKERS

A number of other lymphocyte markers have been described which we have chosen to simply list in this review. The significance of these receptors to leukemia has not yet been extensively studied.

Insulin receptors are present to both T and B lymphocytes which have been activated by stimulation with antigens or mitogens (Helderman and Strom, 1978; Strom et al., 1978; Helderman et al., 1979). Esber and co-workers (1976) reported a difference in the expression of insulin receptors between "null" ALL and T-ALL.

Receptors for catecholamines (Pochet et al., 1979), adenosine (Marone et al., 1978), prostaglandins (Goodwin et al., 1978), C-reactive protein (Croft et al., 1976), and T-cell growth factor (Ruscetti and Gallo, 1981) have been described. These receptors may play an important immunoregulatory role, but have not as yet been related to subclassifications of leukemia.

Lymphocytes of the T and B lineage have been differentiated according to their surface glycoproteins (Wang et al., 1979; Andersson et al., 1976) and according to their electrophoretic mobility (Kaplan and Uzgiris, 1976; Chollet et al., 1977).

Receptors for the Epstein–Barr virus (EBV) are present on B cells and on some "third-population" lymphocytes (Greaves et al., 1975; Jondal and Klein, 1973). A close association between EBV receptors and the C3d receptor was reported by Jondal and co-workers (1976). T-lymphocytes possess a receptor for measles virus (Valdimarsson et al., 1975). Teodorescu and co-workers (1977a,b, 1979) have subdivided peripheral blood lymphocytes into several categories based on their ability to bind certain strains of bacteria. These lymphoid subsets were shown to be different when used in functional assays (Kleinman and Teodorescu, 1979).

TABLE II
ENZYME MARKERS AND ALL

Enzyme	Null cell	T cell	B cell
5-Nucleotidase	Normal	Low	—
Terminal desoxynucleotidase transferable	Increased	Increased	Low
Adenosine deaminase	Low	Increased	Low
Hexoseaminidase I	Increased	Low	Low
Acid phosphatase	Low	Increased	—
Alkaline phosphatase	Increased	Normal	Normal
Alkaline phosphadiesterase I	Increased	Normal	Normal
Acid esterase	Low	Faint localized activity	Low

M. ENZYME MARKERS

The determination of the presence of certain enzymes has been most useful for the differentiation of acute myeloblastic leukemia from acute lymphoblastic leukemia. Many reports have appeared in the literature which have related quantitative changes in a variety of cellular enzymes to the classification of this disease by membrane markers. These data have been reviewed recently (Humphrey et al., 1980; Blatt et al., 1980) and are summarized in Table II.

We are of the opinion that enzyme marker analysis has not yet proven itself to be as useful an immunologic marker analysis for subclassification of acute lymphoblastic leukemia. Enzyme analysis will continue to be of value for differentiation of ALL and AML.

III. Clinical Applications in Acute Lymphoblastic Leukemia

A. BACKGROUND

By the mid 1970s, three major groups within ALL had been identified using two markers: E receptor and surface membrane immunoglobulin (sIg) (reviewed by Humphrey and Lankford, 1976). The definition of these three groups had both therapeutic and prognostic significance. Null cell ALL (E^0 sIg^0) is also commonly referred to as non-T, non-B ALL. It is the most common of the major groups (85% of cases), has the best prognosis, and has no distinguishing clinical features. T ALL (E^+ sIg^0) is less common (10–15% of childhood ALL), has a poor prognosis with most of the patients having relapsed or died by the end of 1 year. Distinctive clinical features characterized patients with T ALL: male predominance, an older age group, and a high percentage of patients presenting a mediastinal mass or a high white count or both. B ALL (1–2%) had the worst prognosis, was characterized in most cases by an unusual morphology similar to that observed with Burkitt cells, and referred to as L3 classification in the FAB system. There are exceptions to these morphological characteristics (Koziner *et al.*, 1980a). This leukemia also is commonly associated with a chromosomal anomaly (14q +) which is also found in cases of Burkitt's lymphoma (Roth *et al.*, 1979; Slater *et al.*, 1979). In fact, B ALL is generally considered to be a leukemic form of Burkitt's lymphoma (Koziner *et al.*, 1980b; Prokocimer *et al.*, 1980).

The prognostic differences observed in these three major groups resulted in some clinical investigators using surface markers to identify patients who were evaluated on therapy other than that commonly used in the treatment of ALL. The treatment of patients with T ALL on non-Hodgkin's lymphoma protocols that generally contain many more multiple agents has resulted in a significant improvement in therapeutic outcome with some patients currently under observation maintaining a 40% disease-free survival rate (Ettinger *et al.*, 1979). Some B ALL cases have been treated on protocols specifically designed for Burkitt's lymphoma or B-cell lymphomas (Hvisdala, 1981).

B. HETEROGENEITY

By the end of the 1970s, considerable heterogeneity within null ALL and T ALL was apparent (reviewed by Humphrey *et al.*, 1980). This heterogeneity is considerable as reflected in Table III and also demonstrates that heterogeneity exists within B ALL. Within null ALL, three subgroups are commonly identified. These include small numbers of cALL^0 cases, sometimes referred to as undifferentiated leukemia, which have been reported to have a poorer response to therapy than cALL$^+$ subgroup and a pre-B-cell subgroup. Within T ALL, a pre-T subgroup (E^{0}T$^+$) and T ALL (mature or late T ALL) (E$^+$T$^+$) are also being recorded or observed (Table III).

In order to tabulate the different subgroups that are being identified by different research groups, we have elected to retain the older designation of null, T, and B ALL. There is one important modification to that original designation in that cases identified as being T antigen positive with or without the E receptor are classified under T ALL. This has been done because many groups have elected to use antisera to define the subgroups and have not measured the E receptor. We have not listed null ALL subgroups that suggest B cell lineage under B ALL. For example, those in-

TABLE III

HETEROGENEITY WITHIN THE MAJOR GROUPS OF ALL: COMMON MARKER STUDIES

| Reference / Percentage population / Adult children / Antisera | Null ($E^0 T^0 sIg^0$) | | T ($E^{+/-}$ and/or T^+) | | B (sIg^+) |
	Pre-B^0 or pre-BND No. phenotype	Pre-B (cIg^+) No. phenotype	Pre-T ($E^0 T^+$) No. phenotype	Periph T (E^+) No. phenotype	No. phenotype
Greaves et al. (1979) A and C Hetero		28 cIg^+ $cALL^+$ 1 cIg^+ $cALL^0$ plus enzyme and morphological heterogeneity			
Greaves et al. (1980a) A and C Mono	71 $cALL^+$ B^+ 3 $cALL^+$ B^0 6 $cALL^0$ B^0			31 T^+ B^0	4 sIg^+ B^+
Greaves et al. (1981a) C and A Hetero	Children 530 $cALL^+$ 85 $cALL^0$ Adults 52 $cALL^+$ 39 $cALL^0$			Children 82 E^+ Adults 10 E^+	Children 4 sIg^+ Adults 2 sIg^+
Thiel et al. (1980) A and C Hetero	119 $cALL^+$ 32 $cALL^0$	$cALL^+$ cIg^+	87 E^0 T^+ $cALL^+$ 47 E^0 T^+ $cALL^0$	48 E^+ T^+ $cALL^0$	6 sIg^+

(Continued)

TABLE III (*Continued*)

Reference Percentage population Adult children Antisera *Hetero*logous *Mono*clonal	Null (E^0 T^0 sIg^0) Pre-B^0 or pre-B^{ND} No. phenotype	Pre-B (cIg^+) No. phenotype	T ($E^{+/-}$ and/or T^+) Pre-T (E^0 T^+) No. phenotype	Periph T (E^+) No. phenotype	B (sIg^+) No. phenotype
Sallen *et al.* (1980) C Hetero	36 Ia^+ $cALL^+$ 7 Ia^+ $cALL^0$ 3 Ia^0 $cALL^0$			11 T^+ Ia^0 $cALL^0$ 1 T^+ Ia^+ $cALL^+$	
Foon *et al.* (1980) C and A Hetero	45 Ia^+ $cALL^+$ 9 Ia^+ $cALL^0$ 2 Ia^0 $cALL^0$	1 E^0 T^+ Ig^0 $cALL^+$	3 E^0 T^+ Ig^0 $cALL^0$ 1 E^0 T^+ Ig^+ $cALL^0$	4 E^+ T^+ Ig^0 $cALL^0$ 2 E^+ T^+ Ig^+ $cALL^0$	1 sIg^+ Ia^+ $cALL^+$ 1 sIg^+ Ia^+ $cALL^0$
Yamanaka *et al.* (1978) C (A) Hetero	8 Fc^0 B^0 7 $Fc^{+/0}$ B^+		1 E^0 T^+ Ig^+ $cALL^+$ 4 E^0 T^0 Thy^0 Fc^0	4 E^+ Thy^+ Fc^0	1 sIg^+ $Fc^{+/0}$ B^+
Pullen *et al.* (1981) C Hetero	78 Ia^+ $cALL^+$ 5 Ia^+ $cALL^0$	19 cIg^+ $cALL^+$ Ia^+ 2 cIg^+ $cALL^0$ Ia^+	5 E^0 T^+ Thy^+ 6 E^I T^+ Thy^0 (2 = $cALL^+$)	11 E^+ T^+ Thy^+ 5 E^+ T^+ Thy^0 (1 = $cALL^+$)	2 sIg^+
Humphrey *et al.* (1981) C Hetero	52 $cALL^+$ C^0 Fc^0 6 $cALL^+$ C^0 Fc^+ 7 $cALL^+$ C^+ Fc^0 7 $cALL^+$ C^+ Fc^+ 4 $cALL^0$ C^0 Fc^0 1 $cALL^0$ C^0 Fc^+ 1 $cALL^0$ C^+ Fc^0 1 $cALL^0$ C^+ Fc^+	12 $cALL^+$ C^0 Fc^0 3 $cALL^+$ C^0 Fc^+ 1 $cALL^+$ C^+ Fc^0 1 $cALL^0$ C^+ Fc^+ 2 $cALL^0$ C^0 Fc^0	7 Thy^0 C^0 Fc^0 1 Thy^+ C^+ Fc^0	2 Thy^0 C^0 Fc^0 4 Thy^+ C^0 Fc^0 1 Thy^+ C^+ Fc^0 2 Thy^+ C^+ Fc^+	sIg^+ $cALL^+$ Fc^0 ND sIg^+ ND Fc^+ ND sIg^+ ND Fc^0 C^0 sIg^+ ND ND C^0 sIg^+ $cALL^+$ ND C^0

Morphological, histochemical, clinical, serum IgG, A, M levels, $C^{+/0}$ and $Fc^{+/0}$ heterogeneity

Reference					
T. Zipf et al. (personal communication) C Mono	126 cALL$^+$ Ia$^+$ 20 cALL$^+$ Ia$^{+/0}$		5 E^0 Thy$^+$ T^0 Ia$^+$ 2 E^0 Thy$^+$ T^0 Ia^0 1 E^0 Thy^0 T$^+$ Ia$^+$ 1 E^0 Thy^0 T$^+$ Ia$^+$	3 E$^+$ Thy$^+$ T$^+$ Ia^0	None detected
Bowman et al. (1981a) C Hetero			14 E^0 T$^+$ (plus 8 T$^{+/-}$ E$^{+/-}$)	11 E$^+$ T$^+$	3 sIg$^+$
A. L. Yu et al. (personal communication) A and C Mono	14 Ia$^+$ cIg^0	1 cIg$^+$ Ia$^+$	2 E^0 T$^+$ Ia^0	4 E$^+$ T$^+$ Ia^0	None detected
Abranson et al. (1981) C Mono	15 Ia$^+$ cALL$^+$ B$^+$ 3 Ia$^+$ cALL$^+$ B^0	cIg$^+$ Ia$^+$ cALL$^+$ B$^+$		6 E$^+$ Ia^0 cALL^0 B^0	
Minowada et al. (1981) A and C Hetero	118 Ia$^+$ cALL$^+$ 4 Ia$^+$ cALL^0 3 Ia^0 cALL^0			13 E$^+$ cALL^0 6 E$^+$ cALL$^+$	4 sIg$^+$ cALL^0 2 sIg$^+$ cALL$^+$
Veit et al. (1980) C Hetero	16 cALL$^+$ 5 cALL^0		3 E^0 Thy$^+$ cALL^0 1 E^0 Thy$^+$ cALL$^+$	4 E$^+$ Thy$^+$ cALL^0	1 sIg$^+$ cALL$^+$

27

vestigators using antisera to find B cell lineage or detect the presence of cytoplasmic immunoglobulin defining the pre-B-cell subgroup have been listed under null ALL because these subgroups do not define groups of patients with an extremely poor prognosis as the sIg^+ B ALL cases.

Before discussing the heterogeneity that is being identified within the major groups and subgroups of ALL, we need to define how we arrived at the phenotypes listed in Table III. As can be seen in the first column, some investigators are using heterologous antisera and others monoclonal antibodies to identify specific phenotypes. Each of these antisera is referred to in the reference by its own code. There is a great deal of variability in what determinants are recognized by these antisera. Rather than use the original code, which in our opinion would have made the table even more confusing, the antisera were identified by the cell lineage or cell type that the investigators felt were determined by their reagents. Thus, antisera identifying B-cell lineage are coded as B + or −, T cell lineage as T + or −, thymic T cells as Thy^+. While it is assumed that there is a wide range of specificity for surface determinants used by those antisera defined by the type of cells used to generate the antisera, there is probably less variability in those antisera that are defined by molecular weight such as the Ia-like antigen and common leukemia antigen (cALL). Finally, it should be noted that the definition of E positivity varies widely from group to group, some individuals classifying a case as E^+ with as few as 10% or greater E^+ marrow lymphoblasts or as high as 50% E^+ bone marrow lymphoblasts.

Without discussing each paper in great detail, some generalities can be drawn from the phenotypes being identified by the investigators listed in Table III. These generalities include the following: (1) there is greater heterogeneity within T ALL than null ALL, (2) the most common phenotype in childhood ALL is Ia^+ $cALL^+$. The second most common subgroup is the pre-B-cell $cALL^+$ group, (3) in adults with null ALL, the $cALL^0$ phenotype is almost as common as the $cALL^+$, (4) the cALL antigen can be expressed on cells isolated from patients in all three major groups: T, B, and null, (5) when T antigenicity is used to identify T ALL, only 30–40% of cases will be E^+, (6) in those cases where a B lineage antisera was used to evaluate null ALL, a portion of these cases will suggest B cell lineage, and (7) within T ALL, there is no common phenotype currently identified.

A number of special marker studies have been reported and are summarized in Table IV. Davey *et al.* (1979) used lymphoblasts as stimulatory cells in the mixed lymphocyte culture. All 10 of these cases were B antigen positive and 9 stimulated in the mixed lymphocyte reaction, again suggesting B-cell lineage for these sIg-negative null cell cases. Minowada *et al.* (1981a) have evaluated 10 cases of ALL with E receptor, cALL anti-

TABLE IV
Heterogeneity within the Major Groups of ALL: Special Marker Studies

Reference	Null	T	B
Davey et al. (1979)	$9\ B^+\ MLR^+$ $1\ B^+\ MLR^0$		
Minowada et al. (1981a) Mono (OKT)		$2\ E^+\ cALL^+\ T_1^+\ T_{10}^+\ T_{3-9}^{Variable}$ $3\ E^+\ cALL^0\ T_1^+\ T_{10}^+\ T_{3-9}^{Variable}$ $3\ E^0\ cALL^+\ T_1^+\ T_{10}^+\ T_{3-9}^{Variable}$ $2\ E^0\ cALL^0\ T_1^+\ T_{10}^+\ T_{3-9}^{Variable}$	
Reinherz et al. (1979a) Hetero		$20\ E^+\ T^+\ TH_2^0$ "Suppressor cell" $5\ E^+\ T^+\ TH_2$ "Helper cell"	
Levin et al. (1980) C none	$8\ PNA^+\ Ia^+$ $9\ PNA^0\ Ia^+$	$3\ E^+\ PNA^+\ Ia^{+/0}$ $1\ E^+\ PNA^0\ Ia^+$	$2\ sIg^+\ PNA^+\ Ia^+$ $2\ sIg^+\ PNA^0\ Ia^+$
Reinherz et al. (1980a) Mono (OKT)		15 early thymocyte $T_9^{+/0}\ T_{10}^+$ 5 common thymocyte $T_9^{+/0}\ T_{10}^+\ T_6^+\ T_8^{+/0}\ T_4^{+/0}$ 1 mature thymocyte $T_9^0\ T_{10}^+\ T_3^+$	
Roper et al. (1981) C Mono (OKT)		$1\ E^+\ T_9^+\ T_{10}^0$ $1\ E^+\ T_9^0\ T_{10}^+$ $3\ E^+\ T_4^+\ T_8^+\ T_{1,3}^{Variable}$ $6\ E^+\ T_4^0\ T_8^0\ T_{1,3}^{Variable}$ $7\ E^+\ T_4^+\ T_8^0\ T_{1,3}^{Variable}$ $2\ E^+\ T_4^0\ T_8^+\ T_{1,3}^{Variable}$	
Russell et al. (1981)			$1\ sIg^+\ Ia^+\ PNA^0\ cALL^+\ Thy^0$ $1\ sIg^+\ Ia^+\ PNA^0\ cALL^0\ Thy^0$ $2\ sIg^+\ Ia^+\ PNA^+\ cALL^0\ Thy^0$ $2\ sIg\ Ia^+\ PNA^+\ cALL^0\ Thy^+$

sera, and 9 different monoclonal antibodies of the OKT series. Four major subgroups are listed based on E receptor, common leukemia antigen, and OKT antigens identified by monoclonals OKT 1 and 10. Using the variability defined by OKT monoclonal antibodies, three through nine allows 10 unique phenotypes to be defined in these 10 cases. Reinherz and co-workers (1979a), using heteroantisera, have identified most T-cell cases as having suppressor cell characteristics and only 5 out of 20 having helper cell characteristics. It should be noted that the suppressor cell nature of these cells is reflected in the phenotype identified by the heteroantisera and not in a suppressor cell or helper cell assay. Levin and co-workers (1980) and Russell and co-workers (1981) have used the peanut agglutinin to demonstrate that positivity can occur in all three major groups. Reinherz et al. (1980a) have used the monoclonal antibodies to demonstrate that 15 out of 21 T-cell cases suggested an early thymocytic phenotype rather than a common thymocyte phenotype or a mature thymocyte phenotype. The cases under evaluation by Roper and co-workers (1981) include both leukemias and lymphomas and only those cases that are E^+ are then evaluated by the monoclonal antibodies. These two differences (evaluation of only E^+ material and the inclusion of non-Hodgkin's lymphoma cases) may account for the difference reported by these two groups of investigators.

C. SPECIAL VARIANTS AND RELAPSE ALL

During the past decade, a number of reports have demonstrated that children and adults with morphologically defined ALL are Philadelphia chromosome positive (Whang-Peng and Knutsen, 1980). The percentage of children presenting this picture is in the range of 3 to 10%, and the morphology may be of the FAB L_1 or L_2 type (Priest et al., 1980; Chessells et al., 1979). Immunological marker studies have demonstrated that Ph^+ chromosome ALL is heterogeneous with cases being classified as null ALL (Crist et al., 1978), $cALL^+$ (Chessells et al., 1979; Priest et al., 1980), pre-B-cell ALL (Vogler et al., 1979, LeBien et al., 1979), and B cell ALL (Priest et al., 1980). While this is a small group of patients, many of these reports emphasize a poor response to therapy. However, an exception has been reported in an infant with Ph' ALL who was disease free 2.5 years after diagnosis (Saffhill et al., 1978).

In 1939, normal and abnormal lymphoid cells having a hand mirror configuration were described. While generally attributed to lymphoid cells, this morphological variant has been described in plasmacytic and myelocytic cells and from cases of CLL, CML, lymphoma, and infectious mononucleosis (reviewed by Whang-Peng and Knutsen, 1980). A minority of patients (19%) with ALL will have this configuration in 40% or greater of their blasts and a good prognosis was suggested in an evaluation of a small series (reported in 1978 and later published, Schumacher *et al.*, 1980), but an analysis of a larger number of cases did not confirm any prognostic significance (reported in 1979 and published in 1979, Schumacher *et al.*, 1979). Hand mirror cell ALL is immunologically heterogeneous with cases being described as null ALL (Stass *et al.*, 1978), B cell (Nix *et al.*, 1978), and T cell (Stern *et al.*, 1979). Because antigen–antibody complexes can induce Hand mirror cell configuration in normal lymphocytes, the plasma and marrow of two cases of Hand mirror cell ALL were recently evaluated for the presence of antigen–antibody complexes. The bone marrow sera were positive, but the peripheral blood was negative. Of particular interest, the antigen(s) in these complexes appear to be immunologically related to the baboon endogenous virus (Stass *et al.*, 1980).

Immunological phenotypic evolution or changes in surface markers at relapse have been reported (Melvin 1981b; Borella *et al.*, 1979; Greaves, 1981). The data from these three series have been pooled and the influence of these phenotypic changes on subgroup definition is presented in Table V. There were a total of 22 patients out of 153 who had a phenotypic shift. this reclassification is of clinical interest as 12 of these were from the relatively good prognostic group, null $cALL^+$ to the poor prognostic subgroup, null $cALL^0$. A decrease in the percentage of blast expressing the cALL antigen at relapse was noted in 6 of the 10 null $cALL^+$ cases in Borella's series, but this decrease resulted in only one case being classified as Null $cALL^+$. While it is tempting to focus on changes at relapse, Greaves and co-workers (1980b) have pointed out that the membrane antigens are stable within leukemic cell populations in the majority of these

TABLE V
SHIFTS IN SUBGROUPS AT RELAPSE[a]

	Diagnosis	First relapse
T-ALL	34	33
		1
N ALL cALL$^+$	94	82
		8
		12
N-ALL cALL^0	21	13
		1
B-ALL	4	3

[a] Pooled data: Borella *et al.* (1979), 17 children; Melvin (1981), 33 children; and Greaves *et al.* (1980), 103 patients, mostly children.

patients. Also, immunological phenotypes are stable in long-term cultures (Greaves *et al.*, 1978).

While ALL in infants is rare, it has been well established that these patients have a poor prognosis. Bowman and co-workers (1981c) encountered seven infants in a childhood ALL patient population of 250 cases. Five of these infants were classified as null cALL^0. Pullen (1981) has collected an additional five infants with ALL, all of whom were classified as null cALL^0. As will be discussed in the next section, the null cALL^0 phenotype is associated with a poor prognosis regardless of age.

D. Prognostic Significance

Some immunological markers may have prognostic significance. The poor prognosis of T ALL (E$^{+/0}$, T$^+$) and B ALL (sIg$^+$) has already been discussed. Several additional markers have been reported to have prognostic significance (see Table VI). But only cALL has both statistical significance and has been confirmed by more than one group of investigators (Greaves and Lister, 1981; Morgan and Clement, 1980; Pullen *et al.*, 1981; Bowman *et al.*, 1981a; Melvin, 1981a; Thiel *et al.*, 1981a). Within T ALL the presence of a Thy antigen has been reported to have poor prognosis (Pincus *et al.*, 1981) and the more common TH$_2$^{0} (suppressor cell) phenotype is also associated with a poor prognosis (Reinherz *et al.*, 1979a). The poor prognosis of the Thy phenotype correlates with a recent clinical observation in a large population of children with ALL. Even after adjustment for the initial leukocyte count by regression analysis, the presence of thymic involvement predicted a poor prognosis (Henze *et al.*, personal communication). The thermal stability of the E rosettes in T ALL and the presence of either a C' or Fc receptor has been reported to be associated with a poor response to therapy in three different patient populations (Humphrey *et al.*, 1979; Richie *et al.*, 1978; Esber *et al.*, 1978). These three studies were of small patient populations and an analysis of over 200 cases suggests that these markers have little or no prognostic significance (Humphrey *et al.*, 1981). A poor prognosis for pre-B-cell leukemia has been suggested by Brouet and co-workers (1979) and Pullen and co-workers (1981). An extended observation on the pre-B ALL cases of Pullen has demonstrated a statistically significant decrease in disease free survival (Crist *et al.*, personal communication).

E. Current and Future Directions

The transition away from the use of heteroantisera and toward monoclonal antibodies for the identification of immunological phenotypes is probably the most important current activity in this field. However, it is

TABLE VI

IMMUNOLOGICAL MARKERS THAT ARE OF POTENTIAL PROGNOSTIC SIGNIFICANCE

Reference	Null		T		B	
	Poor prognosis	Good prognosis	Poor prognosis	Good prognosis	Poor prognosis	Good prognosis
Levin et al. (1980)	PNA^+	PNA^-				
Russel et al. (1981)					PNA^+	PNA^-
Greaves et al. (1981a)	$cALL^-$	$cALL^+$	E^+		sIg^+	
Morgan and Clement (1980)	$cALL^-$	$cALL^+$				
Pullen et al. (1981)	$cALL^-$ cIg^+	$cALL^+$	T^+ and/or E^+		sIg^+	
Bowman et al. (1981a)	$cALL^-$	$cALL^+$	E^+	T^+ $cALL^+$	sIg^+	
Thiel et al. (1980)			E^0 T^+ $cALL^0$ E^+ T^+ $cALL^0$	T^+ $cALL^+$		
Humphrey et al. (1979)			E_4^+ E_{37}^+ (Thermal stable)	E_4^+ E_{37}^0 (Thermal label)		
Crist et al. (personal communication)	cIg^+					
Pincus et al. (1981)			Thy^+ T^+ Th_2^0	Thy^- T^+ TH_2^+		
Reinherz et al. (1979a)	C'^+					
Richie et al. (1978)	C'^+					
Esber et al. (1978)	Fc^+					

important that both heteroantisera and monoclonal antibodies be used for a period of time so that the patients evaluated in the past and who are currently being evaluated for response to therapy can be compared to future patients defined by monoclonal antibodies. This is particularly important for the smaller subgroups within T ALL. For example, Thy antigen positivity defines a subgroup of T ALL of potential prognostic interest, but it has taken more than 3 years to identify 50 cases through a combined effort of Duke University and the Pediatric Oncology Group (Pincus *et al.*, 1981). Furthermore, it will require 2 or more years of further clinical observation before disease-free survival off therapy can be compared between the Thy$^+$ and Thy^0 patient subgroups. The relationship of heteroantisera defined Thy positivity to the OKT series of monoclonal antibodies (Reinherz *et al.*, 1980a) should be established before deleting the use of the Thy heteroantisera. The same argument can be made for TH$_2^{+/0}$ T ALL subsets (Reinherz *et al.*, 1979a). Such an analysis using both heteroantisera and a variety of monoclonal antibodies, including the OKT series, is currently underway (Metzgar and Dowell, personal communication). This study will also avoid an additional pitfall of monoclonal antibody evaluation in that the unique monoclonal antibodies generated in the laboratory of the investigator will be compared both with commercially available OKT series antibodies and unique monoclonal antibodies generated in other research laboratories. No matter how unique an individual monoclonal antibody may be, an evaluation of clinical material that does not also include standard or widely available commercial monoclonal antibodies will result in an isolated study with a generation of phenotypes that cannot be compared to other studies.

Immunologically defined phenotypes should be identified and compared to subgroups identified by other nonimmunological criteria such as those listed in Table I. In the introduction, we commented that a number of vastly different research approaches are currently being used to better define ALL. Immunological evaluation is only one area of research that is identifying heterogeneity and prognostic subgroups. What has not been clearly established is the relative prognostic significance of the various techniques used to define a poor prognostic group. A number of such studies have been recently reported, and examples would include morphological classification of ALL as assessed by FAB group and membrane phenotypes (Bennett *et al.*, 1981); enzyme and membrane markers in ALL (Hoffbrand and Janossy, 1981); TdT, immune markers, morphology, and clinical features in various lymphoid malignancies (Mertelsmann *et al.*, 1979; Beck *et al.*, 1980; Thiel *et al.*, 1981b); enzyme and surface markers in pre-B ALL (Greaves *et al.*, 1979); TdT and the production of a T-cell growth factor, interleukin 2, in various leukemias (Mertelsmann *et al.*, 1981); cytogenetics, clinical characteristics, morphology, and immunological markers in adults and children with ALL (Kaneko and Rowley, 1981b; Smithson *et al.*, 1979); clinical characteristics, immune status as measured by serum immunoglobulins, morphology, cytochemistry, and immune markers (Kersey *et al.*, 1979); immune status, serum inhibitors to mitogenic transformation to the mixed lymphocyte culture, and clinical characteristics in childhood ALL (Leiken *et al.*, 1980); morphological, cytochemical, ultrastructural, and clinical characteristics of T ALL (McKenna *et al.*, 1979); immunological characteristics, proliferation patterns, and prednisone sensitivity (Bakkeren *et al.*, 1979); immunological and clinical characteristics and ultrastructural analysis (Glick *et al.*, 1978). It is beyond the scope of this chapter to detail the implications of the above studies, however, one or two generalities are probably appropriate. Several different groups have compared the FAB morphological classification of childhood and adult ALL with immune markers and have found no correlation with the possible exception of B ALL, which is generally FAB type 3. Clinical characteristics such as age and white count are generally as important, if not more important, than immunological markers. Clearly, additional studies evaluating both the patient and lymphoblasts isolated from that patient need to be undertaken. One such study is currently in progress by the Pediatric Oncology Group (Pullen *et al.*, 1981) in which genetics, immune status, clinical characteristics, morphology, hormone receptors, cytochemistries, cytogenetics, and immune markers are being studied in all patients (Pullen *et al.*, 1981). Another multiparameter study is currently being conducted in the United Kingdom (Greaves, 1981). The importance of immunological markers has been recently questioned (Hammond, 1981; and Aisenberg, 1981). A case for the importance of immunological markers, independent of age and white count, has recently emerged from an analysis of pre-B ALL. Pre-B ALL has no clinical features such as age or white count which distinguish it from null ALL, cALL$^+$, and cIg^0 (Vogler *et al.*, 1981). However, children with pre-B ALL have a statistically significant poor prognosis (Crist *et al.*, personal communication).

A number of investigators have been evaluating nonimmune receptors for hormones such as cortisol, histamine, norepinephrine, and prostaglandin. With the exception of the cortisol receptor, most of this work has been done in animals (Peterson and Palmer, 1980). Some of these receptors are of particular interest in T ALL. The hormone sensitivity of different subpopulations of normal T lymphocytes is quite different in mice and can be used as distinguishing features of specific subgroups. For most of these hormones, their distribution among immunologically defined human subsets of lymphocytes is not known, and we are not aware of any studies underway to determine their prognostic significance. Also, whether these hormones or their antagonists can be used to manipulate tumor growth in man also remains to be determined. As mentioned in the previous section, glucocorticoid receptors have not been evaluated in immunologically defined phenotypes, however, one such study is currently underway (Leventhal, personal communication).

The detection of minimal residual disease, impending relapse, and the differentiation of normal from malignant lymphocytes are other areas that have not been adequately explored using immunological marker technology. Some interesting studies using the enzyme marker, TdT, however, can serve as useful models. A high level of this DNA polymerase is found in most cases of ALL as well as normal thymocytes. In a preliminary report, Bradstock and co-workers (1980) have reported that lymphocytes isolated from the cerebrospinal fluid of three nonleukemic patients with viral CSF leukocytosis were all TdT negative but that a case of ALL with CSF pleocytosis was TdT positive, thus confirming the diagnosis of meningeal leukemia. Currently, many institutions or cooperative groups define meningeal leukemia based on the number of CSF mononuclear cells, thus allowing the potential for aggressive intrathecal therapy or cranial spinal radiotherapy to patients with a virally induced CSF lymphocytosis. In the peripheral blood of normal individuals, TdT-positive cells are present, but in very small numbers, and increased percentages of TdT-positive cells in patients with ALL have been correlated with subsequent bone marrow relapse (Froehlich *et al.*, 1981). The combination of surface antigen detection and the TdT enzyme marker has been successfully applied to the bone marrow to detect residual disease in T ALL (Bradstock *et al.*, 1981). However, the presence of normal TdT-positive cells in normal marrow precludes this approach being applied to non-T ALL (Stass *et al.*, 1981). Recently, immunological markers have been applied to the problems of minimal residual disease. An analysis of cALL$^+$ cells in the peripheral blood indicates that this is a sensitive technique for the detection of leukemia cells in children with cALL$^+$ leukemia (Morgan and Hsu, personal communication). As stated previously, the definition of leukemia and lymphoma is very indistinct, and immunological light chain analysis complements light microscopy detection of bone marrow involvement in patients who clinically present with B cell lymphoma (Sobol *et al.*, 1981).

The functional activity, maturational capacity, or the ability of malignant lymphoblasts to interact with normal lymphocytes has not been extensively investigated; however, a few studies have been done. In one case, T lymphoblasts (E^+T^+) from an 11-month-old boy were demonstrated to depress immunoglobulin production of normal lymphocytes (Broder *et al.*, 1978). Additional studies done on these cells that were cryopreserved at the diagnosis of this infant have demonstrated that these leukemia T suppressor cells are prosuppressor cells and require a subset of cooperating normal T cells to effect maximal suppressive effects (Broder *et al.*, 1981). Kaur and co-workers (1980) have demonstrated that in one case null lymphoblasts were suppressor cells, and in a second case of null ALL, helper activity was demonstrated. Thiel and co-workers (1981c) have demonstrated that pre-B lymphoblasts (cIg$^+$ sIg^0) incubated in diffusion chambers implanted in CBA mice can differentiate to B cells (sIg$^+$), suggesting that the assumed differentiation arrest in the lymphoblast can be overcome. Finally, a number of investigators have suggested that normal immune competent mononuclear cells have infiltrated solid tumor or the bone marrow cavities in cases of leukemia, and that these cells may have biological or prognostic significance. These normal mononuclear and presumed immune competent cells can be detected by marker technology, and one such example of this type of evaluation would be that of Kaszubowski and co-workers (1980b) in their evaluation of T-cell subpopulations in the peripheral blood and tumor tissue of patients with cancer.

One of the most innovative directions in this field of research has been the application of recombinant DNA technology to the study of immunoglobulin genes. As a progeny of stem cells commits to the B-cell lineage, there is a rearrangement of at least one light chain gene. The allelic light chain gene either remains in the germ line configuration, undergoes a second rearrangement, or is lost (Hieter *et al.*, 1981). In those cell lines that have been examined to date, cells expressing the κ light chain gene have the λ light chain gene present in the germ line configuration, but in cells expressing λ light chain genes, the allelic κ gene is either deleted or has undergone rearrangement. These are presumably early events and would precede or occur with the pre-B cell phenotypically defined (cIg$^+$) stage of maturation (Cooper, 1981). When this methodology is applied to non-T non-B ALL, the majority of cells have gene rearrangements characteristic of B cells (Waldmann, personal communication). Thus, for a B ALL lymphoblast expressing a λ light chain, the presumed sequence of events leading to that phenotype would have been: (1) a reorganization of the μ immunoglobulin gene, (2) a deletion of the κ constant region gene, (3) a rearrangement of the λ immunoglobulin gene, (4) the expression of λ μ in the cytoplasma, and finally (5) the expression of λ μ on the cell surface. This proposal, especially step 4, is supported by the observation that in the normal human bone marrow, pre-B cells are more commonly cIg μ^+, λ^0, κ^0 (Kabagawa *et al.*, 1981). The use of recombinant DNA technology should clarify the origins of many of the null cell leukemias. Other approaches to a better characterization of leukemia cells include activation of T lymphoblasts to suppressor cells under the influence of cooperating normal T cells (Broder *et al.*, 1981), enhanced antigen expression by cell incubation (Hsu and Morgan, personal communication), and incubation with thymic hormone factor, resulting in null lymphoblasts becoming functional immunocompetent T cells in a xenogeneic graft-versus-host reaction (Shohat *et al.*, 1979).

During the next decade, there will certainly be some clarification of the heterogeneity that is currently being defined in ALL. It is our bias that immunological markers will be an important methodology leading to a clearer definition of subgroups with prognostic significance within ALL. However, anything that can be done to free us from the subjective limitations of light microscopy can only result in a better definition of leukemic subgroups. Admittedly, there are many subgroups currently being defined that have no clinical relevance, but analysis of large numbers of patients who are well characterized should identify relevant subgroups. To the nonimmunologically oriented oncologist, surgeon, and radiation therapist, the literature on immunological markers is probably very confusing. "God is subtle but not malicious" remarked Albert Einstein and, hopefully, the 1980s will result in appreciation of the subtlety of ALL and result in the elimination of what might be considered malicious and confusing nomenclatures.

F. RECOMMENDATIONS

We feel that determination of immunological markers is required in a diagnostic evaluation of ALL and mandatory for patients who will be entering clinical research protocols. Is there a minimal set of immunological markers that can be recommended? We propose an answer with the knowledge that any recommendations will quickly be out-of-date or inappropriate. At present, we would recommend the following for all cases of ALL: sIg, cIg, cALL, a pan T reagent (OKT 10), and E. For T ALL, additional evaluation with the OKT series, especially OKT 3, 4, 8, and 9, is highly recommended.

Finally, it must be remembered that any major advance in therapy could obliterate the prognostic significance of any of the subgroups being identified within ALL. One such example has recently been reported by Sallen and co-workers (1980). Except for this report, all other investigators have emphasized the prognostic significance of the initial leukocyte count at diagnosis and the poor response of such patients to maintenance therapy. The vast majority of this maintenance therapy has been with methotrexate and 6-mercaptopurine with or without pulses of either vincristine or prednisone or both. Sallen and co-workers do not find the initial leukocyte count to be of any prognostic significance, but their maintenance program contains adriamycin as well as 6-mercaptopurine, vincristine, and prednisone. With any new major change in therapy, a reevaluation of the prognostic significance of immunological markers or any prognostic indicator will have to be undertaken.

Hopefully, this chapter has shed some light on the importance of immunological markers in ALL. This is a very fashionable area of research, however, therapeutic advances will occur, and prevention of ALL is not impossible. For those of us in pursuit of yet another unique immunological phenotype, we must remember "sic transient gloria mundi."

ACKNOWLEDGMENTS

The authors would like to express their deepest appreciation to the following individuals who provided unpublished data or preprints for inclusion in this manuscript: Drs. John Bennett, Ronald Billing, Paul Bowman, D. Catovsky, Curt Civin, Max Cooper, Gerald Crabtree, Jean Dausset, Gideon Goldstein, M. F. Greaves, Toshio Hattori, Ronald Herberman, George Janossy, John Kersey, Kimmo Kontula, Ronald Levy, Alvin Mauer, Susan Melvin, Roland Mertelsmann, Jun Minowada, T. Mohanakumar, Elaine Morgan, Raymond Peterson, Hansjorg Riehm, Ellis Reinherz, Ellen Richie, Jerome Ritz, Janet Rowley, Ivor Royston, Edward Russell, C. S. Scott, H. L. Spielberg, Sanford Stass, E. Thiel, Teruhiko Tsubota, Elisabeth van Wering, and Thomas Waldmann. They are acknowledged in the references as personal communication. Also the authors would like to thank Betty Cameron, Patricia Randall, and Peggy Devinish for secretarial help.

REFERENCES

Abo, T., and Kumagai, K. (1978). *Clin. Exp. Immunol.* **33,** 441–452.

Abramson, C. S., Kersey, J. H., and LeBien, T. W. (1981). *J. Immunol.* p.23.

Acton, R. T., and Barger, B. O. (1981). *In* "Ped. Oncology" (G. B. Humphrey, L. P. Dehner, G. B. Grindey, and R. T. Acton, eds.), Vol. 1, pp. 47–77. Martinus Nighoff, The Hague.

Aisenberg, A. C. (1981). *N. Engl. J. Med.* **304** (6), 331–336.

Aiuti, F., Cerottini, J. C., Coombs, A., Cooper, M., Dickler, H. B., Froland, S., Hudenberg, H. H., Greaves, M. F., Grey, H. M., Kunkel, H. G., Natvig, J., Preud'homme, J. L., Rabellino, E., Ritts, R. E., Rowe, D. S., Selligmann, M., Siegal, F. P., Stjernsward, J., Terry, W. D., and Wybran, J. (1975). *Clin. Immunol. Immunopathol.* **3,** 584.

Alderson, M. (1980). *Adv. Cancer Res.* **31,** 1–76.

Ammann, A. J. Borg, D., Kondo, L., and Wara, D. W. (1977). *J. Immunol. Methods* **17,** 365–371.

Anderson, J. K., and Metzgar, R. S. (1979). *Clin. Exp. Immunol.* **37,** 339–347.

Anderson, R., Glover, A., and Rabson, A. R. (1977). *J. Immunol.* **118,** 1690–1696.

Andersson, L. C., Wasastjerna, C., and Gahmberg, C. G. (1976). *Int. J. Cancer* **17,** 40–46.

Arbeit, R. D., Henkart, P. A., and Dickler, H. B. (1976). *In* "In Vitro Methods in Cell-Mediated and Tumor Immunity" (B. R. Bloom and J. R. David, eds.), pp. 143–154. Academic Press, New York.

Arbeit, R. D., Henkart, P. A., and Dickler, H. B. (1977). *Scand. J. Immunol.* **6,** 873–878.

Avella, J., Binder, H. J., Madsen, J. E., and Askenase, P. W. (1978). *Lancet* **i**, 624–626.

Bakkeren, J. A. J. M., de Vaan, G. A. M., and Hillen, H. F. P. (1979). *Blood* **53** (5), 883–891.

Balch, C. M., Dougherty, P. A., Vogler, L. B., Ades E. W., and Ferrone, S. (1978). *J. Immunol.* **121**, 2322–2328.

Baxley, G., Bishop, G. B., Cooper, A. G., and Wortis, H. H. (1973). *Clin. Exp. Immunol.* **15**, 385–392.

Beck, J. D., Haghbin, M., Wollner, N., Mertelsmann, R., Garrett, T., Koziner, B., Clarkson, B., Miller, D., Good, R. A., and Gupta, S. (1980). *Cancer* **46**, 45–49.

Beck, J. D., Haghbin, M., and Wollner, N. (1981). *Cancer,* in press.

Bennett, J. M., Catovsky, D., Daniel, M. T., Flandrin, G., Galton, D. A. G., Gralnick, H. R., and Sultan, C. (1981). *Br. J. Haematol.* **47**, 553–561.

Berger, R., Bernheim, A., Brouet, J. C., Daniel, M. T., and Flandrin, G. (1979). *Br. J. Haematol.* **43**, 87–90.

Bertoglio, J., Thierry, C., Flores, G., Boucharel, C., Dorej J. F., and Serrou, B. (1977). *Clin. Exp. Immunol.* **27**, 172–177.

Billing, R. J., Foon, K. A., and Linker-Israeli, M. (1981). Personal communication.

Blatt, J., Reaman, G., and Poplack, D. G. (1980). *N. Engl. J. Med.* **303**, 918–922.

Borella, L., and Sen, L. (1974). *Cancer* **34**, 646–654.

Borella, L., Casper, J. T., and Lauer, S. J. (1979). *Blood* **54** (1), 64–71.

Boumsell, L., Bernard, A., Coopen, H., Richard, Y., Penit, C., Rouget, P., Lemerle, J., and Dausset, J. (1979). *J. Immunol.* **123**, 2063–2067.

Boumsell, L., Coppin, H., Pham, D., Raynal, B., Lemerle, J., Dausset, J., and Bernard, A. (1980). *J. Exp. Med.* **152**, 229–234.

Bowman, W. P., and Mauer, A. (1981). Personal Communication.

Bowman, W. P., Melvin, S. L., Aur, R. J. A., and Mauer, A. M. (1981a). *Cancer Res.,* in press.

Bowman, W. P., Melvin, S. L., Kalwinsky, D. K., Dahl, G. V., and Mauer, A. M. (1981b). *Proc. AACR ASCO* **22**, 481.

Boyd, N. F., Clemens, J. D., and Feinstein, A. R., (1979). *Arch. Intern. Med.* **139**, 324–329.

Braathen, L. R., Forre, O., and Natvig., J. B. (1979). *Clin. Immunol. Immunopathol.* **13**, 211–219.

Bradstock, K. F., Papageorigiou, E. S., Janossy, G., Hoffbrand, A. V., Willoughby, M. L., Roberts, P. D., and Bollum, F. J. (1980). *Lancet* **i**, 1144.

Bradstock, K. F., Janossy, G., Hoffbrand, A. V., Ganeshaguru, K., Lewhin, P., Prunon, H. G., and Bollum, F. J. (1981). *Br. J. Haematol.,* in press.

Brandzaeg, P. (1976). *Clin. Exp. Immunol.* **25**, 59–66.

Brian, P., Gordon, J., and Willetts, W. A. (1979). *Clin. Exp. Immunol.* **6**, 681–688.

Broder, S., Poplack, D., Whang-Peng, J., Durm, M., Goldman, C., Muul, L., and Waldmann, T. A., (1978). *N. Engl. J. Med.* **298**, 66–72.

Broder, S., Uchiyama, T., Muul, L. M., Goldman, C., Sharrow, S., Poplack, D. G., and Waldmann, T. A. (1981). *N. Engl. J. Med.* **304**, 1382–1387.

Brouet, J. C., Preud'Homme, J. L., and Seligmann, M. (1975). *Blood Cells* **1**, 81–90.

Brouet, J. C., Valensi, F., Daniel, M. T., Flandrin, G., Preud'homme, J. L., and Seligmann, M. (1976). *Br. J. Haematol.* **33**, 319–328.

Brouet, J. C., and Chevalier, A. (1979). *J. Immunol.* **122**, 260–264.

Brouet, J. C., Preud'homme, J. L., Penit, C., Valensi, F., Rouget, P., and Seligmann, M. (1979). *Blood* **54** (1), 269–273.

Brown, G., Capellaro, D., and Greaves, M. (1975). *J. Natl. Cancer Inst.* **55**, 1281–1289.

Brown, R. A., Potts, R. C., Robertson, A. J., Hayes, P. C., Ramesar, K., and Beck, J. S. (1979). *J. Immunol. Methods* **29**, 117–131.

Burns, G. F., and Cawley, J. C. (1980). *Clin. Exp. Immunol.* **39**, 83–89.
Callihan, T. R., and Berard, C. W. (1980). *Semin. Roentgenol.* **15** (3), 203–218.
Campbell, A. C., and Watter, C. A. (1979). *J. Immunol. Methods.* **26**, 337–344.
Caraux, J., Thierry, C., Esteve, C., Flores, G., Lodise, R., and Serrou, B. (1979). *Cell. Immunol.* **45**, 36–48.
Carrel, S., Gross, N., and Mach, J. P. (1979). *Cancer Res.* **39**, 5171–5176.
Catovsky, D., Papmichail, M., Okos, A., Miliani, E., and Holborrow, J. E. (1975). *Biomedicine* **23**, 81–84.
Cerottini, J. C., and Brunner, K. T. (1971). *In* "In vitro Methods in Cell-Mediated Immunity" (B. O. Bloom and P. R. Glade, eds.), pp. 369–374. Academic Press, New York.
Chao, W., and Yokoyama, M. M. (1977). *Clin. Chim. Acta* **78**, 79–84.
Charreire, J., and Bach, J. F. (1974). *Lancet* **ii**, 299–300.
Chess, L., and Schlossman, S. F. (1977). *Adv. Immunol.* **25**, 213–241.
Chessells, J. M., Janossy, G., Lawler, S. D., and Walker, L. M. S. (1979). *Br. J. Haematol.* **41**, 25–41.
Chiao, J. W., Dowling, M., and Good, R. A. (1978). *Clin. Exp. Immunol.* **32**, 498–503.
Chollet, P., Chassagne, J., Thierry, C., Sauvezie, B., Serrou, B., and Plagne, R. (1977). *Eur. J. Cancer* **13**, 333–339.
Claman, H. N. (1972). *N. Engl. J. Med.* **287**, 388–397.
Clements, P. J., and Levy, J. (1978). *Clin. Exp. Immunol.* **34**, 281–287.
Cobleigh, M. A., Braun, D. P., and Harris, J. E. (1980). *Clin. Immunol. Immunopathol.* **15**, 162–174.
Collins, R. D., Waldron, J. A., and Glick, A. D. (1979). *J. Clin. Pathol.* **72** (Suppl.), 699–707.
Cooke, A., Heppell, L., Hutchings, P., and Roitt, I. M. (1979). *Cell. Immunol.* **47**, 90–99.
Cooper, M. D. (1981). Personal communication.
Cossman, J., Glorioso, J. C., and Adler, R. (1978). *J. Immunol. Methods* **19**, 227–234.
Crabtree, G. R., Munck, A., and Smith, K. A. (1980a). *J. Immunol.* **124**, 2430–2435.
Crabtree, G. R., Munck, A., and Smith, K. A. (1980b). *J. Immunol.* **125**, 13–17.
Crist, W. M., Ragab, A. H., and Ducos, R. (1978). *Pediatrics* **61** (4), 560–563.
Crist, W., Roper, M., Ragab, A., Pullen, J., Humphrey, G. B., Boyett, J., Metzger, R., van Eys, J., Nix, W., and Cooper, M. Personal communication.
Croft, S. M., Mortensen, R. F., and Gewurz, H. (1976). *Science* **193**, 685–687.
Davey, F. R., Dock, N. L., Wolos, J. A., Terzian, J. A., and Gottlieb, A. J. (1979). *Cancer* **44**, 1622–1628.
David, J. R., and David, R. A. (1971). *In* "In Vitro Methods of Cell-Mediated Immunity" (B. R. Bloom and P. R. Glade, eds.), pp. 249–258. Academic Press, New York.
DeWolf, W. C., Schlossman, S. F., and Yunis, E. J. (1979). *J. Immunol.* **122**, 1780–1784.
Diaz, P., Jones, D. G., and Kay, A. B. (1979). *Nature (London)* **278**, 454–456.
Dickler, H. B., Adkinson, N. F., and Terry, W. D. (1974). *Nature (London)* **247**, 213–215.
Dighiero, G., Bodega, E., Mayzner, R., and Binet, J. L. (1980). *Blood* **55**, 93–100.
Duval, D., Dausse, J. P., and Dardenne, M. (1976). *Biochim. Biophys. Acta* **451**, 82–91.
Dwyer, J. M. (1976). *Prog. Allergy* **21**, 178–260.
Eremin, O., Kraft, D., Coombs, R. R. A., Franks, D., Ashby, J., and Plumb, D. (1977). *Int. Arch. Allergy Appl. Immunol.* **55**, 112–125.
Esber, E. C., Buell, D. N., and Leikin, S. L. (1976). *Blood* **48**, 33–39.
Esber, E. C., Movassaghi, N., and Leikin, S. L. (1978). *Clin. Exp. Immunol.* **32**, 523–530.
Espinouse, D., Touraine, F., Schmitt, D., and Touraine, J. L. (1978). *Clin. Exp. Immunol.* **34**, 379–387.
Espinouse, D., Touraine, J. L., Schmitt, D., and Revol, L. (1980). *Clin. Exp. Immunol.* **39**, 756–767.

Ettinger, R., Woods, G. W., Terry, W. F., and Falletta, J. M. (1979). *Clin. Res.* **27**, 815A.
Evans, R. L., Breard, J. M., Lazarus, A., Schlossman, S. F., and Chess, L. (1977). *J. Exp. Med.* **145**, 221–233.
Evans, R. L., Lazarus, H., Penta, A. C., and Schlossman, S. F. (1978). *J. Immunol.* **120**, 1423–1428.
Fanger, M. W., and Lydyard, P. M. (1979). *Clin. Exp. Immunol.* **37**, 495–501.
Feldman, M., and Pepys, M. B. (1974). *Nature (London)* **249**, 159–160.
Felsburg, P. J., and Edelman, R. (1977). *J. Immunol.* **118**, 62–66.
Ferreira, G. G. R., Brascher, H. K. M., Javierre, M. Q., Sassine, W. A., and Lima, A. O. (1976). *Experentia* **32**, 1594–1596.
Foon, K. A., Billing, R. J., Terasaki, P. I., and Cline, M. J. (1980). *Blood* **56**, 1120–1126.
Forbes, I. J., and Zalewski, P. D. (1977). *Clin. Exp. Immunol.* **26**, 99–107.
Fournier, C., and Charreire, J. (1977). *Clin. Exp. Immunol.* **29**, 468–473.
Froehlich, T. W., Buchanan, G. R., Cornet, J. A., Sartain, P. A., and Smith, R. G. (1981). *Blood* **58**, 214–220.
Froland, S. S., and Wisloff, F. (1976). "In Vitro Methods in Cell-Mediated and Tumor Immunity" (B. R. Bloom and J. R. David, eds.), pp. 137–142. Academic Press, New York.
Froland, S. S., Michaelsen, T. E., Wisloff, F., and Natvig, J. B. (1974). *Scand. J. Immunol.* **3**, 509–517.
Fu, S. M., Chiorazzi, N., Wang, C. Y., Montazen, G., Kunkel, H. G., Ko, H. S., and Gottlieb, A. B. (1978). *J. Exp. Med.* **148**, 1423–1428.
Galili, U., and Schlesinger, M. (1976). *J. Immunol.* **117**, 730–735.
Galili, U., Galili, U., Klein, E., Rosenthal, L., and Nordenskjold, B. (1980). *Cell. Immunol.* **50**, 440–444.
Gallinger, L. A., Pross, H. F., and Baines, M. G. (1980). *Int. J. Cancer* **26**, 139–150.
Gathings, W. E., Lawton, A. R., and Cooper, M. D. (1977). *Eur. J. Immunol.* **7**, 804–810.
Gelfand, E. W., Shore, A., Green, B., Lin, M. T., and Dosch, H. M. (1979). *Clin. Immunol. Immunopathol.* **12**, 119–123.
Gilbertsen, R. B., and Metzger, R. S. (1976). *Cell. Immunol.* **24**, 97–108.
Glick, A. D., Vestal, B. K., Flexner, J. M., and Collins, R. D. (1978). *Blood* **52** (2), 311–322.
Glick, B. Chang, T. S., and Japp, R. G. (1956). *Poult. Sci.* **35**, 224–225.
Gluckman, J. C., and Legrain, M. (1975). *Transplant Proc.* **7**, 407.
Gluckman, J. C., and Montambault, P. (1975). *Clin. Exp. Immunol.* **22**, 302–310.
Golightly, M. G., and Golub, S. H. (1980). *Clin. Exp. Immunol.* **39**, 222–232.
Gonzalez-Molina, A., and Spiegelberg, H. L. (1977). *J. Clin. Invest.* **59**, 616–624.
Good, R. A., and Bach, F. H. (1974). *Clin. Immunobiol.* **2**, 65–115.
Goodwin, J. S., Wiik, A., Lewis, M., Bankhurst, A. D., and Williams, R. C., Jr. (1978). *Cell. Immunol.* **43**, 150–159.
Gordon, I. L., Lukes, R. J., O'Brien, R. L., Parker, J. W., Rembaum, A., Russell, R., and Taylor, C. R. (1977). *Clin. Immunol. Immunopathol.* **8**, 51–63.
Gormus, B. J., Woodson, M., and Kaplan, M. E. (1978a). *Clin. Exp. Immunol.* **34**, 268–273.
Gormus, B. J., Woodson, M., and Kaplan, M. E. (1978b). *Clin. Exp. Immunol.* **34**, 274–280.
Gormus, B. J., Basara, M. L., Cossman, J., Arneson, M. A., and Kaplan, M. E. (1980). *Cell. Immunol.* **55**, 94–105.
Greaves, M. F. (1981). *Cancer Res.,* in press.
Greaves, M., and Janossy, G. (1978). *Biochim. Biophys. Acta* **516**, 193–230.
Greaves, M. F., and Lister, T. A. (1981). *N. Engl. J. Med.* **304**, 119–120.
Greaves, M. F., Brown, G., and Rickinson, A. (1975). *Clin. Immunol. Immunopathol.* **3**, 514–524.
Greaves, M. F., Janossy, G., Francis, G., and Minowada, J. (1978). *In* "Differentiation of

nal and Neoplastic Hematopoietic Cells'' (B. Clarkson, P. A. Marks, and J. Till, .), p. 823. Cold Spring Harbor Laboratory, Cold Spring Harbor, New York.

G. ːs, M., Verbi, W., Vogler, L., Cooper, M., Ellis, R., Ganeshaguru, K., Hoffbrand, V., Janossy, G., and Bollum, F. J. (1979). *Leuk. Res.* **3** (6), 353–362.

Greaves, M., Paxton, A., Janossy, G., Pain, C., Johnson, S., and Lister, T. A. (1980a). *Leuk. Res.* **4**, 1–14.

Greaves, M. F., Verbi, W., Kemshead, J., and Kennett, R. (1980b). *Blood* **56** (6), 1141–1144.

Gross, N., and Bron, C. (1978). *Clin. Exp. Immunol.* **33**, 283–291.

Grossi, C. E., Webb, S. R., Zicca, A., Lydyard, P. M., Moretta, L., Mingari, M. C., and Cooper, M. D. (1977). *J. Exp. Med.* **145**, 1405–1417.

Gupta, S., and Good, R. A. (1977). *Cell. Immunol.* **34**, 10–18.

Gupta, S., and Good, R. A. (1978). *Cell. Immunol.* **36**, 263–270.

Gupta, S., and Good, R. A. (1980). *Semin. Hematol.* **17** (1), 1–29.

Gupta, S., and Grieco, M. H. (1975). *Int. Arch. Allergy Appl. Immunol.* **49**, 734–742.

Gupta, S., Goel, Z., and Grieco, M. H. (1976a). *Int. Arch. Allergy Appl. Immunol.* **52**, 273–276.

Gupta, S., Good, R. A., and Siegal, F. P. (1976b). *Clin. Exp. Immunol.* **26**, 204–213.

Gupta, S., Ross, G. D., Good, R. A., and Siegal, F. P. (1976c). *Blood* **48**, 755–763.

Gupta, S., Good, R. A., and Siegal, F. P. (1976d). *Clin. Exp. Immunol.* **25**, 319–327.

Gupta, S., Platsoucas, S. C., Schulof, R. S., and Good, R. A. (1979a). *Cell. Immunol.* **45**, 469–470.

Gupta, S., Platsoucas, C. D., and Good, R. A. (1979b). *Proc. Natl. Acad. Sci. U.S.A.* **76**, 4025–4028.

Haegert, D. G. (1978). *J. Immunol.* **120**, 124–129.

Hammond, D. (1981). *Cancer Res.*, in press.

Harris, C. C., Mulvihill, J. J., Snorri, S., Thorgeirsson, S. S., and Minna, J. D. (1980). *Ann. Intern. Med.* **92** (6), 809–825.

Hattori, T., Uchiyama, T., Takatsuki, K., and Uchino, H. (1980). *Clin. Immunol. Immunopathol.* **17**, 287–295.

Hayward, A. R., Layward, L., Lydyard, P. M., Moretta, L., Dagg, M., and Lawton, A. R. (1978). *J. Immunol.* **121**, 1–5.

Heijnen, C. J., Haag, F. U., Gmelig-Meyling, F. H. J., and Ballieux, R. E. (1979). *Cell. Immunol.* **43**, 282–292.

Helderman, J. H., and Strom, T. B. (1978). *Nature (London)* **274**, 62–63.

Helderman, J. H., Strom, T. B., and Dupuy-D'Angeac, A. (1979). *Cell. Immunol.* **46**, 247–258.

Henze, G., Langermann, H. J., Kaufmann, V., Ludwig, R., Schellong, G., Stollmann, B., and Riehm, H. Personal communication.

Hepburn, B., and Ritts, R. E. (1974). *Mayo Clin. Proc.* **49**, 866–869.

Hieter, P. A., Korsmeyer, S. J., Waldmann, T. A., and Leder, P. (1981). Personal communication.

Hiraoka, A., Yamagishi, M., Ohkubo, T., Yoshida, Y., and Uchiro, H. (1980). *Blood* **56**, 859–865.

Hoffbrand, A. V., and Janossy, G. (1981). *J. Clin. Pathol.* **34**, 254–262.

Horowitz, S., Groshong, T., Albrecht, R., and Hong, R. (1975). *Clin. Immunol. Immunopathol.* **4**, 405–414.

Horwitz, D. A., Cooper, M., and Carvalho, E. (1979). *Clin. Immunol. Immunopathol.* **14**, 159–171.

Hsu, C. C. S., and Morgan, E. R. (1978). *Am. J. Clin. Pathol.* **70**, 741–747.

Hsu, C. C. S., and Morgan, E. R. Personal communication.

Huber, C., Flad, H. D., Nilsson, K., Wigzell, H., Michlmayr, G., Frischauf, H., and Braun-steiner, H. (1978). *Blood* **52**, 911–921.

Huhn, D. (1980). *Cancer Chemother. Pharmacol.* **4**, 237–242.

Humphrey, G. B., and Lankford, J. (1976). *Semin. Oncol.* **3** (3), 243–251.

Humphrey, G. B., Herson, J., Pullen, J., Crist, W., Ragab, A., Falletta, J., and Ped. Div. SWOG. (1978a). *Int. Soc. Exp. Hematol.* **6** (Suppl. 3), 85.

Humphrey, G. B., Falletta, J., Crist, W., and Ragab, A. (1978b). *Proc. AACR ASCO,* **19**, 220.

Humphrey, G. B., Crist, W., Falletta, J., Richie, E., Ragab, A., and Pullen. J. (1979). *Proc. AACR ASCO* **20** (1176), 289.

Humphrey, G. B., Blackstock, R., and Filler, J. (1980). *Ann. Clin. Lab. Sci.* **10** (3), 169–180.

Humphrey, G. B., Blackstock, R., Falletta, J. M., Metzgar, R., van Eys, J., Richie, E. R., Crist, W. M., Cooper, M. D., Pullen, D. J., and Schuster, J. (1981). *Exp. Hematol.* Suppl. **9**, 79 (Abstr.)

Hvizdala, E. (1981). Unpublished results of the Pediatric Oncology Group.

Iacobelli, S., Ranelletti, F. O., Longo, P., Riccardi, R., and Mastrangelo, R. (1978). *Cancer Res.* **38**, 4257–4262.

Indiveri, F., Pellegrino, M. A., Molinaro, G. A., Quaranta, V., and Ferrone, S. (1979). *J. Immunol. Methods* **30**, 317–328.

Isaacson, P. (1979). *J. Clin. Pathol.* **32**, 802–807.

Janossy, G., Francis, G. E., Capellaro, D., Goldstone, A. H., and Greaves, M. F. (1978). *Nature (London)* **276**, 176–178.

Janossy, G., Bollum, F. J., Bradstock, K. F., and Ashley, J. (1980). *Blood* **56** (3), 430–441.

Jondal, M., and Klein, G. (1973). *J. Exp. Med.* **138**, 1365–1378.

Jondal, M., Holm, G., and Wigzell, H. (1972). *J. Exp. Med.* **136**, 207–215.

Jondal, M., Klein, G., Oldstone, M. B. A., Bokish, V., and Yefenof, E. (1976). *Scand. J. Immunol.* **5**, 401–410.

Kabisch, H., Arndt, R., Becker, W. M., Thiel, H. G., and Landbeck, G. (1979). *Leuk. Res.* **3**, 83–91.

Kaji, H., and Parkhouse, R. M. E. (1974). *Nature (London)* **249**, 45–47.

Kaneko, Y., and Rowley, J. D. (1981a). In "Pediatric Oncology" (G. B. Humphrey, L. P. Dehner, G. B. Grindez, and R. T. Acton, eds., Vol. II. Martinus Nighoff, The Hague (in press).

Kaneko, Y., and Rowley, J. D. (1981b). *Proc. AACR ASCO* **22**, 338.

Kaneko, Y., Rowley, J. D., Check, I., Variakojis, D., and Moohr, J. W. (1980). *Blood* **56** (5), 782–785.

Kaplan, J. (1975). *Clin. Immunol. Immunopathol.* **3**, 471–475.

Kaplan, J. H., and Uzgiris, E. E. (1976) *J. Immunol.* **117**, 115–123.

Kaplan, M. E., and Clark, C. (1974). *J. Immunol. Methods* **5**, 131–135.

Kaszubowski, P. A., Goodwin, J. S., and Williams, R. C., Jr. (1980a). *J. Immunol.* **124**, 1075–1078.

Kaszubowski, P. A., Husby, G., Tung, K. S. K., and Williams, R. C., Jr. (1980b). *Cancer Res.* **40**, 4648–4657.

Katoh, G., and Charoensiri, S. (1977). *J. Immunol.* **118**, 2291–2292.

Katoh, A., and Charoensiri, S. (1978). *Immunol. Commun.* **7**, 483–494.

Kaur, P., Miller, D., Good, R., and Gupta, S. (1980). *Proc. AACR ASCO* p. 204.

Kawashima, K., Morishima, Y., Kato, Y., Takeyama, H., Kabayashi, M., Suzuki, K. Veda, R., Yamada, K., Naito, K., Yoshikawa, S., and Sako, F. (1978). *Clin. Exp. Immunol.* **31**, 448–455.

Kay, N. E., Ackerman, S. K., and Douglas, S. D. (1979). *Semin. Hematol.* **16** (4), 252–282.

Kedar, E., and Bonavida, B. (1974). *J. Immunol.* **113**, 1544–1552.

Kerman, R. H., Smith, R., Stefani, S. S., and Ezdinli, E. Z. (1976). *Cancer Res.* **36**, 3274–3278.

Kersey, J., Nesbit, M., Hallgrer, H., Sabad, A., Yunis, E., and Gajl-Peczalska, K. (1975). *Cancer* **36**, 1348–1352.

Kersey, J. H., LeBein, T. W., Hurwitz, R., Nesbit, M. E., Gajl-Peczalska, K. J., Hammond, D., Miller, D. R., Coccia, P. F., and Leikin, S. (1979). *Am. J. Clin. Pathol.* **72**, 746–752.

Kersey, J. H., LeBien, T. W., Abramson, C. S., Newman, R., Sutherland, R., and Greaves, M. (1981). *J. Exp. Med.* **153**, 726–731.

Kleinman, R., and Teodorescu, M. (1979). *Cell. Immunol.* **48**, 43–51.

Ko, H. S., Fu, S. M., Winchester, R. J., Yu, D. T. Y., and Kunkel, H. G. (1979). *J. Exp. Med.* **150**, 246–255.

Kontula, K., Andersson, L. C., Paavonen, T., Myllyla, G., Teerenhovi, L., and Vuopio, P. (1980). *Int. J. Cancer* **26**, 177–183.

Koziner, B., Mertelsmann, R., Filippa, D. A., Good, R. A., and Clarkson, B. D. (1978). *In* "Differentiation of Normal and Neoplastic Hematopoietic Cells" (B. Clarkson, P. A. Miles, and J. E. Till, eds.). 843–857. Cold Spring Harbor Laboratory, Cold Spring Harbor, New York.

Koziner, B., Kempin, S., Passe, S., Gee, T., Good. R. A., and Clarkson, B. D. (1980a). *Blood* **56** (5), 815–823.

Koziner, B., Mertelsmann, R., Andreeff, M., Arlin, Z. Hansen, H., De Harven, E., McKenzie, S., Gee, T., Good, R. A., and Clarkson, B. (1980b). *Blood* **55** (4), 694–698.

Kubagawa, H., Gathings, W. E., Levitt, D., and Cooper, M. D. (1981). *Pediatr. Res.* **15**, 599.

Kung, P. C., Goldstein, G., Reinherz, E. G., and Schlossman, S. F. (1979a). *Science* **206**, 347–349.

Kung, P. C., Talle, M. A., DeMaria, M., Butler, M., Lifter, J., and Goldstein, G. (1979b). *Nat. Workshop Organ Spec. Alloantigens, 1st, Albert Einstein Med. School.*

Lambermont, M., Wybran, J., and Govaerts, A. (1977). *J. Immunol. Methods* **15**, 157–162.

Laurent, G., Gourdin, M. F., and Reyes, F. (1980). *Am. J. Clin. Pathol.* **74**, 265–273.

LaVia, M. F., and LaVia, D. S. (1978). *Cell. Immunol.* **39**, 297–306.

Lay, W. H., Coombs, R. R. A., Gurner, B. W., Wilson, A. B., Holm, G., and Lindgren, B. (1970). *Int. Arch. Allergy* **39**, 658–663.

Lay, W. H., Mendes, N. D., Bianco, C., and Nussenzweig, V. (1971). *Nature (London)* **230**, 531–532.

LeBien, T. W., and Kersey, J. H. (1980). *J. Immunol.* **125**, 2208–2214.

LeBien, T. W., Hozier, J., Minowada, J., and Kersey, J. H. (1979). *N. Engl. J. Med.* **301**, 144.

Lees, O. (1977). *Eur. J. Cancer* **13**, 345–349.

Leikin, S., Miller, D., Sather, H., Albo, V., Vitale, L., Rogentine, N., and Hammond, D. (1980). *Proc. AACR ASCO* p. 372. (Abstr.)

Leimert, J. T., Burns, C. P., Wiltse, C. G., Armitage, J. O., and Clarke, W. R. (1980). *Blood* **56** (3), 510–515.

Leventhal, B. Pediatric Oncology Group, personal communication.

Levin, S., Russell, E. C., Blanchard, D., McWilliams, N. B., Maurer, H. M., and Mohanakumar, T. (1980). *Blood* **55** (1), 37–39.

Limatibul, S., Shore, A., Dosch, H. M., and Gelfand, W. (1978). *Clin. Immunol. Immunopathol.* **33**, 503–513.

Lippman, M. E., Yarbro, G. K., and Leventhal, B. G. (1978). *Cancer Res.* **38**, 4251–4256.

Lohrmann, H. P., and Novikovs, L. (1974). *Clin. Immunol. Immunopathol.* **3**, 99–111.
Lum, L. G., Muchmore, A. V., Decker, J. M., and Blase, R. M. (1979). *Clin. Exp. Immunol.* **37**, 558–561.
Lydyard, P. M., and Fanger, M. W. (1979). *Clin. Exp. Immunol.* **37**, 486–494.
McKenna, R. W., Parkin, J., and Brunning, R. D. (1979). *Cancer* **44**, 1290–1297.
Mahowald, M. L., Handwerger, B. S., Capertone, E. M., and Douglas S. D. (1977). *J. Immunol. Methods* **15**, 239–245.
Mantovani, B., Rabinovitch, M., and Nussenzweig, V. (1972). *J. Exp. Med.* **135**, 780–792.
Marone, G., Plaut, M., and Lichtenstein, L. M. (1978). *J. Immunol.* **11**, 2153–2159.
Mastrangelo, R., Malandrino, R., Riccardi, R., Longo, P., Ranelletti, F. O., and Iacobelli, S. (1980). *Blood* **56** (6), 1036–1040.
Melvin, S. L. (1979). *Blood* **54** (1), 210–215.
Melvin, S. L. (1981a). *Cancer Res.,* in press.
Melvin, S. L. (1981b). *Front. Immunogenet.,* in press.
Mendes, N. F., Tolnai, M. E. A., Silveira, N. P. A., Gilbertson, R. B., and Metzgar, R. S. (1973). *J. Immunol.* **111**, 860–867.
Mendes, N. F., Miki, S. S., and Peixinho, Z. F. (1974). *J. Immunol.* **113**, 531–536.
Mertelsmann, R., Filippa, D. A., Koziner, B., Grossbard, E., Beck, J., Moore, M. A., Lieberman, P. H., Clarkson, B. D., Gupta, S., and Good, R. A. (1979). *Adv. Exp. Med. Biol.* **114**, 553–560.
Mertelsmann, R., Gillis, S., Steinmann, G., Ralph, P., Stiehm, M., Koziner, B., and Moore, M. A. S. (1981). *Blut,* in press.
Mestecky, J., Preud'Homme, J. L., Crago, S. S., Mihaesco, E., Prchal, J. T., and Okos, A. J. (1980). *Clin. Exp. Immunol.* **39**, 371–385.
Metzger, R. S., and Mohanakumar, T. (1977). *Am. J. Clin. Pathol.* **68**, 699–705.
Metzger, R. S., and Mohanakumar, T. (1978). *Semin. Hematol.* **15**, 139–157.
Metzger, R., and Nowell, P. (1981). Personal communication.
Miller, J. F. A. P. (1961). *Lancet* **II**, 748–751.
Miller, J. F. A. P. (1979). *Semin. Hematol.* **16** (4), 283–292.
Miller, J. F. A. P., Doak, S. M. A., and Cross, A. M. (1963). *Proc. Soc. Exp. Biol.* **112**, 785–792.
Minowada, J., Sagawa, K., Lok, M. S., Kubonishi, I., Nakazawa, S., Tatsumi, E., Ohnuma, T., and Goldblum, N. (1980). *In* "International Symposium on New Trends in Human Immunology and Cancer Immunotherapy" (B. Serrou and C. Rosenfeld, eds.), pp. 188–199. Doin, Paris.
Minowada, J., Sagawa, K., Trowbridge, I. S., and Kung, P. D. (1981a). *In* "Third Annual Bristol-Myers on Cancer Research, Advances in Malignant Lymphomas: Etiology, Immunology, Pathology, Treatment" (H. S. Kaplan and S. A. R. Rosenberg, eds.). Academic Press, New York.
Minowada, J., Koshiba, H., Sagawa, K., Kubonishi, I., Lok, M. S., Tatsumi, E., Han, T., Srivastava, B. I. S., and Ohnuma, T. (1981b) *J. Cancer Res. Clin. Oncology,* in press.
Mishell, R. I., and Dutton, R. W. (1966). *Science* **153**, 1004–1005.
Moore, A. L., and Zusman, J. (1978). *J. Immunol. Methods* **23**, 275–284.
Moore, M. A. S., Broxmeyer, H. E., Sheridan, A. P. C., Meyers, P. A., Jacobsen, N., and Winchester, R. J. (1980). *Blood* **55**, 682–690.
Moretta, L., Ferrarini, M., and Durante, M. L. (1975). *Eur. J. Immunol.* **5**, 565–568.
Moretta, L., Ferrarini, M., Mingari, M. C., Moretta, A., and Webb, S. R. (1976). *J. Immunol.* **117**, 2171–2174.
Moretta, L., Webb, S. R., Grossi, C. E., Lydyard, P. M., and Cooper, M. D. (1977). *J. Exp. Med.* **146**, 184–200.

Morgan, E., and Clement, C. S. H. (1980). *Am. J. Pediatr. Hematol. Oncol.* **2** (2), 99–102.

Morgan, E., and Hsu, C. C. S. Personal communication.

Mullink, H., VonBlomberg, M., Wilders, M. M., Drexhage, H. A., and Alons, C. L. (1979). *J. Immunol. Methods* **29**, 133–137.

Nadler, L. M., Reinherz, E. L., and Schlossman, S. F. (1980a). *Cancer Chemother. Pharmacol.* **4**, 11–15.

Nadler, L. M., Reinherz, E. L., Weinstein, H. J., D'Orsi, C. J., and Schlossman, S. F. (1980b). *Blood* **55** (5), 806–810.

Nadler, L. M., Ritz, J., Hardy, R., Pesando, J. M., Schlossman, S. F., and Stashenko, P. (1981). *J. Clin. Invest.* **67**, 134–140.

Nekam, K., Kalamar, L., Gergely, P., Kelemen, G., Fekete, B., Lang, I., Levai, J., and Petranyi, G. Y. (1977). *Clin. Exp. Immunol.* **27**, 416–420.

Netzel, B., Rodt, H., Thiel, E., Haas, R. J., and Thierfelder, S. (1979). *Acta Haematol.* **61**, 177–183.

Nishida, Y., Okudaira, K., Tanimoto, K., and Akaoka, I. (1980). *Exp. Hematol.* **8** (5), 593–598.

Nix, W. L., Mukhopadhyay, N., Steuber, C. P., Shepherd, D. A., and Fernbach, D. J. (1978). *Blood* **52** (Suppl. 1), 267. (Abstr.)

Olisa, E. G., Chandra, R., Jackson, M. A., Kennedy, J., and Williams, A. O. (1975). *J. Natl. Cancer Inst.* **55**, 281–284.

Osband, M. E., Cohen, E. B., McCaffrey, R. P., and Shapiro, H. M. (1980). *Blood* **56**, 923–925.

Paavoner, T., Andersson, L. C., and Kontula, K. (1981). *J. Recept. Res.,* in press.

Palutke, M., and Tabaczka, P. (1980). *Ann. Clin. Lab. Sci.* **10** (4), 269–279.

Pandolfi, F., Kurnick, J. T., Nilsson, K., Forsbeck, K., and Wigzell, H. (1978). *Clin. Exp. Immunol.* **32**, 504–509.

Pandolfi, F., Strong, D. M., and Bonnard, G. D. (1981). In press.

Pape, G. R., Moretta, L., Troye, M., and Perlmann, P. (1979). *Scand. J. Immunol.* **9**, 291–296.

Park, C. H. (1980). *Proc. AACR ASCO* **221**, 56.

Pearl, E. R., Vogler, L. B., Okos, A. J., Crist, W. M., Lawton, A. R., and Cooper, M. D. (1978). *J. Immunol.* **120**, 1169–1175.

Pellegrino, M. A., Ferrone, S., Dierich, M. P., and Reisfeld, R. A. (1975a). *Clin. Immunol. Immunopathol.* **3**, 324–328.

Pellegrino, M. A., Ferrone, S., and Theofilopolous, A. N. (1975b). *J. Immunol.* **115**, 1065–1071.

Pesando, J. M., Ritz, J., Levine, H., Terhorst, C., Lazarus, H., and Schlossman, S. F. (1980). *J. Immunol.* **124**, 2794–2799.

Peterson, R. D. A., and Palmer, G. C. (1980). *Immunopharmacology* **2** (2), 147–155.

Pichler, W. J., and Broder, S. (1978). *J. Immunol.* **121**, 887–890.

Pichler, W. J., Gendelman, F. W., and Nelson, D. L. (1979). *Cell. Immunol.* **42**, 410–417.

Pincus, J. K., Falletta, J. M., Metzgar, R., Pullen, J., Crist, W., Humphrey, G. B., Boyette, J., and van Eys, J. (1981). *Pediatr. Res.* **15**, 584.

Platsoucas, C. D., Good, R. A., and Gupta, S. (1979) *Proc. Natl. Acad. Sci. U.S.A.* **76**, 1972–1976.

Plaut, M., Lichtenstein, L. M., Gillespie, E., and Henny, C. S. (1973). *J. Immunol.* **111**, 389–394.

Plaut, M., Lichtenstein, L. M., and Henney, C. S. (1975). *J. Clin. Invest.* **55**, 856–874.

Pochet, R., Delespesse, G., Gausset, P. W., and Collet, H. (1979). *Clin. Exp. Immunol.* **38**, 578–584.

Priest, J. R., Warkentin, P. I., LeBien, T. W., Lindquist, L. L., Brunning, R. D., Yasmineh, W. G., Kersey, J. H., Nesbit, M. E., and Coccia, F. F. (1979). *Proc. Am. Assoc. Cancer Res.* **20**, 97.

Priest, J. R., Robison, L. L., McKenna, R. W., Lindquist, L. L., Warkentin, P. I., LeBien, T. W., Woods, W. G., Kersey, J. H., Coccia, P. F., and Nesbit, M. E., Jr. (1980). *Blood* **56** (1), 15–22.

Prokocimer, M., Matzner, Y., Ben-Bassat, H., and Polliack, A. (1980). *Cancer* **45**, 2884–2889.

Pullen, D. J. (1981) Unpublished results for the Pediatric Oncology Group.

Pullen, D. J., Falletta, J. M., Crist, W. M., Vogler, L. B., Dowell, B., Humphrey, G. B., Blackstock, R., Van Eys, J., Cooper, M. D., Metzgar, R. S., and Meydrech, E. F. (1981). *Cancer Res.*, in press.

Raff, M. C., Megson, M., Owen, J. J. T., and Cooper, M. D. (1976). *Nature (London)* **259**, 224–228.

Raney, R. B., Jr., Festa, R. S., Waldman, M. T. G., Manson, D., and Hann, H. L. (1979). *Am. J. Hematol.* **6**, 27–34.

Reaman, G. H., Pichler, W. J., Broder, S., and Poplack, D. G. (1979). *Blood* **54**, 285–291.

Reaman, G. H., Lum, L. G., and Poplack, D. G. (1980). *Cell. Immunol.* **52**, 218–222.

Reinherz, E. L., and Schlossman, S. F. (1979). *J. Immunol.* **122**, 1335–1341.

Reinherz, E., and Schlossman, S. F. (1980). *Cell* **19**, 821–827.

Reinherz, E. L., and Schlossman, S. F. (1981). *Immunol. Today*, in press.

Reinherz, E. L., Nadler, L. M., Sallan, S. E., and Schlossman, S. F. (1979a). *J. Clin. Invest.* **64**, 392–397.

Reinherz, E. L., Strelkauskas, A. J., O'Brien, C., and Schlossman, S. F. (1979b). *J. Immunol.* **123**, 83–85.

Reinherz, E. L., Kung, P. C., Goldstein, G., and Schlossman, S. F. (1979c). *J. Immunol.* **123**, 1312–1317.

Reinherz, E. L., Kung, P. C., Pesando, J. M., Ritz, J., Goldstein, G., and Schlossman, S. F. (1979d). *J. Exp. Med.* **150**, 1472–1482.

Reinherz, E. L., Kung, P. C., Goldstein, G., Levey, R. H., and Schlossman, S. F. (1980a). *Proc. Natl. Acad. Sci. U.S.A.* **77** (3), 1588–1592.

Reinherz, E. L., Moretta, L., Roper, M., Breard, J. M., Mingari, M. C., Cooper, M. D., and Schlossman, S. F. (1980b). *J. Exp. Med.* **151**, 969–974.

Reisner, Y., Linker-Israeli, M., and Sharon, N. (1976). *Cell. Immunol.* **25**, 129–134.

Reisner, Y., Itzicovitch, L., Meshorer, L., and Sharon, N. (1978). *Proc. Natl. Acad. Sci. U.S.A.* **75**, 2933–2936.

Reisner, Y., Biniaminov, M., Rosenthal, E., Sharon, N., and Ramot, B. (1979). *Proc. Natl. Acad. Sci. U.S.A.* **76**, 447–451.

Rich, R. R., and Rich, S. S. (1975), *J. Immunol.* **114**, 1112–1115.

Richie, E., and Patchen, M. (1978). *Clin. Immunol. Immunopathol.* **11**, 88–97.

Richie, E. R., Culbert, S. J., Sullivan, M. P., and van Eys, J. (1978). *Cancer Res.* **38**, 3616–3620.

Ridway, J. C., Taylor, G. M., and Harris, R. (1979). *J. Immunol. Methods* **29**, 271–277.

Rigal, D., Monier, J. C., and Souweine, G. (1979). *Cell. Immunol.* **46**, 360–372.

Ritz, J., Pesando, J. M., Notis-McConarty, J., Lazarus, H., and Schlossman, S. F. (1980a). *Nature (London)* **283**, 583–585.

Ritz, J., Pesando, J. M., Notis-McConarty, J., and Schlossman, S. F. (1980b). *J. Immunol.* **125**, 1506–1514.

Ritz, J., Pesando, J. M., Notis-McConarty, J., Clavell, L. A., Sallan, S. E., and Schlossman, S. F. (1981). *Cancer Res.*, in press.

Rivero, I., Abaca, H. E., Valles, R., Vannucci, J. D., Diumengo, M. S., and Moravenik, M. B. (1979). *Scand. J. Immunol.* **9,** 9–14.

Roberts, M., Greaves, M., Janossy, G., Sutherland, R., and Pain, C. (1978). *Leuk. Res.* **2,** 105–114.

Rocklin, R. E. (1976). *J. Clin. Invest.* **57,** 1051–1058.

Rocklin, R. E. (1977). *J. Immunol.* **118,** 1734–1738.

Rocklin, R. E., Greineder, D. K., and Melmon, K. L. (1979). *Cell. Immunol.* **44,** 404–415.

Romagrani, S., Maggi, E., Biagiotti, R., Giudizi, G. M., Amadori, A., and Ricci, M. (1978). *Clin. Exp. Immunol.* **82,** 324–332.

Romagnani, S., Maggi, E., Lorenzini, M., Giudizi, G. M., Biagiotti, R., and Ricci, M. (1979). *Clin. Exp. Immunol.* **36,** 502–510.

Roper, M., Crist, W., Metzgar, R., Nix, W., Smith, S., Pullen, J., Ragab, A., and Cooper, M. D. (1981). *Proc. AACR ASCO*, in press.

Rosenszajn, L. A., Gutman, A., Radnay, J., David, E. B., and Shoham, D. (1976). *Am. J. Clin. Pathol.* **66,** 432–441.

Ross, G. D. (1979). *Blood* **53** (5), 799–811.

Ross, G. D., and Polley, M. J. (1975). *J. Exp. Med.* **141,** 1163–1180.

Roth, D. G., Cimino, M. C., Variakojis, D., Golomb, H. M., and Rowley, J. D. (1979). *Blood* **53** (2), 235–243.

Rothbarton, P. H., Tanke, H., Gmelig-Meyling, F., Ballieux, R. E., and Stoop, J. W. (1978). *J. Immunol. Methods* **19,** 111–118.

Royston, I., Omary, M. B., and Trowbridge, I. S. (1981). *Transplant Proc.* **13,** 761–766.

Rudders, R. A., Andersen, J., and Fried, R. (1980). *J. Immunol.* **124,** 2347–2351.

Ruscetti, F. W., and Gallo, R. C. (1981). *Blood* **57,** 379–394.

Russell, E. C., Mohanakumar, T., McWilliams, N. B., Dunn, N. L., and Maurer, H. M. (1981) *Pediatr. Res.* **15,** 586.

Saffhill, R., Dexter, T. M., Testa, N., Morris-Jones, P. H., and Hann, I. M. (1978). *Br. Med. J.* **6104,** 49.

Sallen, S. E., Ritz, J., Pesando, J., Gelber, R., O'Brien, C., Hitchcock, S., Coral, F., and Schlossman, S. F. (1980). *Blood* **55** (3), 395–400.

Sandilands, G. P., Gray, K. G., Coone, A. E., Browning, J. D., and Anderson, J. R. (1975). *Clin. Exp. Immunol.* **22,** 493–501.

Saxon, A., Morledge, D., and Bonavida, B. (1977). *Clin. Exp. Immunol.* **28,** 394–399.

Saxon, A., Stevens, R. H., and Golde, D. W. (1979). *N. Engl. J. Med.* **300,** 700–704.

Schlesinger, M., and Kertes, T. (1979). *Clin. Immunol. Immunopathol.* **12,** 1–11.

Schmidt, T. J., and Thompson, E. B. (1978). *Prog. Canc. Res. Ther.* pp. 263–290.

Schreiber, A. B., Hoebeke, J., Bergman, Y., Haimovich, J., and Strosberg, A. D. (1978). *J. Immunol.* **121,** 19–23.

Schumacher, H. R., Champion, J. E., Thomas, W. J., Pitts, L. L., and Stass, S. A. (1979). *Am. J. Hematol.* **7,** 11–17.

Schumacher, H. R., Clapp, W. L., Thomas, W. J., Mandavia, S. G., and Pitts, L. L. (1980). *Arch. Pathol. Lab. Med.* **104,** 134–136.

Scribner, D. J., and Fahrney, D. (1976). *J. Immunol.* **116,** 892–897.

Segal, D. M., and Horowitz, E. (1977). *J. Immunol.* **118,** 1338–1339.

Sen, L., and Borella, L. (1975). *N. Engl. J. Med.* **292,** 828–832.

Sen, L., Mills, B., and Borella, L. (1976). *Cancer Res.* **36,** 2436–2441.

Shannon, E. J., and Hastings, R. C. (1977). *J. Immunol. Methods* **18,** 321–336.

Shaw, G. M., Levy, P. C., and Lobuglio, A. F. (1979a). *Clin. Exp. Immunol.* **36,** 496–501.

Shaw, S., Pichler, W. J., and Nelson, D. L. (1979b). *J. Immunol.* **122,** 599–604.

Shearer, G. M., Melmon, K. L., Weinstein, Y., and Sela, M. (1972). *J. Exp. Med.* **136,** 1302–1307.

Shen, L., Lydyard, P. M., Penfold, P., and Roitt, I. M. (1979). *Clin. Exp. Immunol.* **35,** 276–285.

Shohat, B., Wolach, B., and Trainin, N. (1979). *Cell. Immunol.* **45,** 255–260.

Shore, A., Dosch, H. M., and Gelfand, E. W. (1978). *Nature (London)* **274,** 586–587.

Slater, R. M., Philip, P., Badsberg, E., Behrendt, H., Hansen, N. E., and van Heerde, P. (1979). *Int. J. Cancer* **23,** 639–647.

Slease, R. B., Gadek, J. E., Frank, M. M., and Scher, I. (1980). *Blood* **56,** 792–797.

Smith, K. A., Crabtree, G. R., Kennedy, S. J., and Munck, A. U. (1977). *Nature (London)* **267,** 523–526.

Smithson, W. A., Li, C. Y., Pierre, R. V., Ritts, R. E., Jr., Burger, E. O., Jr., Gilchrist, G. S., Ilstrup, D. M., and Hoffman, A. D, (1979). *Med. Pediatr. Oncol.* **7,** 83–93.

Sobol, R. E., Chisari, F., and Royston, I. (1981). Personal communication.

Spiegelberg, H. L. (1981). Personal communication.

Spiegelberg, H. L., and Dainer, P. M. (1979). *Clin. Exp. Immunol.* **35,** 286–295.

Stass, S. A., Perlin, E., Jaffe, E. S., Simon, D. R., Creegan, W. J., Robinson, J. J., Holloway, M. L., and Schumaker, H. R. (1978). *Am. J. Hematol.* **4,** 67–77.

Stass, S. A., Phillips, T. M., Weislow, O. S., Perlin, E., and Schumacher, H. R. (1980). *Blood* **56** (4), 661–666.

Stass, S. A., McGraw, T. P., Folds, J. D., Odle, B., and Bollum, F. J. (1981). *Am. J. Clin. Pathol.* **75,** 838–840.

Stathopoulos, G., and Elliott, E. V. (1974). *Lancet* **i,** 600–601.

Stern, R., Widirstky, S. T., Wurster-Hill, D. H., Allen, R. D., Smith, K. A., Cornwell, G. G., III, and Cornell, C. J., Jr. (1979). *Blood* **54** (3), 703–712.

Stevens, R. H., and Saxon, A. (1978). *Clin. Immunol. Immunopathol.* **10,** 438–445.

Stratton, J. A., and Byfield, P. E. (1977). *Cell. Immunol.* **28,** 1–14.

Strelkauskas, A. J., Schauf, V., Wilson, B. S., Chess, L., and Schlossman, S. F. (1978a). *J. Immunol.* **120,** 1278–1282.

Strelkauskas, A. J., Callery, R. T., McDowell, J., Borel, Y., and Schlossman, S. F. (1978b). *Proc. Natl. Acad. Sci. U.S.A.* **75,** 5150–5154.

Strom, T. B., Helderman, J. H., and Williams, R. M. (1978). *Immunogenetics* **7,** 51–56.

Stuart, A. E., Young, G. A., and Grant, P. F. (1976). *Br. J. Haematol.* **34,** 457–464.

Sutherland, R., Smart, T., Niaudet, P., and Greaves, M. (1978). *Leuk. Res.* **2,** 115–126.

Taetle, R., and Royston, I. (1980). *Blood* **56,** 943–946.

Tartakovsky, B., Segal, S., Shanis, A., Hellerstein, S., Weinstein, Y., and Bentwich, 2. (1979). *Clin. Exp. Immunol.* **38,** 166–174.

Taub, R. N., Baker, M. A., and Madyastha, K. R. (1980). *Blood* **55,** 294–298.

Teodorescu, M., Mayer, E. P., and Dray, S. (1977a). *Cell. Immunol.* **29,** 353–362.

Teodorescu, M., Mayer, E. P., and Dray, S. (1977b). *Cancer Res.* **37,** 1715–1718.

Teodorescu, M., Bratescu, A., and Mayer, E. P. (1979). *Clin. Immunol. Immunopathol.* **13,** 194–210.

Thiel, E., Rodt, H., Huhn, D., Netzel, B., Grosse-Wilde, H., Ganeshaguru, K., and Thierfelder, S. (1980). *Blood* **56,** 759–772.

Thiel, E., Rodt, H., and Thierfelder, S. (1981a). *Haematologica,* in press.

Thiel, E., Rodt, H., Huhn, D., Stunkel, K., Gutensohn, W., and Thierfelder, S. (1981b). *In* "Leukemia Markers" (W. Knapp, ed.). Academic Press, New York.

Thiel, E., Lau, B., Rodt, H., Jager, G., and Pachmann, K. (1981c). *Blut* **42,** 315–322.

Tilz, G. P. (1978). *Clin. Exp. Immunol.* **32,** 366–369.

Traycoff, R. B., Wortsman, J., Myers, W. L., and Rogers, W. (1979). *Clin. Immunol. Immunopathol.* **13,** 383–393.

Trucco, M. M., Stocker, J. W., and Ceppellini, R. (1978). *Nature (London)* **273**, 666–668.

Tsubota, T., Miyoshi, I., Uno, J., Hiraki, S., Kobayashi, T., Sato, U., and Kimura, I. (1980). *Clin. Exp. Immunol.* **41**, 130–135.

Tsukimoto, I., Wong, J. Y., and Lampkin, B. C. (1976). *N. Engl. J. Med.* **294**, 245–248.

Turesson, I., Berntorp, E., and Zettervall, O. (1979). *Acta Med. Scand.* **206**, 31–36.

Valdimarsson, H., Agnarsdottir, G., and Lachmann, P. J. (1975). *Nature (London)* **255**, 554–556.

van Eys, J. (1977). *Cancer Res.* **37**, 2457–2461.

Veit, B. C., Melvin, S. L., and Bowman, W. P. (1980). *J. Natl. Cancer Inst.* **64** (6), 1321–1328.

Vogler, L. B., Crist, W. M., Bockman, D. E., Pearl, E. R., Lawton, A. R., and Cooper, M. D. (1978). *N. Engl. J. Med.* **298**, 872–878.

Vogler, L. B., Crist, W. M., Vinson, P. C., Sarrif, A., Brattain, M. G., and Coleman, M. S. (1979). *Blood* **54** (5), 1164–1170.

Volger, L. B., Crist, W. M., Sarrif, A. M., Pullen, D. J., Bartolucci, A. A., Falletta, J. M., Dowell, B., Humphrey, G. B., Blackstock, R., van Eys, J., Metzgar, R. S., and Cooper, M. D. (1981). *Blood* **58**, 135–140.

Wahl, S. M., Rosentreich, D. L., and Oppenheim, J. J. (1976). *In* "In Vitro Methods in Cell-Mediated and Tumor Immunology" (B. R. Bloom and J. R. David, eds.), pp. 231–240. Academic Press, New York.

Waldman, T. Personal communication.

Waller, M., and Lawler, S. D. (1962). *Vox Sang. (Basel)* **7**, 591–606.

Wang, C. Y., Fu, S. M., and Kunkel, H. G. (1979). *J. Exp. Med.* **149**, 1424–1437.

Weiner, M. S., Bianco, C., and Nussenzweig, V. (1973). *Blood* **42**, 939–946.

Wernet, P., Betsch, C., Barth, P., Jaramillo, S., Schunter, F., Waller, H. D., and Wilms, K. (1977). *Scand. J. Immunol.* **6**, 563–574.

Whang-Peng, J., and Knutsen, T. (1980). *Clin. Haematol.* **9** (1), 87–127.

Whitehead, R. H., Roberts, G. P., Hughes, L. E., and Thatcher, J. (1978). *Br. J. Cancer* **37**, 28–32.

Winchester, R. J., Hoffman, T., Ferrarini, A., Ross, G. D., and Kunkel, H. G. (1979). *Clin. Exp. Immunol.* **37**, 126–133.

Wybran, J., and Fudenberg, H. H. (1973). *N. Engl. J. Med.* **288**, 1072–1073.

Wybran, J., and Govaerts, A. (1978). *Clin. Immunol. Immunopathol.* **9**, 240–247.

Wybran, J., Carr, M. C., and Fudenberg, H. H. (1972). *J. Clin. Invest.* **51**, 2537–2543.

Wybran, J., Levin, A. S., Spitler, L. E., and Fudenberg, H. H. (1973). *N. Engl. J. Med.* **288**, 710–713.

Wybran, J., Spitler, L. E., Lieberman, R., and Fudenberg, H. H. (1976). *Cancer Immunol. Immunother.* **1**, 153–156.

Yamanaka, N., Ishii, Y., Koshiba, H., Mikuni, C., Konno, M., and Kikuchi, K. (1978). *Cancer* **42**, 2641–2647.

Yarbro, G. S. K., Lippman, M. E., Johnson, G. E., and Leventhal, B. G. (1977). *Cancer Res.* **37**, 2688–2695.

Yodoi, J., and Ishizaka, K. (1979). *J. Immunol.* **122**, 2577–2583.

Yu, A. L. Leung, K. L., Kung, F. H., Sobol, R. E., and Royston, I. (1981). *Proc. AACR ASCO* **22**, 409.

Yu, D. T. Y. (1975). *Clin. Exp. Immunol.* **20**, 311–322.

Zech, L., Hagland, U., Nilsson, K., and Klein, G. (1976). *Int. J. Cancer* **17**, 47–56.

Zighelboim, J., Gale, R. P., Chiu, A., Bonivida, B., Ossorio, R. C., and Fahey, J. L. (1974). *Clin. Immunol. Immunopathol.* **3**, 193–200.

Zipf, T. F., Fox, R. I., Dilley, J., and Levy, R. (1981). Personal communication.

Zola, H. (1977). *J. Immunol. Methods* **18**, 387–389.

CHAPTER II

CELL SURFACE GLYCOPROTEIN MARKERS FOR NEOPLASIA

V. P. BHAVANANDAN AND E. A. DAVIDSON

I. Introduction

It is generally recognized that events which occur at the surface of eukaryotic cells can regulate a variety of phenotypic characteristics. These include essential functions such as transport of key metabolites and response to external stimuli which may allow a cell to move from a quiescent or resting state through the cell cycle to mitosis. These events are modulated by a wide variety of receptor molecules which are either integrally or transiently associated with the plasma membrane and provide specific recognition sites for appropriate ligand interactions. It is not surprising, therefore, that cells which have undergone malignant transformation or otherwise lost aspects of growth control have associated with their external membrane, either continually or intermittently, molecules unique to their particular growth characteristics; (for reviews see Wallach, 1968; Burger, 1973; Emmelot, 1973; Hughes, 1973, 1976; Warren *et al.*, 1974; Glick and Santer, 1978; Yamada and Pouyssegur, 1978; Hynes, 1979). In some situations these serve as do other cell surface molecules, in a receptor capacity to respond to external signals in such a fashion as to promote cell division or regulate other metabolic events. The binding of molecules (such as insulin, steroid hormones, epinephrine, etc.) can induce either conformational changes within the membrane leading to altered activities or to internalization of the receptor ligand complex with eventual targeting for the nucleus of the cell thus regulating expression of particular genes. The immense diversity of signals to which a cell must respond requires the presence on its surface, therefore, of a broad variety of receptor type molecules. Most, if not all, of these are glycoproteins for reasons which are physiologically and biologically appealing. There are a diversity of carbohydrate molecules available. The hydrophilic nature of the sugars provides the necessary directionality for these molecules ensuring that the appropriately substituted regions of the polypeptide are directed toward the outer environment. In addition, there is sufficient opportunity for structural variation to provide the level of selectivity and specificity necessary to discriminate among a broad variety of external signals. Normally there are only a few sugars found in mammalian glycoproteins but the opportunities for branching and for differing distributions on any given polypeptide backbone provide an enormous number of possible structures. For a trisaccharide containing three different sugars, for example, there are well over a thousand possible structures whereas for a comparable tripeptide only six structures exist.

II. Glycoprotein Structures

In the sense that a genetic control is exerted over the structures of surface macromolecules, the glycosyl or saccharide portion of these is constructed by addition of mono- or oligosaccharides to a growing polypeptide chain at specific attachment sites. As a rule, only two types of carbohydrate–peptide linkage are found in glycoproteins associated with the plasma membrane (Marshall and Neuberger, 1970; Spiro, 1970; Marshall, 1974).

The first is linkage between the amide nitrogen of asparagine and a carbohydrate chain wherein the initial sugar attached to the polypeptide is N-acetylglucosamine. Such oligosaccharide attachments are formed by a complex biosynthetic pathway involving the addition of a 14 unit oligosaccharide (dolichol-P-P-N-acetylglucosamine$_2$ mannose$_9$ glucose$_3$) *en bloc* to specific asparagine residues within the polypeptide chain (Struck and Lennarz, 1980). Partial sequence studies have indicated that asparagine residues are candidates for glycosylation when they are separated from serine or threonine residues by one amino acid whose structure appears not to be regulated (Asn-X-Ser). Other asparagine residues are not glycosylated, and even those meeting sequence requirements may not be glycosylated; regulation in this area is still a matter of continuing study. Processing of the 14 member oligosaccharide unit takes place first by removal of the glucosyl moieties followed by trimming of the mannose structure and subsequent elongation to provide one of two types of final structures: either an oligomannosyl (so-called simple) type or the lactosaminyl (complex) types which generally terminate in a sequence of N-acetylglucosamine-galactose-sialic acid (see Fig. 1). The branching possibilities allow for the latter group to have as many as four such end terminal units attached to a single glycosyl core. Thus, the oligosaccharide structures may

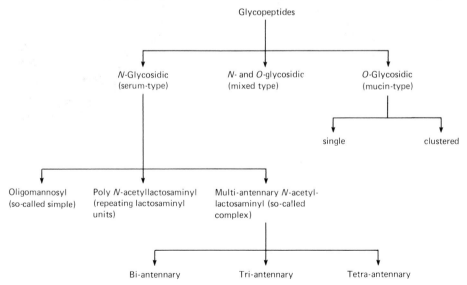

FIG. 1. Types of cell surface glycopeptides presently known.

contain up to about 20 monosaccharide units, with single or multiple an-
tennary structures giving a wide diversity of possible products. As a general rule, sialic acid (and fucose) residues are terminal nonreducing ends
and provide a stop signal for further glycosylation. The diversity of glycosyltransferases required for the elongation of processed oligosaccharide
chains is considerable and few of them have been studied in detail. Regulation is not thoroughly understood and it is believed, at least by some
investigators, that the control is imperfectly established and that considerable microheterogeneity exists in the end product carbohydrate chains,
especially with regard to completeness of glycosylation at the outer periphery.

A second type of carbohydrate peptide linkage that is found in these
glycoproteins is that between the hydroxyl group of either serine or
threonine residues and N-acetylgalactosamine which serves as the initiat-
ing residue for oligosaccharide chain assembly. In this case, the glycosyl
transfer appears to take place by sequential addition of monosaccharides
from nucleotidyl sugars with galactose usually the next sugar and sialic
acid commonly present. The structures found for this class of oligosaccharides may be rather simple as are present in erythrocyte glycophorin
wherein two sialic acids, one galactose and one N-acetylgalactosamine,
comprise the entire oligosaccharide unit (Lisowska, 1969; Thomas and
Winzler, 1969), to those found in epithelial secretions of intestinal muco-
sal cells or lung cells wherein large complex oligosaccharide chains containing up to 15 sugars are present. It is not uncommon for the O-glycosidically linked carbohydrate chains to bear blood group determinants, especially if the individual is a secretor. However, these are less frequently
found on cell surfaces than they are in secretory products. There is little
or nothing known about the regulation of the end product structure for the
O-glycosidically linked glycoproteins. Thus, structural diversity or heterogeneity is the norm and a single family of molecules may be derived from
a common polypeptide chain with a considerable diversity of carbohydrate substitution. The recognition of appropriate serine and threonine
residues by the glycosyltransferases is not understood nor is the control
of oligosaccharide chain length. It is generally believed that this is a kinetic regulation involving transit time in the Golgi apparatus for the incompletely glycosylated protein and availability of the nucleotidyl substrates to the appropriate membrane-bound glycosyltransferases. Thus, at
a given serine or threonine residue in such a glycoprotein, glycosyl substitution may or may not have taken place and the chain may be completed to different sizes.

Accordingly, isolation techniques must compromise in terms of purity
criteria, generally accepting overall compositional analyses as representa-

tive rather than applying the standards usually employed for simple proteins. Single molecule purity probably does not exist in this class of compounds and structural analyses represent probability statements rather than specific details. The methodologic problems involved are discussed later in this chapter but are formidable in terms of defining both the oligosaccharide and polypeptide structures in detail (see Section VII).

III. Qualitative and Quantitative Changes

Association with the transformed state can be expressed in several ways. Descriptive changes involving, for example, the interaction of lectins with cell surfaces provide qualitative or crude information about some alteration in surface properties (Nicolson, 1974). Whether this represents the expression of new molecules, modification of old ones, total or local bilayer fluidity change, or some cryptic phenomenon whereby previously available macromolecules are now physically reorganized within the membrane structure such that the external probes no longer can find them has generally not been defined. The same type of problem applies to surface alterations detected by electron microscopy using, for example, ferritin-conjugated lectins or antibodies. There is an element of qualitative information that is definitely available from such studies but it is impossible to translate such observations to the presence or absence of specific molecular species. Similarly, changes in biologic properties have been correlated with the presence or absence of specific types of macromolecules on the cell surface. A well-studied example is the mouse mammary carcinoma TA3 system wherein transplantability across species boundaries is associated with the presence on the cell surface of an unusual glycoprotein (epiglycanin) whose apparent function is to mask otherwise responsive cell surface antigens (Codington, 1975; Codington *et al.*, 1978, 1979a,b; Cooper *et al.*, 1979). Properties such as adhesion to substrate, metastatic potential, and immunogenicity of whole cells as well as masking have been correlated with the presence on the cell surface of particular types of macromolecules (Hudson and Kunz, 1925; Hynes, 1976; Codington, 1978). Specific molecules have not been identified and structural information not forthcoming to define their nature.

A type of quantitative change that has been widely associated with malignancy is the loss of a large glycoprotein from the cell surface. This macromolecule, originally described about 10 years ago (Hynes, 1973, 1976), has been the subject of intensive study. A variety of names have been used including fibronectin, LETS (large, external, trypsin or transformation sensitive), cell surface protein, and galactoprotein A among others (Yamada and Weston, 1974; Vaheri and Ruoslahti, 1975; Hakomori, 1975; Engvall and Ruoslahti, 1977; Hynes *et al.*, 1979). The near identity of this material with a previously described circulating glycoprotein, cold insoluble globulin, has also been well documented and the relationship between the surface glycoprotein and the circulating form has been examined in some detail (Mosesson and Umfleet, 1970; Ruoslahti and Vaheri, 1974; Mosesson *et al.*, 1975; Mosher, 1975). The generality of the loss of fibronectin from transformed cell surfaces is broad but not total and may well be related to the generally increased protease activity associated with malignant tumors (Unkeless *et al.*, 1973; Rifkin *et al.*, 1974; Lang *et al.*, 1975). This field has been extensively reviewed in recent years and insofar as fibronectin represents a cell surface glycoprotein marker for neoplasia, it can only be said to represent a negative marker since it is a normal component of all fibroblastic cells and a number of other cell types that have been studied.

The specific associations of glycoproteins with discrete types of malignant cells have been under intensive study for well over a decade. The literature is frequently and extensively reviewed and the following discussion does not claim to be exhaustive but rather representative. The topical subdivision is arbitrary and other means of classification could well have been employed. We will discuss initially studies with virus-transformed cells, second, animal cells and animal tumor models, data available from studies with human systems, and finally the methodology.

IV. Virus-Transformed Cells

The association of viruses with animal tumors has been known since the description of Rous sarcoma virus nearly 70 years ago (Rous, 1911). That virus-directed transformation would be an excellent model to study virtually every event associated with cellular metabolism is also well recognized and a wide variety of systems has been studied. Reviews have been published recently by Montagnier and Torpier (1976) and on RNA tumor viruses by Kurth (Kurth and Bauer, 1975; Kurth, 1976; Kurth *et al.*, 1979).

Early studies with Rous sarcoma virus transformed cells indicated that glycopeptides derived from such cells had increased molecular size primarily due to either increased fucosylation or increased sialylation and that there was an increase in sialyltransferase levels associated with the transformed cell (Warren *et al.*, 1972a,b). At least one glycosyltransferase was demonstrated to be externally directed as contrasted with the same activity in nontransformed cells (Bosmann 1972; Bosmann *et al.*, 1974) suggesting that accessibility of the external glycoproteins to this enzyme could result in altered glycosylation patterns. The problem of substrate availability in terms of nucleotidyl sugars has rarely been addressed in any of these studies. The loss of LETS glycoprotein from Rous sarcoma virus-transformed cells has also been studied in some detail. It is generally agreed that the levels of this glycoprotein are sharply reduced when chick embryo fibroblasts are transformed with Rous sarcoma virus (Hynes and Wyke, 1975; Parry and Hawkes, 1978). In an attempt to define tumor-specified cell surface changes more closely, transformed fibroblasts have been examined by both metabolic labeling and labeling of cell surface components by lactoperoxidase catalyzed iodination (see Section VII).

Early experiments carried out by Warren with control and Rous sarcoma virus transformed BHK 21 cells indicated that although the glycopeptides present in the latter cells appeared to be of somewhat larger size, treatment with sialidase converted these to a size pattern characteristic of the controls (Warren et al., 1972a). Accordingly, it was concluded that the major difference found in the transformed cell population could be ascribed to the increased sialylation of normally present glycoproteins; these results were later shown to be due to an increase in multiantennary saccharide substitution. A number of related experiments have subsequently been carried out along these lines including examinations of fucosylated glycopeptides with comparisons made between the pattern of glycopeptides obtained from metabolically labeled material (tritiated sugar material) and molecules accessible on the cell surface by one of several labeling procedures such as lactoperoxidase catalyzed iodination, periodate oxidation–sodium borotritide reduction, or galactose oxidase–sodium borotritide reduction with or without prior neuraminidase treatment (Critchley et al., 1976, Gahmberg et al., 1976). The primary observations can be summarized as follows: in general, the glycopeptides of the transformed cells appear to be larger. The size differences are attributable in part to increased sialylation but the fucose-containing glycopeptides appear to be somewhat larger as well even after neuraminidase treatment (Glick, 1979). Both N- and O-linked glycopeptides appear to be present with the latter group clearly less prevalent in the untransformed cells (Santer and Glick, 1979; Hunt et al., 1981). Examination of radiolabeled material either from metabolic labeling experiments or by cell surface labeling indicates substantially identical patterns although Flowers has reported some change in molecular size and an increase in a 150,000 molecular weight glycoprotein (Flowers and Glick, 1980), and new surface antigens have been described (Phillips and Perdue, 1978). Increased sialic acid is generally present after transformation but explicit isolation of altered or modified glycoproteins has rarely been carried out. It is believed that the virus-transformed cells show an increased turnover of cell surface glycoproteins, including not only fibronectin but others more tightly associated with the plasmalemma. Rieber has indicated that although the general turnover of cell surface proteins in transformed cells is increased, there are variations within this group and that the changed rates are not all uniform (Rieber *et al.*, 1975).

Similar studies have been carried out with a wide variety of virally transformed cells including polyoma (Chiarugi and Urbano, 1972; Gahmberg *et al.*, 1974; Ogata *et al.*, 1976; Koide *et al.*, 1979), SV40 (Wu *et al.*, 1969; Meezan *et al.*, 1969; Onodera and Sheinin, 1970; Culp and Black, 1972; Sheinin and Onodera, 1972; Ceccarini, 1975; Smets *et al.*, 1976; Luborsky *et al.*, 1976; Onodera *et al.*, 1976; Duksin and Bornstein, 1977; Aoi and Yokota, 1980), and murine sarcoma viruses (Fishman *et al.*, 1976; Van Nest and Grimes, 1977; Kamm and Grimes, 1978), mouse mammary tumor viruses (Yang *et al.*, 1977; Teramoto *et al.*, 1977), leukemia viruses (Smart and Hogg, 1976; Ledbetter and Nowinski, 1977; Troy *et al.*, 1977; Murray and Kabat, 1979), and Epstein–Barr virus (Strnad *et al.*, 1981). In virtually every case, some alteration in surface labeling patterns has been observed including the appearance of viral envelope glycoproteins. Many of the recent studies depend on surface accessibility of glycoproteins using either the periodate–borotritide or galactose oxidase techniques. It should be noted that these procedures, especially the latter, will label only available surface glycoproteins and that those components which are masked or rapidly shed may appear to have been altered when in fact their physical configuration in association with the plasma membrane may be that which is changed.

Several studies have indicated the obverse of these general conclusions noted above. It was reported that polyoma virus-transformed BHK cells have associated with the plasma membrane, glycoproteins which tend to be less glycosylated than those found in the control population whereas those released into the medium appear to be more heavily glycosylated (Chiarugi and Urbano, 1972). Conversely, using the same system and cells metabolically labeled with mannose, the mannose-containing oligosaccharides were isolated after pronase digestion, separation of glycopeptides, and cleavage of the oligosaccharides with endoglycosidase H. It was concluded that the oligomannosyl fragments were substantially the same in the normal and transformed cells (Koide *et al.*, 1979).

In a study with polyoma-transformed cells, the differences in the transformed glycopeptides were shown to involve more than simply sialic acid as observed by affinity chromatography on Con A–Sepharose (Koide *et al.*, 1979). The different patterns of affinity chromatographic behavior indicated that although the core structures of the glycopeptides were similar, the outer branches of the transformed cells were more complex. This result is in keeping with those generally obtained with Rous sarcoma virus-transformed cells which indicate that the glycosylation pattern tends to become more complete or extensive yielding glycopeptides which are both fully sialylated and of a higher molecular size.

A number of investigators have examined SV40-transformed cells utilizing basic strategies very similar to those employed in other systems. Two types of studies indicate differences between control (3T3) cells and their SV40 transformed counterparts: the first involves affinity chromatography utilizing as ligand antibodies elicited by whole cells or plasma membranes. As a rule, cells are either metabolically or surface labeled and glycoproteins that adsorb to the affinity matrix eluted by appropriate measures and examined by polyacrylamide gel electrophoresis. Glycoproteins have been identified with molecular weights in the 50,000–60,000 range; these appear to be associated with SV40 transcription, although detailed characterization has not been carried out (Luborsky *et al.*, 1976). One report has indicated that exposure of SV40-transformed cells to tunicamycin affects surface glycosylation patterns resulting in a marked reduction of glycoprotein affinity for Con A–Sepharose. This is not surprising since tunicamycin inhibits an early step in the assembly of the dolichol oligosaccharide which serves as the precursor for all of the *N*-glycosidically linked oligosaccharides found on glycoproteins. A second approach involves genetic analysis. The gene A of SV40 was shown to be related to a sialyltransferase and thus to associated changes in glycosylation (Onodera *et al.*, 1976). The implication from these data is that the expression of a new type of sialyltransferase in the transformed cells allows modification of preexisting glycoproteins to take place with associated increased sialylation—a frequently observed result and one consonant with alterations in both chromatographic mobility and lectin affinity behavior.

Work with mouse mammary tumor virus-transformed cells has indicated the presence of a 52,000 molecular weight externally directed glycoprotein which appears to be uniquely associated with the transformed cell (Yang *et al.*, 1977; Teramoto *et al.*, 1977). This glycoprotein has been identified both by immunologic means and also by direct visualization following lactoperoxidase catalyzed iodination and gel chromatography. It is not known if this protein arises as a result of expression of a viral gene or due to a secondary circumstance wherein a normally quiescent host gene is expressed following viral transformation. Tumor-specific antigens have also been described for spontaneous or chemically transformed cells (Invernizzi *et al.*, 1977; Natori *et al.*, 1977, 1978).

V. Animal Tumors and Derived Cell Clones

A. NEUROBLASTOMA

A number of laboratories have studied the C 1300 mouse neuroblastoma in cell culture (Brown, 1971; Glick *et al.*, 1976b; Glick, 1976). Differences in glycopeptide patterns between more and less differentiated cells have been indicated using metabolic labeling with tritiated glucosamine followed by trypsinization of membranes or whole cells, and chromatography on diethylaminoethyl cellulose. A study with cloned C 1300 cells involved prior induction of neurite expression with dimethyl sulfoxide or hexamethylene bis-acetamide. The cells were labeled with tritiated fucose or glucosamine and glycoproteins examined following neurite isolation from plasma membranes by shearing and discontinuous sucrose gradient ultracentrifugation. At least one qualitative difference was observed in a 200,000 molecular weight protein which appeared to be reduced in undifferentiated cell membranes but then appeared in the growth medium. This was distinct from fibronectin on the basis of molecular weight, trypsin sensitivity, and lack of growth relatedness but was a glycoprotein since it was well labeled by carbohydrate and poorly stained with Coomassie Blue (Littauer *et al.*, 1980). Further characterization of this component has not been reported.

In analogy to other studies, it has been shown that the turnover kinetics of plasma membrane components in the neuroblastoma system differ considerably for individual components (Mathews *et al.*, 1976). These studies involve carbohydrate labels such as fucose followed by gel chromatographic examination of products. As a rule, high turnover components appear to be more sensitive to protease cleavage from the plasma membrane. An increased complexity of the neuroblastoma glycopeptides as compared to those of less differentiated cells has been suggested, and in addition Glick (1976) has indicated a structural homology between both mouse and human membrane glycoproteins derived from this type of cells.

B. MELANOMA

A large number of laboratories have studied the B16 mouse melanoma system as a model for cell surface expression (Warren *et al.*, 1975; Bhavanandan *et al.*, 1977; Evans *et al.*, 1977; Yogeeswaran *et al.*, 1978; Bystryn, 1978; Gersten and Marchalonis, 1979). Early work indicated the same general pattern for these cells as observed with others in that an increased content of sialic acid and fucose as well as higher molecular weight oligosaccharides was found when compared to normal tissues. It should be noted that finding appropriate controls for melanoma cells is difficult since primary cultures of readily available melanocytes (e.g., from iris), while possessing the characteristic of melanin production are not identical to the skin melanocytes; established lines of normal melanocytes are generally not available. A study of the glycopeptides produced by B16 mouse melanoma cells has indicated that an unusual sialoglycopeptide is present in these cells which has a molecular weight of approximately 10,000–12,000 and an affinity for wheat germ agglutinin–Sepharose (Bhavanandan et al., 1977). The saccharide portion of this glycopeptide is analogous or identical to that found in human glycophorin and contains galactose, N-acetylgalactosamine, and sialic acid. The parent glycoprotein which contains this glycopeptide was also identified both from cultured cells and from the solid B16 tumor grown in vivo (Fareed et al., 1978). An interesting feature of this glycopeptide is that its affinity for the wheat germ agglutinin–Sepharose column is completely dependent on the presence of sialic acid since digestion with neuraminidase results in cleavage of the sialic acid with concomitant loss of affinity. This is an example of lectin lack of specificity in that the glycopeptide is free of N-acetylglucosamine which is not only the nominal ligand for wheat germ agglutinin but also can be used as a haptenic displacer to remove the bound glycopeptide from a WGA–Sepharose column (Bhavanandan and Katlic, 1979).

The availability of sublines of the B16 with high and low metastatic potential has prompted a number of studies designed to examine the relationship between cell surface components and metastatic behavior. In general, the more metastatic lines have been found to have increased concentrations of sialoglycopeptides and possibly some additional glycoproteins which are not present in low metastatic lines (Warren et al., 1975; Nicolson et al., 1977; Raz et al., 1980b). Electron microscopic visualization of high and low metastatic lines of B16 has been carried out using cationic ferritin derivatives. Qualitative differences were observed although it was reported in these studies that the same level of sialic acid was present in both lines (Raz et al., 1980a). The difference between total sialic acid content and the rather descriptive nature of the electron microscopic visualization makes it difficult to interpret these data further. As a rule, the glycoproteins in high and low metastatic lines were similar but at least one (78,000 molecular weight) sialoglycoprotein was reported to be related to the ability of these cells to colonize in the lung (Jumblatt et al., 1980). Glycoproteins from these same cells showed a reduced affinity for wheat germ agglutinin–Sepharose. There appeared to be no differences in membrane fluidity, substrate adhesion properties, or ganglioside patterns. A directly contrasting report has indicated that increased levels of sialic acid are well correlated with metastatic potential for these cells and that this increased level of sialic acid is related to increased lectin affinity. In a continuation of this type of study, an examination was made of B16 cells which are resistant to wheat germ agglutinin. Variants were selected by growth in high concentrations of the lectin and the surface glycopeptide patterns examined by conventional techniques. There is a reduction in sialic acid containing glycopeptides both of the *N*- and *O*-glycosidic type with an apparent increase in fucose-containing glycopeptides (Finne *et al.*, 1980b). It was concluded that the glycopeptide patterns indicate that more than one receptor for wheat germ agglutinin is present on the surface of these cells and that in different variants one or another such receptor might be present in reduced quantity. In addition, it was suggested that a certain minimal number of wheat germ agglutinin molecules must bind to the surface of such cells before a toxic threshold is crossed. Thus, reduction in a single type of glycoprotein receptor might be sufficient to render cells resistant to the lectin (Lin and Davidson, 1981). There was some suggestion that the resistant cells had less metastatic and tumor-forming potential than did the parent lines but the *in vivo* studies were insufficient to allow general conclusions to be drawn. It should be noted that studies in other laboratories have indicated, at least intermittently, that alteration of cell surface sialic acid content by pretreatment with neuraminidase may render such cells either more immunogenic or less tumorigenic depending on the nature of the host response (Currie *et al.*, 1968; Simmons and Rios, 1971).

C. Ascites

Detailed studies have been done on the general profile of plasma membrane glycoproteins obtained from cells grown in ascites form including Ehrlich ascites carcinoma (Nachbar *et al.*, 1976), sarcoma 180 (Shin and Carraway, 1973), and mouse mammary carcinoma (Codington *et al.*, 1979a,b; Sherblom and Carraway, 1980). As a rule, plasma membranes have been isolated utilizing the zinc chloride procedure developed by Warren (Warren *et al.*, 1966; Colombini and Johnstone, 1973) and proteins solubilized from such preparations with detergents such as deoxycholate, lithium diiodosalicylate, or by sequential extraction with high salt followed by detergent. The solubilized materials are then subjected to affinity chromatography on lectin Sepharose columns utilizing lectins such as *Ricinus communis*, wheat germ agglutinin, concanavalin A, soybean lectin, and limulin. Glycoproteins have been identified from Ehrlich ascites cells ranging in molecular weight from 35,000 to 200,000 (Nachbar *et al.*, 1976). However, there was no comparison of such material with any control cell so it is impossible to tell whether any qualitative or even quantitative changes occurred. A second study with sarcoma 180 cells utilized lactoperoxidase-catalyzed iodination of plasma membranes followed by their isolation and solubilization. Glycoproteins were identified which ranged in molecular weight from 33,000 to 300,000 (Shin and Carraway, 1973). Utilizing the AH 66 hepatoma, proteins were isolated from the plasma membrane of these by lithium diiodosalicylate extraction followed by phenol partitioning. A protein was identified with a molecular weight of 165,000 which had approximately 50% carbohydrate, most if not all of which was *O*-glycosidically linked (Funakoshi and Yamashina, 1976; Nakajo *et al.*, 1979); it was indicated that the glycoprotein was glycophorin-like. It should be noted that glycophorin-like macromolecules have now been reported to be surface components of a number of cells and at least in the case of the B16 mouse melanoma, the saccharide structures have been sufficiently well identified to confirm this similarity (Bhavanandan *et al.*, 1977). The immunologic reactivity of cell surface glycoproteins with antiglycophorin antibodies has been examined and our group has indicated the presence of reactive surface molecules using indirect immunofluorescent techniques (Barsoum and Bhavanandan, 1981, unpublished results).

D. HEPATOMA

A number of hepatoma lines have been examined for glycoprotein alterations; most studies relied on general descriptions. In Reuber and Novikoff hepatoma cells, neuraminidase-sensitive sialic acid is increased in these cells as compared to control liver cells, as is the overall level of sialic acid and glycopeptide size (Glenney and Walborg, 1979). These data are generally consistent with reports from other cell studies. An early report indicated that treatment of AH 62 hepatoma cells with either concanavalin A or neuraminidase affected the electrophoretic mobility of these cells (Yamada and Yamada, 1973). This simply indicates that charged moieties responsible for electrical migration are either available to the lectin and thus masked by its presence or susceptible to enzymatic cleavage, since removal of sialic acid from cell surface macromolecules would be expected to influence mobility.

In studies with Novikoff hepatoma cells, descriptive profiles have been developed following lactoperoxidase-catalyzed iodination and lectin affinity chromatography. More detailed studies were performed following labeling of sialic acid residues by periodate treatment and borotritide reduction followed by examination of detergent solubilized glycoproteins on SDS–polyacrylamide gels. A variety of proteins ranging in molecular weight from 25,000 to 240,000 was detected with representatives at 120,000 and 92,000 which contain both sialic acid and N-acetylgalactosamine as indicated by affinity of those macromolecules for soybean lectin following neuraminidase treatment (Glenney et al., 1979).

Morris hepatoma cells in contrast to normal liver have increased plasma membrane fucose (4-fold) as well as an increase in the number of fucose-labeled glycoproteins (Vischer and Reuter, 1978). Specific macromolecules, however, were not identified in these studies. In still other hepatoma work, trypsin-sensitive membrane glycoprotein fragments were isolated from HTC cells following either cell surface labeling with lactoperoxidase or metabolic labeling using leucine and fucose. A heavily sialylated product of molecular weight 55,000 was identified and noted to contain approximately 17 sialic acid residues per mole (Baumann and Doyle, 1979). This was apparently a fragment derived from an 85,000 molecular weight precursor containing about 40% carbohydrate. Although both of these were purified, further characterization was not carried out. The relation of these to specific surface markers of hepatoma remains to be defined. In related work, AS 30D hepatoma cell glycoproteins were examined by several labeling techniques followed by affinity chromatography on *Ricinus communis* lectin–Sepharose and two-dimensional gel electrophoresis. Three galactoproteins were identified which possess charge heterogeneity due to varying levels of sialic acid. One of these was cleaved to a 63,000 molecular weight fragment by papain but the relationship, if any, of this to the above mentioned 55,000 molecular weight component was not defined (Glenney et al., 1980).

E. Mammary Carcinoma

A detailed study of the surface properties of a mouse mammary carcinoma (TA3) system has been carried out by Codington and co-workers. Two variants of this mammary carcinoma differ in their ability to be transplanted into allogeneic hosts. It has been found that the transplantable form contains on its cell surface, a carbohydrate-rich glycoprotein called epiglycanin which is not present in the nontransplantable line. This protein has a molecular weight of approximately 500,000 and contains about 80% carbohydrate, essentially all of which is O-glycosidically linked. There are approximately 500 to 600 carbohydrate substitution sites on the polypeptide chain with most of the subsituents being disaccharide units. The apparent function of this macromolecule, which is broadly distributed over the cell surface, is to mask surface antigenic structures which may permit immune response of the host and thus rejection of the tumor cells. The saccharide units are free of fucose and it has been shown that removal of sialic acid results in a decrease in transplantability of the tumor cells (Sanford, 1967). This is probably the best studied of the cell surface glycoprotein markers and its function is reasonably well established. There is some saccharide heterogeneity so that structural data represent composite information but the overall features are quite clear and have been confirmed by direct electron microscopic visualization (Slayter and Codington, 1973; Miller *et al.*, 1977).

A related study using a rat mammary carcinoma (13762) grown in ascites form has focused on membrane glycoproteins solubilized either by detergent extraction or by treatment with guanidine hydrochloride. Purification included cesium chloride density gradient centrifugation and led to the isolation of one mucin type glycoprotein which may serve a masking function as does epiglycanin in the mouse system (Sherblom *et al.*, 1980). It was noted that within the membrane system, this component and a second glycoprotein were associated to give a complex with a molecular weight of approximately 600,000 (Sherblom and Carraway, 1980). One subunit bound to concanavalin A and one did not. The nature of the association was not covalent since the two species were separable in the presence of guanidinium chloride; the overall data suggest that the association is primarily hydrophobic.

F. LUNG CARCINOMA

Studies with a murine lung carcinoma revealed the presence of a surface glycoprotein with a molecular weight of 180,000 which is not present on normal cells (Kennel, 1979; Kennel *et al.*, 1980). The protein was identified by metabolic labeling, isolated, and a radioimmunoassay developed. The data suggest that the protein is shed from the surface of the cells at some regular rate and eventually appears in the serum as the tumor burden in the animal increases. Lactoperoxidase-catalyzed iodination of the cell surface indicated that the molecule was expressed at least transiently at that locus; comparable macromolecules were identified in several lung carcinoma lines. There was some suggestion that charge heterogeneity was present based on isoelectric focusing studies but apparently this was not due exclusively to variations in sialic acid (Eisinger and Kennel, 1981).

G. LEUKEMIAS AND LYMPHOMAS

Mouse leukemia cells (GRSL) were shown to contain a glycoprotein with apparent N-acetylgalactosaminyl residues, a conclusion based on interaction with a lectin from *Dolichos biflorus* (Muramatsu *et al.*, 1980). This glycoprotein had a molecular weight of 100,000, contained O-linked oligosaccharides, and had properties somewhat reminiscent to one described by Bramwell and Harris (Bramwell and Harris, 1978a,b). In a number of other studies on leukemic cell lines, properties of glycopeptides have been described. Increased size and fucose content was generally noted and interaction with lectins defined (Hourani *et al.*, 1973).

An interesting report suggested that antigenic determinants of membrane glycoproteins derived from a mouse plasma cell line may involve N-acetylneuraminic acid (Prat *et al.*, 1975; Prat and Comiglio, 1976). These studies were based on immunologic methods with alterations in immune reactivity observed following treatment with neuraminidase. In spite of these observations, the interpretation is unlikely to be correct. As a rule, sialic acid does not function as an antigenic determinant although its presence in a molecule can confer specific conformations which make one or another antigenic determinant site unique and accessible. Thus, although removal of sialic acid from a given glycoprotein may alter immune properties (similar to studies carried out with MM and NN glycophorin) (Springer and Desai, 1975; Lisowska and Wasniowska, 1978; Sadler *et al.*, 1979) this does not necessarily mean that the sugar itself is recognized by the antibody but rather that its removal occasions a conformational change which results in altered immune properties.

H. VIRAL GLYCOPROTEINS

A number of laboratories have been concerned with the possible expression of viral glycoproteins on the surface of infected cells (Nilsson *et al.*, 1977; Snyder and Fleissner, 1980; Kurth *et al.*, 1977; Kurth and Mikschy, 1978; Krakower and Aaronson, 1978; Krakower *et al.*, 1978; Mesa-Tejada *et al.*, 1978). Attempts have been made to define such components immunologically as well as by direct analysis of labeled macromolecules. Although the results are suggestive, perhaps the clearest data have come from studies with Epstein–Barr virus glycoproteins. Two types of glycoproteins have been identified, one on a human lymphoma line and one as a membrane antigen from infected cells (Nilsson *et al.*, 1977). The labeling techniques involved either galactose oxidase or neuraminidase and then galactose oxidase; glycoproteins of molecular weight 71,000 or 69,000 and 236,000 were identified. The latter was characterized on the basis of lectin affinity and subsequently isolated on a preparative scale by polyacrylamide gel electrophoresis.

I. GENERAL PHENOMENA

A provocative series of studies has been carried out by Bramwell and Harris on several murine lines, including hybrid lines with suppressed malignancies (Bramwell and Harris, 1978a,b). Plasma membranes were isolated from these cells by treatment with zinc chloride followed by discontinuous sucrose gradient centrifugation. The membranes were extracted with Triton and the glycoprotein patterns examined by lectin-binding properties and gel chromatographic behavior. A membrane-associated glycoprotein with a molecular weight of approximately 100,000 and an isoelectric point of approximately 4 was found with high consistency in the tumorigenic cells. The level of this component was reduced in the relatively less malignant hybrid lines. It may be present in the cell membrane as a dimer; there was some suggestion, not confirmed, that this molecule is associated with glucose transport.

VI. Human Cells

A number of human cell lines have been examined for specific membrane-associated glycoproteins (Table I).

A. MELANOMA

Early work conducted with a line of melanoma cells adopted the following strategy: rabbits were immunized with inactivated human melanoma cells and the elicited antibodies used as a primary fractionation tool. Screening was conducted on extracts of solid tumors and on urine of patients for proteins which reacted with the rabbit antibodies. The reactive molecules were examined by gel electrophoresis and melanoma associated antigens identified in the 40,000–60,000 molecular weight range (Carrel and Theilkaes, 1973).

Evidence was developed for membrane-associated melanoma antigens by use of a delayed hypersensitivity reaction utilizing extracts of melanoma cell membranes. A number of active fractions were identified although none was purified (Hollinshead et al., 1974). In comparable studies using immunologic approaches, melanoma patients were screened for the presence of circulating antibodies directed against cell surface anti-

TABLE I

GLYCOPROTEINS OF HUMAN TUMOR CELL SURFACES[a]

Source	Methodology	Properties
Melanoma cells	Immunoadsorbent (patient serum)	20,000–50,000 MW; affinity for *Lens culinaris* lectin
Melanoma cells	Monoclonal antibody	97,000 MW
Mammary ductal carcinoma	Membrane isolation, extraction; immuno-adsorbent	20,000 MW; PCA-soluble, 38–57% carbohydrate; p*i* 4.45–5.35
Lung adenocarcinoma	Standard biochemical	77,000 MW; cross reacts with α_1-antichymotrypsin
Colon adenocarcinoma	Surface labeling, lectin affinity	Carcinoembryonic antigen
Renal cancer cells	Metabolic labeling, two-dimensional gels	27,500 MW; p*I* 5.7, 5.3, 4.9
Neuroblastoma cells	Monoclonal antibody	20,000 MW; fucose, glucosamine label
Ovarian tumor	Immunoadsorbent	70,000 MW; PCA-soluble

[a] See text for references.

gens of cultured melanoma cells (Carey *et al.*, 1976; Leong *et al.*, 1977a,b). In one study, a particular patient with a high titer was identified and serum from that patient utilized as a screening tool for the presence of melanoma associated cell surface antigens in a variety of cell sources (Carey *et al.*, 1979). A group of proteins in the molecular weight range of 20,000–50,000 was identified by this technique. An indication that they were glycoproteins was derived from their interaction with *Lens culinaris* lectin. However, structural details were not reported in these studies.

Surface labeling of several lines of cultured melanoma cells indicated that galactosyl residues were sterically hindered. Common features included proteins with molecular weights of 90,000 and 110,000 as well as two glycoproteins with the characteristics of Ia antigens (Lloyd *et al.*, 1979).

A putative melanoma associated antigen was identified by radioimmunoassay and a molecular weight of 97,000 was assigned (Brown *et al.*, 1981a). However, the specificity of this to melanoma was not defined, nor were any structural details reported.

Several laboratories have utilized hybridomas to develop panels of monoclonal antibodies directed against cell lines derived from human melanoma and other malignant cells (Carrel *et al.*, 1980; Dippold *et al.*,

1980). A number of common antigens have been identified but relatively few specific components. The release of antigens from melanoma cell lines has been examined but in contrast to studies with virus-transformed lines, no apparent change in antigen secretion rate was observed when data were compared to that from control cell populations (Bystryn *et al.*, 1981).

B. Mammary Carcinoma

Studies carried out with human mammary tumors utilizing both chemical and surface localization techniques have identified tumor-related glycoproteins of approximately 20,000 molecular weight; these were distinct from carcinoembryonic antigen (Kuo *et al.*, 1973). The glycoproteins are soluble in perchloric acid and contain between 40 and 60% carbohydrate; isoelectric focusing identified a p*I* of 4.45 for one component and 5.35 for another. It was not known if these were related by differences in sialic acid content although both components contained sialic acid (Leung *et al.*, 1978; Leung and Edgington, 1980).

An association of human breast cancer with T antigen which is a precursor of the MN blood groups has been described (Springer *et al.*, 1976; Howard and Batsakis, 1980).

C. Lung Carcinoma

An antigen associated with lung tumor has been identified as a 76,000 molecular weight, sialic acid-containing glycoprotein (Gaffar *et al.*, 1979; Braatz *et al.*, 1978). The protein was isolated by direct extraction from lung tumor and was shown to have some structural homology with α_1-antichymotrypsin on the basis of immunologic cross reactivity; the two molecules were not identical (Gaffar *et al.*, 1980).

D. Colon Carcinoma

The interest in carcinoembryonic antigen has prompted a number of studies with colonic carcinoma lines. Surface labeling of one such with galactose oxidase indicated the presence of at least five glycoproteins; the major one had a molecular weight of 200,000 and properties similar to those of carcinoembryonic antigen (Tsao and Kim, 1978). Soluble antigens from colonic carcinomas have been studied by the usual techniques and a number of glycoproteins identified but other than similarities to CEA, no structural details have been reported. The appearance of carcinoembryonic antigen on the cell surface of cultured colon adenocarcinoma cells requires protein synthesis and can be inhibited by the presence of bromouracil deoxyriboside (Rosenthal *et al.*, 1980). Internalization of the surface antigen was accomplished by exposure of the cells to antibody and the subsequently denuded cells were allowed to recover under conditions which permit reexpression of the CEA.

E. OVARIAN CARCINOMA

A perchloric acid-soluble glycoprotein with a nominal molecular weight of 70,000 has been purified from extracts of human ovarian tumor (Knauf and Urbach, 1974, 1976). The development of a satisfactory radioimmunoassay has permitted discrimination between this molecule and carcinoembryonic antigen and the lack of association of this molecule with lung cancer; cross reactive material was present in colon carcinoma. The generality of this particular antigen has yet to be defined but the authors suggest that it may be common to certain types of cyst adenocarcinomas (Knauf and Urbach, 1981). Screening for the presence of this macromolecule in plasma indicates an association with advanced disease (Knauf and Urbach, 1977, 1978).

F. NEUROBLASTOMA

Studies on human neuroblastoma glycopeptides have shown that they have the same general features associated with those found in other transformed cells in that they tend to be more complex and perhaps more highly fucosylated (Glick *et al.*, 1976a). An unusual linkage has been identified in glycopeptides from these cells with fucose linked 1-3 or 1-4 to *N*-acetylglucosamine (Santer and Glick, 1980). At least one membrane glycoprotein with a molecular weight of approximately 20,000 has been identified from human neuroblastoma utilizing monoclonal antibodies as the detecting tool (Momoi *et al.*, 1980). Glycopeptides derived from this glycoprotein had some antigenic activity, although reactivity with glycolipids was not found. It is of interest to note that there was cross reactivity with extracts of fetal but not adult brain.

G. MISCELLANEOUS

Physical studies have indicated surface changes in cultured lines of bladder epithelial cells associated with transformations (Kahan *et al.*,

1977). A similar analysis compared renal cancer and normal kidney epithelial cells; protein components of molecular weights 27,500 and isoelectric points ranging from 5.7 to 4.9 were uniquely present in the malignant cells (Ogata *et al.*, 1981).

VII. Methodology

The general approaches toward defining the nature of cell surface glycoproteins can be subdivided into metabolic or biochemical procedures as contrasted to immunologic procedures. In most cases that have thus far been described, few of the glycoproteins have been isolated in sufficient quantity to permit detailed biochemical characterization. Most studies have been performed with either metabolic or chemically labeled material and identification of unusual products by means of polyacrylamide gel electrophoresis or more recently, monoclonal antibodies. Considerable work has been done with proteolytic digests of crude fractions isolated from plasma membranes or whole cells to examine glycopeptide profiles. Progress in this field will remain limited until techniques are worked out for isolating native glycoproteins and providing at least minimal structural details for them, including immunologic behavior, so that a library of defined surface glycoproteins can be established. There are many indications that malignancies both of animal and human origin have associated with their cell surfaces glycoproteins that are either immunologically or otherwise unique; a vast amount of work remains to be done to provide adequate characterization profiles.

A. PREPARATION OF CELLS

A major reason for the relatively slow progress in this field is that the cells utilized for studies are available in limited quantities. Developments in cell culture techniques such as growth of cells on microbeads (Levine *et al.*, 1977), in multi-plate culture systems (Schleicher, 1973), large volume fermentors and spinner cultures (Chee *et al.*, 1976), and the use of serum-free medium (Barnes and Sato, 1980a,b) should alleviate the primarily economic aspects of this shortcoming. An associated problem is the requirement of normal cells of the same cell lineage and comparable cell growth characteristics; these are not always available. When available, it is best to carry out the comparative studies of cancer and control cells at the same cell cycle phase, since growth-dependent changes of cellular glycopeptides have been documented (Buck *et al.*, 1971; Sakiyama and Burge, 1972; Muramatsu *et al.*, 1973).

B. Metabolic Labeling of Cellular Glycoproteins

In this approach, a suitably labeled precursor sugar is added to culture medium containing metabolically active cells, organs, or tissue slices. The injection of isotopes into animals is uneconomical because the extensive dilution results in extremely poor incorporation into the desired tissue products. A number of precursor sugars can be utilized, the most commonly employed is glucosamine ([6-^{3}H] or [1-^{14}C]). This is the preferred sugar since all known animal glycoconjugates, with the exception of glycogen and collagen, contain at least one of the three sugars (N-acetylglucosamine, N-acetylgalactosamine, sialic acid) biosynthetically derived from it. Further, the major part of the added precursor is utilized in synthetic pathways (Kohn et al., 1962). Recent studies in our laboratory, however, have shown that a significant proportion of glucosamine may be used by certain cultured cells for energy metabolism (O'Connor and Davidson, unpublished results).

L-Fucose is another precursor widely used for the metabolic labeling of glycoproteins. The use of this sugar was suggested by the pioneering studies of Bekesi and Winzler (1967) which indicated that it is exclusively incorporated as such into tissue glycoproteins and is not extensively metabolized. However, the subsequent isolation of various fucoglycolipids (Hakomori, 1975; McKibbin, 1978), fucose-containing glycosaminoglycans (Bray et al., 1967), and fucose-free glycopeptides (Tai et al., 1975; Bhavanandan et al., 1977, 1981; Li and Kornfeld, 1979; Van den Eijnden et al., 1979), and fucose-free glycoproteins (Spiro, 1973; Kawasaki and Ashwell, 1976a; Montreuil, 1980), does not support the earlier claim of exclusivity of fucose incorporation into glycoproteins. Nevertheless, this sugar as well as isotopically labeled mannose, galactose, and N-acetylmannosamine are useful for obtaining specific information on the carbohydrate composition and structure of cell surface glycoproteins (Yurchenco et al., 1978). Metabolic labeling with a precursor sugar (for example, [6-^{3}H]glucosamine) and a precursor amino acid ([^{14}C]leucine) or [^{35}S]sulfate will help in subsequent purification since the second isotope serves to screen for nonglycosylated proteins or sulfated glycosaminoglycans, respectively.

C. In Vitro Cell Surface Labeling of Glycoproteins

All of the carbohydrate moieties of the cell membrane glycoproteins (intrinsic and extrinsic) and portions of the protein are present on the outer surface of the intact cell. This arrangement makes it possible to isotopically label these glycoproteins by in vitro techniques and allows their visualization after treating with carbohydrate-specific dyes, lectins, or antibodies (see Section VII,F).

Isotopic labeling of the exposed (available) sugar or amino acid on intact cells involves chemical modification using isotopic reagents under conditions that do minimal damage to the cells. The available methods include labeling of sialic acid residues by brief periodate treatment and tritiated borohydride reduction (Liao *et al.*, 1973; Gahmberg and Andersson, 1977) labeling of galactose residues by galactose oxidase oxidation followed by reduction with tritiated borohydride (Gahmberg and Hakomori, 1973) or coupling with methionine [^{35}S]sulfone hydrazide (Itaya *et al.*, 1975); labeling of available tyrosine by iodination with $^{125}I_2$ generated by treatment of Na^{125}I with lactoperoxidase and H_2O_2 (Phillips and Morrison, 1971; Hunt and Brown, 1975); and coupling of exposed $-NH_2$ (lysine) with pyridoxal phosphate to form a Schiff base which is stabilized by reduction with tritiated borohydride (Rifkin *et al.*, 1972). Labeling techniques including some not widely tested are summarized in Table II.

All of the above procedures attempt, not always successfully, to label only the surface-exposed molecules by employing either reagents that are too large (for example, lactoperoxidase, galactose oxidase) or highly charged (pyridoxal-5'-phosphate, formyl methionylsulfonemethyl phosphate) so that they do not penetrate the hydrophobic interior of the membrane. The exclusivity of these techniques has been questioned (Schmidt-Ullrich *et al.*, 1973; Juliano and Beher-Bennelier, 1975) but they are still suitable for preliminary studies. The periodate–borotritide labeling procedure was initially applied to erythrocytes (Liao *et al.*, 1973) and subsequently extended to lymphoid and other cell systems (Gahmberg and Andersson, 1977; Flowers and Glick, 1980; Brown *et al.*, 1981b). In our own preliminary work on various nucleated cultured cells (hepatoma, melanoma), it was found that 60–90% of the cells were permeable to Trypan Blue at the end of the labeling period (Bhavanandan, unpublished results).

It is thus clear that some of these techniques should be used judiciously and appropriate controls carried out, particularly if it is essential that *only* externally exposed residues are labeled. If it is critical to establish the surface localization of a glycoprotein, additional evidence should be obtained by independent criteria involving visualization techniques or by initial isolation of plasma membranes. Failure to label a molecule does not necessarily mean that it is absent at the surface since cryptic (sterically unavailable loci) molecules may not be acted upon by enzymes or other reagents. A serious disadvantage of the *in vitro* labeling technique is that glycoproteins adsorbed to the cell surface are not distinguished from true cell surface components. Strong adsorption of fetal calf serum components to the cell surface has been reported (Phillips and Perdue, 1977).

TABLE II
CELL SURFACE LABELING TECHNIQUES

Reagents	Group(s) labeled	Reference
Sodium periodate and sodium [³H]boro-hydride	Sialic acid	Liao et al. (1973); Gahm-berg and Andersson (1977)
Galactose oxidase-sodium [³H]borohydride	Galactose; N-acetyl-galactosamine (pre-ferentially non-reducing terminals)	Gahmberg and Hakomori (1973)
Lactoperoxidase–H_2O_2 or glucose oxidase and glucose and radioactive iodide	Tyrosine	Phillips and Morrison (1971); Hunt and Brown (1975)
Pyridoxal phosphate and sodium [³H]boro-hydride	$-NH_2$ (ϵNH_2 group of lysine, aminoterminal)	Rifkin et al. (1972)
Galactose oxidase–methionine [³⁵S]sulfone hydrazide	Galactose, N-acetyl-galactosamine	Itaya et al. (1975)
4,4′-Diisothiocyano-2,2′-ditritiostilbene disulf-onate ([³H]DIDS)	$-NH_2$	Cabantchik and Rothstein (1974)
[³⁵S]Formylmethionyl sulfone methyl phos-phate ([³⁵S]FMMP)	$-NH_2$	Bretscher (1971)
Diazobenzene [³⁵S]sulf-onate (DABS)	$-NH_2$; tyrosine; histidine	Bender et al. (1971)

Despite these limitations the *in vitro* labeling procedures, particularly the lactoperoxidase iodination and the galactose oxidase $-NaB^3H_4$ technique in conjugation with prior neuraminidase treatment, are very useful. At the present time, these techniques are of primary value in providing radioactive handles for the purification and preliminary characterization of minute quantities of glycoproteins (Fareed *et al.*, 1978). Improvements in application as well as development of newer methods can be expected to broaden the usefulness of this approach to the study of cell surface glycoproteins.

D. ISOLATION AND PURIFICATION OF CELL SURFACE GLYCOPEPTIDES

Different strategies have been used for the isolation of cell surface glycopeptides of malignant cells. The two types discussed in this chapter are those involving mild protease treatment of intact cells and exhaustive proteolysis of isolated plasma membranes.

1. Mild Proteolysis of the Cell Surface Components

Information on the nature of cell surface glycoproteins may be obtained by limited proteolysis of intact labeled or unlabeled cells resulting in controlled release of fragments. It is important to choose conditions of pH, ionic concentration of buffer, time, and temperature of incubation such that cell viability is not affected. Several investigators have used trypsin to release glycopeptides (and glycosaminoglycans) from the cell surface (Langley and Ambrose, 1967; Codington et al., 1972; Saito et al., 1977; Nakada and Yamashina, 1978; Debray and Montreuil, 1978). Codington et al. (1972) were able to release significant quantities of cell surface sialic acid in the form of glycopeptides from TA3 mammary adenocarcinoma cells. Using similar conditions, we were able to release mucin-type glycopeptides from B16 mouse melanoma cells metabolically labeled with [^{14}C]glucosamine (Bhavanandan et al., 1977).

Walborg et al. (1969) and Robinson et al. (1976) were successful in solubilizing several glycoproteins from rat hepatoma cells by the use of papain. Papain seems capable of releasing larger glycoprotein fragments, which sometimes retain biological activity. Thus, biologically active antigens have been released from several cell types by treatment with papain (Shimada and Nathenson, 1969; Baldwin et al., 1973; Viza and Phillips, 1975; Clemetson et al., 1976; Ishii et al., 1980). However since the conditions for maintaining cell viability are not optimal for papain activity, the yields of released glycopeptides are poor. Ficin (Langley and Ambrose, 1967) and bromelain are two other narrow spectrum proteases which may be useful for the release of cell surface components. In contrast to the above mentioned proteases, Pronase, which is a mixture of broad spectrum proteases, is generally not suitable for the release of surface components without affecting cell viability. The mildest conditions tried resulted in loss of viability of cultured cells (Bhavanandan, unpublished observations). However Ceccarini et al. (1975) and Ceccarini and Atkinson (1977) were able to isolate mannose-containing glycopeptides from monolayers of cultured human cells.

Mild proteolysis of intact cells probably results in the release of a selective rather than a representative population of surface glycopeptides. This is illustrated by the preferential release of epiglycanin (a peripheral glycoprotein) compared to other intrinsic membrane glycoproteins of TA3 cells. Further, this approach seems to work better on cells grown in suspension or Ascites form than on detached monolayer cultured cells since the latter have an already altered surface.

2. Total Proteolytic Fragmentation of Isolated Membranes

A majority of the studies on cell-associated glycoproteins have been carried out on limit protease (Pronase) digestion products of isolated plasma membranes (Meezan *et al.*, 1973; Glick and Buck, 1973; Nakada *et al.*, 1975; Warren *et al.*, 1978; Glick, 1979) or whole cells (Bhavanandan *et al.*, 1977, 1981; Muramatsu *et al.*, 1978; Li *et al.*, 1980; Takasaki *et al.*, 1980). This procedure has the advantage of yielding water-soluble fragments of membrane glycoproteins most of which have amphiphatic characteristics rendering them not readily soluble in aqueous systems. In addition, it is possible to obtain information on total carbohydrate changes at the cell surface without concern for the protein moiety; the latter is likely to influence solubilization, purification, and analytical procedures. Major disadvantages of this approach are that it does not provide information on changes of discrete glycoproteins and it is difficult to determine the relationship between observed differences and malignancy.

3. Purification of Glycopeptides

Glycopeptides derived from the proteolytic treatment of intact cells or plasma membranes can be broadly classified as illustrated in Fig. 1. Within each class, wide structural variations are possible; incompleteness of chains, mode and number of branches, linkage positions, etc. In addition to glycopeptides, glycosaminoglycans are present in digests of plasma membranes, a fact which has not always been previously considered. Several methods are available to separate glycosaminoglycans from glycopeptides. We have generally used cetyl pyridinium chloride to precipitate the glycosaminoglycans from the Pronase digests (Bhavanandan *et al.*, 1977, 1981; Chandrasekaran and Davidson, 1979). This procedure works well except for small losses of glycopeptides which occur during the precipitation of excess cetyl pyridinium chloride with KSCN followed by dialysis of the supernatant. An alternative technique, used in our studies on nuclear glycoconjugates, is fractionation by ion exchange chromatography on DEAE-cellulose or Sephadex columns (Bhavanandan and Kemper, unpublished results). This approach was only partially successful due to overlap of the elution of certain sialoglycopeptides and the non- or low-sulfated glycosaminoglycans (hyaluronic acid, chondroitin). If information on the nature of the glycosaminoglycans is not required, then it is possible to use enzymes and/or chemicals to selectively degrade these molecules. For example, hyaluronic acid and the chondroitin sulfates could be degraded by using hyaluronidases (Meyer, 1971) and chondroitinases (Suzuki, 1972), and the heparan sulfates by either heparitinase (Linker and Hovingh, 1972) or nitrous acid (Cifonelli, 1968). This approach has not been widely used apparently due to the difficulty in obtaining the requisite saccharases free of exoglycosidase activity. A recent study described the use of *Flavobacterium heparinum* culture filtrates to degrade chondroitin sulfates and heparan sulfates (Gill *et al.*, 1981).

Standard techniques such as gel filtration, ion exchange chromatography, and lectin affinity chromatography are then employed to fractionate the complex mixture of glycopeptides (Smith *et al.*, 1973; Bhavanandan *et al.*, 1977, 1981; Debray and Montreuil, 1978; Santer and Glick, 1979; Finne *et al.*, 1980a). In view of the intrinsic microheterogeneity of the oligosaccharide portion of glycopeptides and because the starting material consists of a pool of glycopeptides derived from a large number of individual glycoproteins, only mixtures of closely related glycopeptides rather than single species can be expected. For example, in work involving extensive purification, apparently homogeneous glycopeptides were obtained from metabolically labeled RSV-BHK cells (Santer and Glick, 1979) and HM7 human melanoma cells (Bhavanandan *et al.*, 1981). Structural investigation of these purified glycopeptides suggested reasonable homogeneity of the carbohydrate portions. However, it cannot be excluded that the isolated fractions contain glycopeptides of near-identical carbohydrate composition and array derived from several different glycoproteins or different areas of the same glycoproteins. A corollary to this is that amino terminal analysis cannot be used as a purity criterion for glycopeptides.

E. ISOLATION OF INTACT CELL SURFACE GLYCOPROTEINS

To understand the relationship between cell surface glycoproteins and malignancy, it will be essential to isolate individual components, ideally, with retention of biological activity. Membrane glycoproteins can be grouped into two categories: peripheral or extrinsic glycoproteins which interact minimally with other membrane components and integral or intrinsic glycoproteins which are partly buried in the bilayer. The possibility of extracting the extrinsic glycoproteins without damaging the intact cell has not been fully investigated. The only extrinsic protein extracted in this manner is cellular fibronectin (LETS glycoprotein) which was solubilized by treatment of cell monolayers with urea (Yamada and Weston, 1974).

The solubilization of intrinsic glycoproteins presents technical problems due to the partial hydrophobic nature of these molecules. In general, these amphipathic glycoproteins can be extracted only after prior purification of plasma membranes. The membranes are then treated with detergents to disrupt the lipid bilayer in essence substituting the hydrophobic lipid surrounding the glycoprotein by hydrophobic detergents.

1. Plasma Membrane Isolation

A variety of techniques are available for the isolation of plasma membranes; as a rule, procedures are continually being improved in terms of speed, yield, and purity (Steck and Wallach, 1970; Brunette and Till, 1971; Warren, 1974; Perdue, 1974; Neville, 1976). Some of these methods have been adapted for zonal centrifugation and therefore can be used for large scale preparations. A rapid method for the isolation of surface membranes from tissue culture cells involves cell lysis in hypoosomotic borate buffer–EDTA followed by differential centrifugation (Thom et al., 1977). The method of Barland and Schroeder (1970) involving the stripping of membrane from monolayer cells with fluorescein mercuric acetate is rapid and simple but may result in selective loss of some membrane components (Quissel et al., 1977). Two novel methods described for the isolation of erythrocyte plasma membranes involve (1) the use of polylysine coupled to glass beads (Jacobson et al., 1978) and (2) the introduction of polydeoxythymidylic acid chains to the membrane followed by hybridization to polyadenylic acid–agarose (Wennogle and Berg, 1978). The applicability of these methods to other cell membranes has not been reported.

2. Solubilization of Plasma Membranes

Prior to solubilization of the glycoprotein, extraction of the membranes with chloroform–methanol mixtures helps to remove lipids and glycolipids (Hakomori and Murakami, 1968). If this is done, then consideration should be given to the possibility that certain glycoproteins may partition, in part, in the organic phase (Watanabe et al., 1980). This could be due to either an overall hydrophobic nature or to strong binding of lipids. This treatment is likely to denature many membrane glycoproteins resulting in the loss of biological activity, if any.

The glycoproteins that are interacting with the lipid bilayer by electrostatic interactions may be solubilized with suitable changes in the ionic strength and/or pH of the extracting medium. Sodium chloride of varying molarity has been used to extract membrane proteins (Rosenberg and Guidotti, 1969; Fairbanks et al., 1971; Braatz et al., 1978). In these and other similar extractions involving 3 M KCl (Reisfeld et al., 1971; Leonard et al., 1975; Chee et al., 1976) the role of endogenous proteases should be considered since some activation by salt solutions appears to occur (Mann, 1972). Therefore, if undegraded glycoproteins are to be obtained, it is essential to include protease inhibitors such a toluene sulfonyl fluoride, diisopropyl fluorophosphate, pepstatin, aprotinin, and iodoacetamide in the extracting medium. Extraction of whole cells with 3 M KCl gave active histocompatibility antigens (Reisfeld *et al.*, 1971) and active melanoma-associated antigen (Bhavanandan *et al.*, 1980) indicating that limited autoproteolysis may not always be undesirable. Treatment with chelating agents such as EDTA (Wise *et al.*, 1975; Dunn *et al.*, 1975) or with the hydrogen-bond breaking agents, urea (Tanner and Gray, 1971) or guanidine hydrochloride (Gwynne and Tanford, 1970), are other methods for extracting extrinsic membrane proteins. If high concentrations (4–8 M) of urea or guanidine HCl are used, the effect of the high density of these solutions should be taken into account in evaluating results. Protein –lipid complexes are small vesicles and are likely to float during centrifugation of the extracts giving the false impression of effective solubilization (Maddy and Dunn, 1976).

Solubilization of intrinsic membrane glycoproteins requires the use of chaotropic agents (potassium or sodium thiocyanate, lithium diiodosalicylate) or organic solvents (butanol, pyridine, phenol) or detergents. Lithium diiodosalicylate introduced by Marchesi and Andrews (1971) for the purification of glycophorin from human erythrocyte membranes has been successfully used for the extraction of glycoproteins from plasma membranes of AH66 rat hepatoma (Funakoshi and Yamashina, 1976; Nakajo *et al.*, 1979) of BHK cells (Tuszynski *et al.*, 1978) and HM7 human melanoma (Umemoto *et al.*, 1981). The strong affinity of lithium diiodosalicylate to glycophorin and probably other membrane glycoprotein was demonstrated by Segrest *et al.* (1979) who recommended the use of sodium deoxycholate for the purification of glycophorin. Butanol, pyridine, and phenol have been used by several investigators to solubilize erythrocyte ghosts (Maddy, 1966; Zwaal and van Deenan, 1968; Blumenfeld and Zvilichovsky, 1972; Howe *et al.*, 1972) but have not been applied to other animal cell membranes. Extraction with chloroform–methanol to partition the lipid and protein components of the erythrocyte membrane used by Hamaguchi and Cleve (1972) was recently adapted for the extraction of glycoproteins from thyroid plasma membranes (Okada and Spiro, 1980).

The most popular agents for solubilizing membranes are detergents. Both nonionic (Triton X-100, Nonidet P-40, octyl glucoside, Triton CF-54, Tween 20) and ionic (sodium deoxycholate, sodium dodecyl sulfate, sodium dodecyl sarcosinate) detergents have been used (Maddy and Dunn, 1976). In general, the former category is preferable since these appear to cause the least alterations in the structure and conformation of the glycoproteins as illustrated by the absence of their influence on the activities of antibodies (Dimitriadis, 1979) and lectins (Lotan *et al.*, 1977) at concentrations of about 1%. These detergents can also be expected to have minimal effect on enzyme and receptor activities. In contrast, the ionic detergents bind strongly to proteins (Reynolds and Tanfold, 1970) and can thus cause irreversible conformational changes. They also interfere in the interaction of antibodies and lectins with glycoproteins (Lotan et al., 1977; Dimitriadis, 1979). Although the nonionic detergents have obvious advantages, the use of ionic detergents is still valuable under special circumstances because of their ability to cause complete solubilization of most membrane glycoproteins.

Once the proteins are solubilized the detergents may, in some instances, be removed without causing precipitation. For example, glycophorin remains in aqueous solution after removal of detergents, probably due to its high carbohydrate content. However, in most cases this procedure is likely to cause aggregation or insolubilization of the glycoproteins (Kawasaki and Ashwell, 1976b; Dorst and Schubert, 1970; Bhavanandan et al., 1980). Thus, an optimum concentration of the detergent should be maintained throughout purification and subsequent studies to ensure that the component of interest remains in solution. The nonionic detergents are usually removed by extensive dialysis, treatment with resins such as BioRad Sm-2 (Holloway, 1973), or by extraction with ice-cold ethanol, or acetone (Funakoshi and Yamashina, 1976; Kawasaki and Ashwell, 1976b). The removal of unbound detergents from proteins is discussed in a recent review (Furth, 1980).

3. Fractionation of the Solubilized Gycoproteins

Generally it is advisable to include protease inhibitors in the buffers during purification procedures. The direct and simplest method of purifying a cell surface glycoprotein is by affinity chromatography on an antibody–Sepharose column, a technique obviously dependent on the availability of an appropriate antibody directed against the glycoprotein of interest. In view of recent advances in the production of monoclonal antibodies, future widespread use of this method can be expected (Goding, 1980; Schlom et al., 1980; Mitchell et al., 1980; St. Groth and Scheidegger, 1980). Several investigators have successfully employed monoclonal antibodies for the purification of cell surface glycoproteins. Thus, Brown et al. (1981b) isolated a glycophorin-like molecule from rat thymocytes; Hellstrom and co-workers (Yeh et al., 1979; Woodbury et al., 1980) isolated a glycoprotein (P97) from human melanoma cells and Momoi et al. (1980) isolated a membrane glycoprotein from human neuroblastoma cells by this technique.

Affinity chromatography on lectin columns is another useful technique for purifying membrane glycoproteins. Because of the wide carbohydrate specificities of lectins such as concanavalin A, wheat germ agglutinin, and the *Ricinus communis* agglutinins, affinity chromatography using these lectins will result in the separation of classes of glycoproteins rather than individual components. If the glycoprotein under investigation binds to an immobilized lectin, then this property can be used successfully to remove all nonglycosylated proteins as well as the nonbinding glycoproteins. In some cases, a specific glycoprotein may entirely bind to a lectin column, as in the case of 5'-nucleotidase of pig lymphocyte membrane (Hayman and Crumpton, 1972). In other cases, it is possible that portions of the same glycoprotein may bind incompletely to one lectin or to different lectin columns due to carbohydrate heterogeneity. Subfractionation of the class of glycoproteins binding to a particular immobilized lectin may be possible by gradient elution with appropriate sugars. In the case of wheat germ agglutinin, subfractionation should also be possible by using a series of columns packed with lectin–Sepharose of varying concentration of lectin per milliliter gel (Bhavanandan and Katlic, 1979).

A note of caution must be introduced regarding the use of affinity chromatography as a structural tool. The characteristics of affinity chromatographic behavior will indicate only general structural information and, within that restriction, only those saccharide moieties which are accessible to and recognized by the affinity ligand. Affinity will also differ depending on the nature and preparation of the glycopeptides. For example, it is quite likely that a fragment with two saccharide units will have quite different behavior on a given lectin affinity column than one with a single saccharide unit. Furthermore, the density of the lectin on the supporting matrix is a critical factor in evaluating chromatographic behavior. Thus, comparisons from one laboratory to another, even with identical cell systems, are very difficult to make.

The nominal structural basis for lectin specificities are often inaccurate. Adsorption to and elution from a particular lectin column with a haptenic monosaccharide eluent (for example utilization of N-acetylglucosamine with wheat germ agglutinin–Sepharose columns) does not at all mean that such sugars are present in the glycoprotein under investigation (Bhavanandan and Katlic, 1979). This kind of oversimplification is frequently encountered and can lead to mistaken identification of saccharide residues on glycoproteins. Most lectins have specificities which either encompass oligosaccharide units or have sufficiently broad specificities that saccharides of more than one structure can be accommodated within the binding site. Nonetheless, with these caveats in mind, the profile of interaction of glycopetides or glycoproteins derived from given cell lines can be quite revealing and indicate changes in accessible carbohydrate associated with transformation.

Due to this lack of strict specificity of most lectins and the inherent microheterogeneity of the oligosaccharides of glycoproteins, it is essential to first test the lectin columns used for purification with glycoproteins and glycopeptides of known structures. In addition it is also important to assess the yield of the glycoprotein from lectin affinity steps because irreversible interaction between the lectin and the ligand is known to occur. Affinity chromatography on immobilized antibody or lectin columns can usually be performed in the presence of a number of detergents (Lotan *et al.*, 1977; Lotan and Nicolson, 1979).

Purification of cell surface glycoproteins can also be carried out by a combination of conventional techniques. Gel filtration on several supports (Sepharose CL, Sephacryl, Controlled Pore Glass beads) can be carried out in the presence of nonionic detergents (Triton X-100; Ammonyx; Nonidet P-40), ionic detergent (sodium dodecyl sulfate), or hydrogen bond breaking solvents (urea, guanidine–HCl). It is necessary, however, to determine the influence (interference) of the buffer additives on the spectrophotometric, colorimetric or isotope counting procedures used for analysis of the fractions. Ion exchange chromatography on DEAE- or CM-Sepharose is usually carried out by gradient elutions which NaCl or LiCl in buffers containing nonionic detergents. Volatile buffers such as pyridinium acetate, widely used for the fractionation of glycopeptides, are not suitable for membrane glycoproteins because of their poor solubility. The purification of mouse melanoma-associated antigen (Bhavanandan *et al.*, 1980) and a 100K glycoprotein from human melanoma cells (Umemoto *et al.*, 1981) was accomplished by repeated ion exchange chromatography on DEAE-Sepharose columns using buffers containing 0.1% Triton X-100. Isoelectric focusing in neutral detergents and urea (Merz *et al.*, 1972; Zechel, 1977; Baumann and Doyle, 1979) has also been used for purification of glycoproteins. A limitation of this method is that the high sensitivity usually results in separation based on microheterogeneity of the oligosaccharides. Thus, a given glycoprotein may given rise to several peaks based on single differences in sialic acid or other charged residues. Preparative polyacrylamide gel electrophoresis in the presence or absence of sodium dodecyl sulfate has also been used for the purification of glycoproteins even though the recoveries in such experiments are usually low (Baldwin *et al.*, 1973; Dunn *et al.*, 1975; Braatz *et al.*, 1978).

F. Mapping the Organization of Cell Surface Glycoproteins

An evaluation of the role of cell surface glycoproteins in malignancy requires more than information on individual glycoproteins. It is possible that the altered properties of cancer cells such as proliferative growth, metastasis, altered recognition, and adhesion may not be due to changes in individual cell surface components but rather to a composite influence of several "new" components. Thus any study on cell surface glycoprotein should also assess the supramolecular organization of these and of other related molecules (glycolipids and glycosaminoglycans). Useful tools for these studies are (1) specific chemical stains, (2) lectins of well-defined specificities, (3) antibodies produced against known oligosaccharide structures, and (4) highly purified exo- and endoglycosidases. The gross distribution of cell surface carbohydrates can be determined by the help of light or electron microscopy after treatment of the cells with the first three classes of the above reagents.

1. Studies with Chemical Stains

Typical chemical reagents used include periodate–Schiff (Rambourg *et al.*, 1966; Ito, 1969; Martinez-Palamo, 1970; Luft, 1976), ruthenium red (Vorbradt and Koprowski, 1969; Luft, 1971), and colloidal iron (Hale, 1946; Gasic and Berwick, 1963; Rambourg *et al.*, 1966; Benedetti and Emmelot, 1967). Treatment of the intact cells with enzymes (neuraminidase, hyaluronidase) as well as carrying out the staining reactions at varying pH would help to distinguish between glycosaminoglycans and sialoglycoproteins or sialoglycolipids (Gasic and Berwick, 1963; Huet and Herzberg, 1973; Kim *et al.*, 1975). For example, at pH 2.0 only about 10% of the sialic acid carboxyl is ionized whereas sulfate ester groups are fully dissociated.

2. Studies with Lectins

Lectins are proteins (or glycoproteins) from plant or other sources which can bind noncovalently to specific carbohydrate groups but are known not to be enzymes, transport proteins, or immunoglobulins. Because of the abundance of carbohydrates on the cell surface (glycocalyx), the multivalent lectins are able to cause agglutination of erythrocytes and other cells, sometimes after prior enzymatically catalyzed modification of the cells. The findings that wheat germ agglutinin caused differential agglutination of normal and transformed cells stimulated a great deal of research on lectins (Aub *et al.*, 1965; Burger and Goldberg, 1967). Subsequently several other lectins (concanavalin A, soybean agglutinin, *Ricinus communis* agglutinins) were found to agglutinate cancer cells at much lower concentrations than control (normal) cells (Brown and Hunt, 1978). It was also noted that mild proteolysis rendered normal cells as agglutinable as transformed cells (Inbar *et al.*, 1969).

Lectins have been used in several additional ways to explore cellular glycoconjugates. The binding of lectins to cell surfaces can be quantitated by the use of isotopically labeled lectins (see reviews by Nicolson, 1974, 1976), preferably the monovalent subunits such as succinylated Con A (Gunther *et al.*, 1973). The topographical distribution of sugars can also be assessed by one of several methods: (1) direct immunofluorescence using lectin conjugated to fluorescent dyes such as fluorescein isothiocyanate or rhodamine (Inbar and Sachs, 1973); (2) indirect immunofluorescence using lectin and a fluorescein-conjugated antibody to the lectin (Mallucci, 1971); (3) electron microscopic visualization of lectins conjugated with ferritin (Nicolson and Singer, 1971, 1974; Marchesi *et al.*, 1972); (4) electron or light microscopic autoradiography using isotopically labeled lectins (Rapin and Burger, 1974); (5) histochemical studies with covalent conjugates of lectins and peroxidase (Bernhard and Avramaes, 1971; Huet and Garrido, 1972; Martinez-Paloma *et al.*, 1972).

3. Studies Using Antibodies against Oligosaccharides

Because most lectins lack strict or defined saccharide specificity other, better defined tools are desired. Antibodies directed against known oligosaccharides have great potential since they can be used to probe cell surface glycoconjugate organization in the same manner as that discussed above for lectins. Antibodies against neuramin 2→3 and 2→6 lactose and other sialyloligosaccharides (Smith and Ginsburg, 1980); lacto-*N*-fucopentaose III, lacto-*N*-tetraose, and mannotetraose (Zopf *et al.*, 1975, 1978); galactose and lactose (Pazur *et al.*, 1978); galactose and Lewis-a-b and -d determinants (Lemieux *et al.*, 1981) have all been prepared. Antibodies against specific oligosaccharides of both the *N*-glycosidically and *O*-glycosidically linked types known to be present on normal and transformed cells can be expected as a result of the rapidly expanding technology of monoclonal antibody.

4. Studies Using Glycosidases

The use of glycosidases to probe the cell surface distribution of saccharides has been largely confined to the use of sialidases (Hughes *et al.*, 1972; Barton and Rosenberg, 1973; Simmons and Rios, 1973; Weiss *et al.*, 1974). The availability of other highly purified exo- and endoglycosidases of known substrate specificities which are active at near physiological pH and ionic conditions should make further studies possible. The applicability of this approach is also limited since most of the presently available glycosidases do not effectively hydrolyze high-molecular-weight glycoprotein substrates (Flowers and Sharon, 1979). The endo β-*N*-acetylglucosaminidases (Muramatsu, 1978; Tarentino *et al.*, 1978), endo-β-galactosidases (Takasaki and Kobata, 1976; Nakagawa *et al.*, 1980), a glycopeptidase acting on aspartylglycosylamine linkages (Takahashi and Nishibe, 1978, 1981), and endo-α-N-acetylgalactosaminidase (Umemoto *et al.*, 1977; Glasgow *et al.*, 1977) are enzymes which satisfy some of the above requirements (Fukuda *et al.*, 1979).

It is important to consider the effect of the cell surface glycosaminoglycans in these studies. The results of experiments on cells before and after treatment with hylauronidase, chondroitinase (Nakada *et al.*, 1977), and heparitinase should be compared. The degradation of cell surface heparan sulfate by heparitinase was recently reported (Ohkubo *et al.*, 1981).

G. Structural Analysis of the Isolated Glycopeptides and Glycoproteins

Before embarking on structural studies, it is essential to establish homogeneity of the component under investigation. This has proved difficult because of the heterogeneous nature of the carbohydrate chains (Horowitz, 1977). In the case of homogeneous preparations of nonglycosylated proteins, techniques such as gel filtration, ion-exchange chromatography, gel electrophoresis, and isoelectric focusing can be expected to give single sharp symmetrical peaks or single sharp bands. In contrast, a pure preparation of glycoprotein, because of variations in the intra- and intermolecular carbohydrates, cannot be expected to yield similar results. An additional complication in the case of membrane glycoproteins is the ability of these molecules to aggregate resulting in either discrete bands as in the case of glycophorin (Silverberg and Marchesi, 1978) or a broad spectrum of aggregates (Kawasaki and Ashwell, 1976b; Dorst and Schubert, 1979; Bhavanandan *et al.*, 1980). This difficulty might be overcome by determining the homogeneity of the protein which carries the saccharide chains. If sufficient (microgram) quantities are available, NH_2 or COOH terminal amino acid determination may provide this information.

A second approach which can be used at tracer levels provided the protein is isotopically labeled (either *in vivo* for example, [^{14}C]leucine or *in vitro* by reductive methylation with $H^{14}CHO$) is chemical or enzymatic deglycosylation followed by examination of the resultant polypeptide. Unfortunately, this method is not widely applicable since complete enzymatic deglycosylation with the available exo- and endoglycosidases can be seldom achieved. The applicability of chemical deglycosylation with hydrogen fluoride (Mort and Lamport, 1977; Glassman *et al.*, 1978) as a general method for all glycoproteins has yet to be established.

Structural studies are usually not carried out on intact glycoproteins. The presence of more than one type of carbohydrate chain on the same molecule makes it difficult to interpret the results and the large quantity of amino acid interferes in many of the analytical procedures. Thus, glyco-proteins are usually subjected to proteolysis with broad spectrum pro-teases such as Pronase and the products fractionated by a combination of techniques (gel filtration, ion exchange chromatography, lectin affinity chromatography, etc.) to yield individual, homogeneous glycopeptides. The few amino acids present on Pronase generated glycopeptides mini-mally influence fractionation. This is in contrast to differences in sac-charide composition, where a difference of just one sugar particularly if it is charged, has a significant effect on chromatographic and electrophore-tic properties. The aim of the fractionation approach should be to separate the different classes of glycopeptides (Fig. 1) rather than to separate on the basis of minor variations. Lectin affinity chromatography appears to be specifically useful for this purpose (Ogata *et al.*, 1975; Krusius *et al.*, 1976; Narasimhan *et al.*, 1979; Rasilo, 1980; Bhavanandan *et al.*, 1981).

1. Isolation of Peptide-Free Oligosaccharides

An alternative approach, for the determination of carbohydrate struc-ture of glycoproteins involves the release of all carbohydrate chains from the protein thus totally eliminating the influence of the protein (or peptide) during fractionation (Finne *et al.*, 1980a). The mild alkaline–borohydride treatment conditions established for the release of O-glycosidically linked saccharides with minimum degradation (Carlson, 1968; Spiro, 1972) have been used extensively for this purpose. The release of the N-glycosidi-cally linked saccharides without destruction is best achieved by hydra-zinolysis (Yosizawa *et al.*, 1966). The use of this technique for structural elucidation has recently been reported by several investigators (Fukuda *et al.*, 1976; Reading *et al.*, 1978; Takasaki *et al.*, 1980; Yoshima *et al.*, 1980). The degradation of the oligosaccharides thus released appears to be mini-mal provided strictly anhydrous conditions are used. Strong alkaline–borohydride treatment recommended for the release of such carbohydrate chains (Lee and Scocca, 1972) was found to cause extensive degradation of the released saccharides of α_1-acid glycoprotein and fetuin (Bhavana-dan, unpublished results). On a limited scale, endoglycosidases can be used to release oligosaccharides from glycoproteins (Flowers and Sharon, 1979; Kobata, 1979).

The oligosaccharides derived from chemical or enzymatic cleavage are then fractionated into different classes. This can be done by gel filtration on fine and superfine gels (Etchison *et al.*, 1977; Van den Eijnden *et al.*, 1979; Natowicz and Baenziger, 1980) ion exchange chromatography (Finne, 1975; Fukuda *et al.*, 1976), thin-layer chromatography (Holmes and O'Brien, 1979), paper chromatography (Bhavanandan *et al.*, 1977,

1981; Fukuda and Hakomori, 1979; Li and Kornfeld, 1979), high voltage paper electrophoresis (Li and Kornfeld, 1979; Takasaki et al., 1980; Yoshima et al., 1980), high-pressure liquid chromatography (Wells and Lester, 1979), and lectin affinity chromatography (Blake and Goldstein, 1980). Reduction of the oligosaccharide with sodium borotritide facilitates the fractionation and analysis of trace amounts.

Once homogeneous preparations of glycopeptides or oligosaccharides are available, one can proceed with the determination of the following: (1) the nature of linkage of carbohydrate to peptide, (2) the sugar composition, (3) the sequence of the sugars, (4) the anomeric configuration of each of the glycosidic bonds, (5) the linkage positions, that is, which hydroxyl groups other than the glycosidic hydroxyls are involved in the linkages. The details of the methods used to obtain this information can be found in prior reviews (Spiro, 1972; Marshall and Neuberger, 1972a; Montreuil, 1975). Thus, only a brief description of the approach is given below.

2. Nature of Carbohydrate–Peptide Linkage

This information can be obtained by mild alkaline treatment in the presence of borohydride, hydrazinolysis, and by the use of glycosidases. The β-elimination reaction with mild alkali, however, is very slow if the glycosylated amino acid is either NH_2 or COOH terminal and can be made more efficient by prior blocking of these groups (Neuberger et al., 1972). β-Elimination in the presence of sodium borohydride in addition to identifying O-glycosidically linked oligosaccharides also permits the determination of the proportion of serine and threonine substituted by estimating the increase in alanine and appearance of α-aminobutyric acid. Further, by carrying out the elimination reaction in the presence of sodium sulfite instead of sodium borohydride it is possible to convert the hydroxyamino acids involved in the linkage to sugar to cysteic acid and α-amino-β-sulfonylbutyric acid (Harbon et al., 1968; Simpson et al., 1972; Spiro and Bhoyroo, 1974). Use of $Na^{35}SO_3$ and sequencing of the peptides would provide information on the location of the sugar-linked hydroxy amino acid in the protein (Simpson et al., 1972; Isemura and Ikenaka, 1975).

3. Determination of Sugar Composition

Several colorimetric methods, including modifications for microdeterminations, are available for quantitating hexoses, hexosamines, deoxyhexoses, and sialic acid (Ashwell, 1966; Spiro, 1966a; Marshall and Neuberger, 1972b). The currently preferred approach however, is gas liquid chromatographic analysis which is more sensitive and rapid. A very useful procedure is methanolysis of the glycopeptide or oligosaccharide followed by trimethylsilylation of the methyl glycosides; this permits determination in one analysis of the total sugar composition (Clamp *et al.*, 1971; Laine *et al.*, 1972; Clamp, 1977). Trifluoroacetylation of methyl glycosides, instead of trimethylsilylation (Montreuil, 1975) is a good alternative since the use of electron capture detection would increase the sensitivity of the analysis several fold (Pritchard and Niedermeier, 1978). However, this procedure has not been widely tested. Alternatively one may analyze the sugars (except sialic acid) as alditol acetates (Lehnhardt and Winzler, 1968; Sloneker, 1972; *et al.*, 1972). Another technique with good potential which needs further development is high-pressure liquid chromatographic separation of underivatized sugars following acid hydrolysis (Tikhomirov *et al.*, 1978; Binder, 1980). This method would permit the recovery of the sugars for further analysis and confirmation of identify. For identification and quantitation of hexosamines the amino acid analyzer has been widely used. The micro amino acid analyzers presently available make it possible to analyze picomole quantities of hexosamines present in hydrolysates of glycopeptides and glycoproteins.

These chromatographic procedures can be adapted to quantitate isotopically labeled sugars by stream-splitting the column effluent and collection of fractions for scintillation counting. Prehm and Scheid (1978) were able to quantitate 0.2 nmoles of monosaccharide by gas liquid chromatography of ^{3}H-labeled alditol acetates. We have made extensive use of this technique in conjunction with the amino acid analyzer to quantitate the distribution of label in glucosamine and galactosamine (Bhavanandan and Davidson, 1976; Bhavanandan *et al.*, 1977, 1981).

Several other techniques for the determination of trace amounts of sugars have been published (Takasaki and Kobata, 1974; Knutson, 1975; Roll and Conrad, 1977; Hase *et al.*, 1978; Hara *et al.*, 1979; Barr and Nordin, 1980).

4. Determination of Structure

There is no single method available that will provide information on the sequence, anomeric configuration, and linkages of sugars in glycoproteins and glycopeptides. The three widely used techniques are methylation analysis (Lindberg, 1972; Montreuil, 1975), treatment with glycosidases and periodate oxidation (Smith Degradation) (Hay *et al.*, 1965; Goldstein *et al.*, 1965). The enzymatic method provides the most information since all glycosidases have sugar and anomeric specificity and in addition certain glycosidases also have linkage and aglycon specificity. Thus it is possible to distinguish (a) between Galβ1 → 4GlcNAc and Galβ1 → 3GlcNAc and Galβ1 → 6GlcNAc by using the appropriate β-galactosidase (Li *et al.*, 1975; Paulson *et al.*, 1978), (b) between manα1 → 2 man,

manα1 → 3 man, and manα1 → 6 man using *Aspergillus saitei* α-manno-sidase (Yamashita *et al.*, 1980), and (c) between NeuNAc 2 → 3 Gal and NeuNAc 2 → 6 Gal using influenza virus neuraminidase (Drzeniek, 1967; Bhavanandan *et al.*, 1977). It can be hoped that the discovery of additional glycosidases (particularly from mammalian sources), the elucidation of the exact specificity of the existing and newly described glycosidases, and their ready availability would widen the use of this approach. For information on currently available glycosidases and their use in structural elucidation, readers are referred to recent reviews (Li and Li, 1977; Flowers and Sharon, 1979; Kobata, 1979).

At present, the most productive approach for structure elucidation is the combination of sequential degradation of the sugar chain from the nonreducing end with glycosidases and methylation (Hakomori, 1964) of the residual portion. This is followed by total hydrolysis and identification of the methylated sugars by GC/MS analysis (Bjorndal *et al.*, 1970). The application of this has been described in several recent studies (Kornfeld, 1978; Fukuda and Hakomori, 1979; van den Eijnden *et al.*, 1979; Finne *et al.*, 1980b; Irimura *et al.*, 1981).

Periodate oxidation is useful in obtaining information on linkage position, branching (Goldstein *et al.*, 1965; Spiro, 1966b), and the substitution position of *N*-acetyl hexosaminitols (Spiro, 1972; van den Eijnden *et al.*, 1976). Because of the differences in the rate of hydrolysis of different glycosidic bonds and of different sugars, partial degradation of carbohydrate chains can be achieved by mild acid hydrolysis (Wolfrom and Franks, 1965; Painter, 1965), acetolysis (Bayard and Montreuil, 1972; Bayard *et al.*, 1975), or hydrazinolysis followed by nitrous acid treatment (Isemura and Schmid, 1971; Montreuil, 1975; Aspinall *et al.*, 1980; Strecker *et al.*, 1981). The resulting fragments can then be sequenced and based on overlapping fragments the structure of the complete carbohydrate chain reduced.

A technique which is being increasingly applied to structural elucidation of saccharides is high resolution (360 to 500 MHz) ^{1}H NMR spectroscopy, as illustrated by the studies of Fournet *et al.* (1978) and Montreuil and Vliegenthart (1979).

VIII. General Recapitulation

Insofar as generalizations can be made regarding the presence of unusual glycoproteins on the surfaces of transformed cells, it appears that such are likely to be found. The most common properties appear to be related to both increased complexity and increased glycosylation of the saccharide moieties of the glycoproteins. Studies conducted by utilization of tritiated sugar precursors or by labeling of saccharide residues in whole cells or membrane preparations followed by glycopeptide isolation have supported the generality of these conclusions. What is much less clear is the tissue-specific origin of the polypeptide portion of these macromolecules. Recent work, which is rather heavily dependent on modern immune technology (production of monoclonal antibodies by the hybridoma technique), has provided strong suggestive evidence showing that the tissue-specific antigen is present in all tumors of a particular type or that it is not present in a variety of tumors of another cell type, as well as adult or fetal cells. One difficulty with the immune technique is that alterations in the carbohydrate moiety of the glycoprotein can easily result in sufficient conformational changes to evoke new antigenic determinants from common polypeptide precursors. Thus, even the sophisticated hybridoma technology may be led astray in presuming that totally new structures are being formed. Without the essential chemical evidence regarding the primary structure of glycoprotein products, it will be impossible to define them as unique and specific products of tumor cell metabolism. It is quite likely that the transformation event results in expression of new genes but it may also result in the modification of preexisting membrane associated glycoproteins and their subsequent appearance as new bands on gels or new antigens in immune screening procedures.

Modern genetic technology would presume that appearance of new phenotypic characteristics would, if associated with a new genotype, be detectable by appropriate techniques. Thus, the presence of a new messenger RNA could be detected if an appropriate library of cloned fragments were available for the necessary hybridization studies. It should be noted that most of the surface components mentioned are present in extremely small quantities, have been detected primarily if not exclusively by isotopic tracer techniques, and the prospect of fishing out the appropriate genetic information must be accorded as relatively remote.

A second problem in dealing with tumor-related cell surface glycoproteins involves their length of residence on the cell surface. It has been reported by a number of laboratories that transformed cells exhibit an elevated level of surface protease activity. This may well account for the apparent loss of fibronectin from the surface of fibroblasts following viral transformation. The altered behavior of the cell surface glycoproteins may arise from the fact that localized processing of intrinsic membrane proteins can occur under circumstances where this event would not have taken place prior to transformation. Furthermore, the putative proteolytic activity could be responsible for the loss from the cell surface of membrane components at a much higher rate (observations confirmed by direct experimentation) than is found in normal cells. As a result of this, increased levels of membrane proteins may appear in the circulation. At least one report has appeared of a circulating glycoprotein associated with malignancy although its identification with the cell surface has not been made (Bolmer and Davidson, 1981). The generality of this observation, that is, the association of this glycoprotein with a variety of malignancies, suggests that origin within a specific tumor cell is less likely than is modification of a preexisting component by a common feature associated with cells that have lost growth control.

IX. Prognosis

The general trend in recent years has indicated that a very large variety of tumor-related glycoprotein antigens will continue to be described. Most of the descriptive material will rely on either metabolic or surface labeling approaches followed by identification of unusual components by gel electrophoretic or immunologic techniques. Sophisticated refinement such as the use of two-dimensional gels or isoelectric focusing gels and monoclonal antibodies are likely to improve the number of qualitative changes that are identifiable but are not likely to provide an understanding of the nature of these differences or the relationship between the characteristics of the transformed cell and the expression of the unusual component. By quite a different route, descriptive material will continue to be acquired based largely on techniques such as lectin affinity chromatography and electron microscopic visualization of surface features utilizing either lectin or other probes derivatized to provide localization information. Here, differences may well be established, but their chemical nature will be very difficult to interpret. Thus, changes in lectin affinity chromatographic profiles can arise from alterations in the carbohydrate composition of glycoproteins or loss of one or another component from the cell surface, and so on. The relationship of these observations to the more explicit ones derived by direct biochemical techniques, will rarely be accomplished in the same laboratories. A key problem that remains has been alluded to above and relates to the explicit chemical definition of observed alterations. It is necessary to isolate sufficient material from any system to define the chemistry and the origin of the macromolecule involved. The next step will be to associate these changes with specific gene expression and to document the generality of such a change with the transformed phenotype. The latter is perhaps the most difficult problem and its solution one that has thus far eluded researchers. The fact remains that the fundamental biologic problem in malignancy has yet to be defined in spite of, for example, a complete knowledge of the gene architecture of a transforming virus. Those events which result in loss of growth control, perhaps the initial problem, followed by selection from within that population of cells that have the ability to metastasize, the life threatening event, is still far from understood. The best information that is likely to derive from continued studies on cell surface glycoproteins has to do with either diagnostic or immunologic approaches to the management of the disease.

REFERENCES

Aoi, Y., and Yokota, M. (1980). *Tohoku J. Exp. Med.* **131,** 95–96.
Ashwell, G. (1966). *In* "Methods in Enzymology" (E. F. Neufeld and V. Ginsburg, eds.), Vol. 8, pp. 85–95. Academic Press, New York.
Aspinall, G. O., Gharia, M. M., Ritchie, G. S., and Wong, C. O. (1980). *Carbohydr. Res.* **85,** 73–92.
Aub, J. C., Sanford, B. H., and Cote, M. N. (1965). *Proc. Natl. Acad. Sci. U.S.A.* **54,** 396–399, 400–402.
Baldwin, R. W., Harris, J. R., and Price, M. R. (1973). *Int. J. Cancer* **11,** 385–397.
Barland, P., and Schroeder, E. A. (1970). *J. Cell. Biol.* **45,** 662–668.
Barnes, D., and Sato, G. (1980a). *Analyt. Biochem.* **102,** 255–270.
Barnes, D., and Sato, G. (1980b). *Cell* **22,** 649–655.
Barr, J., and Nordin, P. (1980). *Analyt. Biochem.* **108,** 313–319.
Barton, N. W., and Rosenberg, A. (1973). *J. Biol. Chem.* **248,** 7353–7358.
Baumann, H., and Doyle, D. (1979). *J. Biol. Chem.* **254,** 3935–3946.
Bayard, B., and Montreuil, J. (1972). *Carbohydr. Res.* **24,** 427–443 and 445–456 (in French with abstract in English).
Bayard, B., Strecker, G., and Montreuil, J. (1975). *Biochimie* **57,** 155–160.
Bekesi, J. G., and Winzler, R. J. (1967). *J. Biol. Chem.* **242,** 3873–3879.
Bender, W. W., Garan, H., and Berg, H. C. (1971). *J. Mol. Biol.* **58,** 783–797.
Benedetti, E. L., and Emmelot, P. (1967). *J. Cell Sci.* **2,** 499–512.
Bernhard, W., and Avramaes, S. (1971). *Exp. Cell Res.* **64,** 232–236.
Bhavanandan, V. P., and Davidson, E. A. (1976). *Biochem. Biophys. Res. Commun.* **70,** 139–145.
Bhavanandan, V. P., and Katlic, A. W. (1979). *J. Biol. Chem.* **254,** 4000–4008.
Bhavanandan, V. P., Umemoto, J., Banks, J. R., and Davidson, E. A. (1977). *Biochemistry* **16,** 4426–4437.
Bhavanandan, V. P., Kemper, J. G., and Bystryn, J.-C. (1980). *J. Biol. Chem.* **255,** 5145–5153.
Bhavanandan, V. P., Katlic, A. W., Kemper, J. G., Banks, J. R., and Davidson, E. A. (1981). *Biochemistry,* in press.
Binder, H. (1980). *J. Chromatogr.* **189,** 414–420.
Bjorndal, H., Hellerquist, C. G., Lindberg, B., and Svensson, S. (1970). *Angew. Chem. (Int. Ed)* **9,** 610–619.
Blake, D. A., and Goldstein, I. J. (1980). *Analyt. Biochem.* **102,** 103–109.
Blumenfeld, O. O., and Zvilichovsky, B. (1972). *In* "Methods in Enzymology" (V. Ginsburg, ed.), Vol. 28, pp. 245–252. Academic Press, New York.
Bolmer, S. D., and Davidson, E. A. (1981). *Biochemistry* **20,** 1047–1054.
Bosmann, H. B. (1972). *Biochem. Biophys. Res. Commun.* **49,** 1256–1262.
Bosmann, H. B., Case, K. R., and Morgan, H. R. (1974). *Exp. Cell Res.* **83,** 15–24.

Braatz, J. A., McIntire, K. R., Princler, G. L., Kortright, K. H., and Herberman, R. B. (1978). *J. Natl. Cancer Inst.* **61**, 1035–1046.
Bramwell, M. E., and Harris, H. (1978a). *Proc. R. Soc. London (Biol.)* **201**, 93–99.
Bramwell, M. E., and Harris, H. (1978b). *Proc. R. Soc. London (Biol.)* **203**, 87–106.
Bray, B. A., Lieberman, R., and Meyer, K. (1967). *J. Biol. Chem.* **242**, 3373–3380.
Bretscher, M. S. (1971). *J. Mol. Biol.* **58**, 775–781.
Brown, J. C. (1971). *Exp. Cell Res.* **69**, 440–442.
Brown, J. C., and Hunt, R. C. (1978). *Int. Rev. Cytol.* **52**, 277–349.
Brown, J. P., Woodbury, R. G., Hart, C. E., Hellstrom, I., and Hellstrom, K. E. (1981a). *Proc. Natl. Acad. Sci. U.S.A.* **78**, 539–543.
Brown, W. R. A., Barclay, A. N., Sunderland, C. A., and Williams, A. F. (1981b). *Nature (London)* **289**, 456–460.
Brunette, D. M., and Till, J. E. (1971). *J. Membr. Biol.* **5**, 215–224.
Buck, C. A., Glick, M. C., and Warren, L. (1971). *Biochemistry* **10**, 2176–2180.
Burger, M. M., (1973). *Fed. Proc. Fed. Am. Soc. Exp. Biol.* **32**, 91–101.
Burger, M. M., and Goldberg, A. R. (1967). *Proc. Natl. Acad. Sci. U.S.A.* **57**, 359–366.
Bystryn, J.-C. (1978). *J. Immunol.* **120**, 96–101.
Bystryn, J.-C., Tedholm, C. A., and Heaney-Kieras, J. (1981). *Cancer Res.* **41**, 910–914.
Cabantchik, Z. I., and Rothstein, A. (1974). *J. Membr. Biol.* **15**, 207–226 and 227–248.
Carey, T. E., Takahashi, T., Resnick, L. A., Oettgen, H. F., and Old, L. J. (1976). *Proc. Natl. Acad. Sci. U.S.A.* **73**, 3278–3282.
Carey, T. E., Lloyd, K. O., Takahashi, T., and Travassos, L. R. (1979). *Proc. Natl. Acad. Sci. U.S.A.* **76**, 2898–2902.
Carlson, D. M. (1968). *J. Biol. Chem.* **243**, 616–626.
Carrel, S., and Theilkaes, L. (1973). *Nature (London)* **242**, 609–610.
Carrel, S., and Accolla, R. S., Carmagnola, A. L., and March, G. P. (1980). *Cancer Res.* **40**, 2523–2528.
Ceccarini, C. (1975). *Proc. Natl. Acad. Sci. U.S.A.* **72**, 2687–2690.
Ceccarini, C., and Atkinson, P. H. (1977). *Biochim. Biophys. Acta* **500**, 197–207.
Ceccarini, C., Muramatsu, T., Tsang, J., and Atkinson, P. H. (1975). *Proc. Natl. Acad. Sci. U.S.A.* **72**, 3139–3143.
Chandrasekaran, E. V., and Davidson, E. A. (1979). *Biochemistry* **18**, 5615–5620.
Chandrasekaran, E. V., Mendicino, A., Garver, F. A., and Mendicino, J. (1981). *J. Biol. Chem.* **256**, 1549–1555.
Chee, D. O., Boddie, A. W., Roth, J. A., Holmes, E. C., and Morton, D. L. (1976). *Cancer Res.* **36**, 1503–1509.
Chiarugi, V. P., and Urbano, P. (1972). *J. Gen. Virol.* **14**, 133–140.
Cifonelli, J. A. (1968). *Carbohydr. Res.* **8**, 233–242.
Clamp, J. R. (1977). *Biochem. Soc. Trans.* **5**, 1693–1695.
Clamp, J. R., Bhatti, T., and Chambers, R. E. (1971). In "Methods of Biochemical Analysis" (D. Glick, ed.), Vol. 19, pp. 229–344. Wiley, New York.
Clemetson, K. J., Bertschmann, M., Widmer, S., and Luscher, E. F. (1976). *Immunochemistry* **13**, 383–388.
Codington, J. F. (1975). "Cellular Membranes and Tumor Cell Behavior," pp. 399–419. Williams & Wilkins, Baltimore, Maryland.
Codington, J. F. (1978). *Am. Chem. Soc. Symp.* **80**, 277–294.
Codington, J. F., Sanford, B. H., and Jeanloz, R. W. (1972). *Biochemistry* **11**, 2559–2564.
Codington, J. F., Klein, G., Cooper, A. G., Lee, N., Brown, M. C., and Jeanloz, R. W. (1978). *J. Natl. Cancer Inst.* **60**, 811–818.
Codington, J. F., Cooper, A. G., Miller, D. K., Slayter, H. S., Brown, M. C., Silber, C., and Jeanloz, R. W. (1979a). *J. Natl. Cancer Inst.* **63**, 153–161.

Codington, J. F., Kelin, G., Silber, C., Linsley, K. B., and Jeanloz, R. W. (1979b). *Biochemistry* **18**, 2145–2149.

Colombini, M., and Johnstone, R. M. (1973). *Biochim. Biophys. Acta* **323**, 69–86.

Cooper, A. G., Codington, J. F., Miller, D. K., and Brown, M. C. (1979). *J. Natl. Cancer Inst.* **63**, 163–169.

Critchley, D. R., Wyke, J. A., and Hynes, R. O. (1976). *Biochim. Biophys. Acta* **436**, 335–352.

Culp, L. A., and Black, P. H. (1972). *Biochemistry* **11**, 2161–2172.

Currie, G. A., Doornich, W. J., and Bagshawe, K. O. (1968). *Nature (London)* **219**, 191–192.

Debray, D., and Montreuil, J. (1978). *Biochimie* **60**, 697–704.

Dimitriadis, G. J. (1979). *Analyt. Biochem.* **98**, 445–451.

Dippold, W. G., Lloyd, K. O., Li, L. T. C., Ikeda, H., Oettgen, H. F., and Old, L. J. (1980). *Proc. Natl. Acad. Sci. U.S.A.* **77**, 6114–6118.

Dorst, H.-J., and Schubert, D. (1979). *Hoppe Seylers Z. Physiol. Chem.* **360**, 1605–1618.

Drzeniek, R. (1967). *Biochem. Biophys Res. Commun.* **26**, 631–638.

Duksin, D., and Bornstein, P. (1977). *Proc. Natl. Acad. Sci. U.S.A.* **74**, 3433–3437.

Dunn, M. J., McBay, W., and Maddy, A. H. (1975). *Biochim. Biophys. Acta* **386**, 107–119.

Emmelot, P. (1973). *Eur. J. Cancer* **9**, 319–333.

Engvall, E., and Ruoslahti, E. (1977). *Int. J. Cancer* **20**, 1–5.

Eisinger, R. W., and Kennel, S. G. (1981). *Cancer Res.* **41**, 877–881.

Etchison, J. R., Robertson, J. S., and Summers, D. F. (1977). *Virology* **78**, 375–392.

Evans, I., DiStefano, P., Case, K. R., and Bosmann, H. B. (1977). *FEBS Lett.* **78**, 109–112.

Fairbanks, G., Steck, T. L., and Wallach, D. F. H. (1971). *Biochemistry* **10**, 2606–2617.

Fareed, V. S., Bhavanandan, V. P., and Davidson, E. A. (1978). *Carbohydr. Res.* **65**, 73–83.

Finne, J. (1975). *Biochim. Biophys. Acta* **412**, 317–325.

Finne, J., Krusius, T., and Jarnefelt, J. (1980a). *Proc. Int. Cogr. Pure Appl. Chem., 27th* pp. 147–159.

Finne, J., Tao, T.-W., and Burger, M. M. (1980b). *Cancer Res.* **40**, 2580–2587.

Fishman, P. H., Brady, R. O., and Aaronson, S. A. (1976). *Biochemistry* **15**, 201–208.

Flowers, H. M., and Glick, M. C. (1980). *Cancer Res.* **40**, 1550–1557.

Flowers, H. M., and Sharon, N. (1979). *Adv. Enzymol.* **48**, 29–95.

Fournet, B., Montreuil, J., Strecker, G., Dorland, L., Haverkamp, J., Vliegenthart, J. F. G., Binette, J., and Schmid, K. (1978). *Biochemistry* **17**, 5206–5214.

Fukuda, M., and Hakomori, S.-I. (1979). *J. Biol. Chem.* **254**, 5451–5457.

Fukuda, M., Kondo, T., and Osawa, T. (1976). *J. Biochem. (Tokyo)* **80**, 1223–1232.

Fukuda, M. N., Fukuda, M., and Hakomori, S.-I. (1979). *J. Biol. Chem.* **254**, 5458–5465.

Funakoshi, I., and Yamashina, I. (1976). *J. Biochem. (Tokyo)* **80**, 1185–1193.

Furth, A. J. (1980). *Analyt. Biochem.* **109**, 207–215.

Gaffar, S. A., Braatz, J. A., Kortright, K. H., Princler, G. L., and McIntire, R. K. (1979). *J. Biol. Chem.* **254**, 2097–2102.

Gaffar, S. A., Princler, G. L., McIntire, K. R., and Braatz, J. A. (1980). *J. Biol. Chem.* **255**, 8334–8339.

Gahmberg, C. G., and Andersson, L. C. (1977). *J. Biol. Chem.* **252**, 5888–5894.

Gahmberg, C. G., and Hakomori, S.-I. (1973). *J. Biol. Chem.* **248**, 4311–4317.

Gahmberg, C. G., Kiehn, D., and Hakomori, S.-I. (1974). *Nature (London)* **248**, 413–415.

Gahmberg, C. G., Itaya, K., and Hakomori, S.-I. (1976). *Methods Membr. Biol.* **7**, 179–210.

Gasic, G., and Berwick, L. (1963). *J. Cell Biol.* **19**, 223–238.

Gersten, D. M., and Marchalonis, J. J. (1979). *Biochem. Biophys. Res. Commun.* **90**, 1015–1024.

Gill, P. J., Adler, J., Silbert, C. K., and Silbert, J. E. (1981). *Biochem. J.* **194**, 299–307.

Glasgow, L. R., Paulson, J. C., and Hill, R. L. (1977). *J. Biol. Chem.* **252**, 8615–8623.

Glassman, J. N. S., Todd, C. W., and Shively, J. E. (1978). *Biochem. Biophys. Res. Commun.* **85**, 209–216.

Glenney, Jr., J. R., and Walborg, Jr., E. F. (1979). *J. Supramol. Struct.* **11**, 493–502.

Glenney, Jr., J. R., Allison, J. P., Hipson, D. C., and Walborg, Jr., E. F. (1979). *J. Biol. Chem.* **254**, 9247–9253.

Glenney, Jr., J. R., Kaulfus, P. J., McIntyre, B., and Walborg, Jr., E. F. (1980). *Cancer Res.* **40**, 2853–2859.

Glick, M. C. (1976). *J. Natl. Cancer Inst.* **57**, 653–658.

Glick, M. C. (1979). *Biochemistry* **12**, 2525–2532.

Glick, M. C., and Buck, C. A. (1973). *Biochemistry* **12**, 85–90.

Glick, M. C., and Santer, U. (1978). *In* "Cell Surface Carbohydrate Chemistry" (R. E. Harmon, ed.), pp. 13–26. Academic Press, New York.

Glick, M. C., Kimbi, Y., and Littauer, U. Z. (1976a). *Nature (London)* **259**, 230–232.

Glick, M. C., Schlesinger, H., and Hummeler, K. (1976b). *Cancer Res.* **36**, 4520–4524.

Goding, J. W. (1980). *J. Immunol. Methods* **39**, 285–308.

Goldstein, I. J., Hay, G. W., Lewis, B. A., and Smith, F. (1965). *In* "Methods in Carbohydrate Chemistry" (R. L. Whistler, ed.), Vol. 5, pp. 361–370. Academic Press, New York.

Gunther, G. R., Wang, J. L., Yahara, I., Cunningham, B. A., and Edelman, G. M. (1973). *Proc. Natl. Acad. Sci. U.S.A.* **70**, 1012–1016.

Gwynne, J. T., and Tanford, C. (1970). *J. Biol. Chem.* **245**, 3269–3271.

Hakomori, S.-I. (1964). *J. Biochem. (Tokyo)* **55**, 205–208.

Hakomori, S.-I. (1975). *Biochim. Biophys. Acta* **417**, 55–89.

Hakomori, S.-I., and Murakami, W. T. (1968). *Proc. Natl. Acad. Sci. U.S.A.* **59**, 254–261.

Hale, C. W. (1956). *Nature (London)* **157**, 802.

Hamaguchi, H., and Cleve, H. (1972). *Biochem. Biophys. Res. Commun.* **47**, 459–464.

Hara, S., Ikegami, H., Shono, A., Mega, T., Ikenaka, T., and Matsushima, Y. (1979). *Analyt. Biochem.* **97**, 166–172.

Harbon, S., Herman, G., and Clauser, H. (1968). *Eur. J. Biochem.* **4**, 265–272.

Hase, S., Ikenaka, T., and Matsushima, Y. (1978). *Biochem. Biophys. Res. Commun.* **85**, 257–263.

Hay, G. W., Lewis, B. A., and Smith, F. (1965). *Methods Carbohydr. Chem.* **5**, 357–361.

Hayman, M. J., and Crumpton, M. J. (1972). *Biochem. Biophys. Res. Commun.* **47**, 923–930.

Hollinshead, A. C., Herberman, R. B., Jaffurs, W. J., Alpert, L. K., Minton, J. P., and Harris, J. E. (1974). *Cancer* **34**, 1235–1243.

Holloway, P. W. (1973). *Analyt. Biochem.* **53**, 304–308.

Holmes, E. W., and O'Brien, J. S. (1979). *Analyt. Biochem.* **93**, 167–170.

Horowitz, M. I. (1977). *In* "The Glycoconjugates" (M. I. Horowitz and W. Pigman, eds.), Vol. I, pp. 15–34. Academic Press, New York.

Hourani, B. T., Chace, N. M., and Pincus, J. H. (1973). *Biochim. Biophys. Acta* **328**, 520–532.

Howard, D. R., and Batsakis, P. (1980). *Science* **210**, 201–203.

Howe, C., Lloyd, K. O., and Lee, L. T. (1972). *In* "Methods in Enzymology" (V. Ginsburg, ed.), Vol. 28, pp. 236–245. Academic Press, New York.

Hudson, C. S., and Kunz, A. (1925). *Am. Chem. J.* **47**, 2052–2055.

Huet, Ch., and Garrido, J. (1972). *Exp. Cell Res.* **75**, 523–527.

Huet, Ch., and Herzberg, M. (1973). *J. Ultrastruct. Res.* **42**, 186–199.

Hughes, R. C. (1973). *Prog. Biophys. Mol. Biol.* **26**, 191–268.

Hughes, R. C. (1976). "Membrane Glycoproteins." Butterworth, London.

Hughes, R. C., Sanford, B., and Jeanloz, R. W. (1972). *Proc. Natl. Acad. Sci. U.S.A.* **69**, 942–945.

Hunt, R. C., and Brown, J. C. (1975). *J. Mol. Biol.* **97**, 413–422.

Hunt, L. A., Lamph, W., and Wright, S. E. (1981). *J. Virol.* **37**, 207–215.

Hynes, R. O. (1973). *Proc. Natl. Acad. Sci. U.S.A.* **70**, 3170–3174.

Hynes, R. O. (1976). *Biochim. Biophys. Acta* **458**, 73–107.

Hynes, R. O., ed. (1979). "Surfaces of Normal and Malignant Cells." Wiley, New York.

Hynes, R. O., and Wyke, J. A. (1975). *Virology* **64**, 492–504.

Hynes, R. O., Destree, A. T., Perkins, M. E., and Wagner, D. D. (1979). *J. Supramol. Struct.* **11**, 95–104.

Inbar, M., and Sachs, L. (1973). *FEBS Lett.* **32**, 124–128.

Inbar, M., Rabinowitz, Z., and Sachs, L. (1969). *Int. J. Cancer* **4**, 690–696.

Invernizzi, G., Carbone, G., Mochini, A., and Parmiani, G. (1977). *J. Immunogenet.* **4**, 115–125.

Irimura, T., Tsuji, T., Tagami, S., Yamamoto, K., and Osawa, T. (1981). *Biochemistry* **20**, 560–566.

Isemura, M., and Ikenaka, T. (1975). *Biochim. Biophys. Acta* **404**, 11–21.

Isemura, S., and Schmid, K. (1971). *Biochem. J.* **124**, 591–604.

Ishii, Y., Goldhofer, W., and Mavligit, G. G. (1980). *GANN* **71**, 881–888.

Itaya, K., Gahmberg, C. G., and Hakomori, S.-I. (1975). *Biochem. Biophys. Res. Commun.* **64**, 1028–1035.

Ito, S. (1969). *Fed. Proc. Fed. Am. Soc. Exp. Biol.* **28**, 12–25.

Jacobson, B. S., Cronin, J., and Branton, D. (1978). *Biochim. Biophys. Acta* **506**, 81–96.

Juliano, R. L., and Behar-Bannelier, M. (1975). *Biochim. Biophys. Acta* **375**, 249–267.

Jumblatt, J. E., Tao, T.-W., Schlup, V., Finne, J., and Burger, M. M. (1980). *Biochem. Biophys. Res. Commun.* **95**, 111–117.

Kahan, B. D., Rutzky, L. P., Kahan, A. V., Oyasu, R., Wiseman, F., and LeGrub, S. (1977). *Cancer Res.* **37**, 2866–2871.

Kamm, A. R., and Grimes, W. J. (1978). *Proc. Natl. Acad. Sci. U.S.A.* **75**, 5912–5916.

Kawasaki, T., and Ashwell, G. (1976a). *J. Biol. Chem.* **251**, 5292–5299.

Kawasaki, T., and Ashwell, G. (1976b). *J. Biol. Chem.* **251**, 1296–1302.

Kennel, S. J. (1979). *Cancer Res.* **39**, 2934–2939.

Kennel, S. J., Lankford, P. K., Foote, L. J. Tsakeres, F. S., Adams, L. M., and Ullrich, R. L. (1980). *Cancer Res.* **40**, 2143–2159.

Kim, U., Baumbler, A., Carruthers, C., and Bielat, K. (1975). *Proc. Natl. Acad. Sci. U.S.A.* **72**, 1012–1016.

Knauf, S., and Urbach, G. I. (1974). *Am. J. Obstet. Gynecol.* **119**, 966–970.

Knauf, S., and Urbach, G. I. (1976). *Gynecol. Oncol.* **4**, 167–175.

Knauf, S., and Urbach, G. I. (1977). *Am. J. Obstet. Gynecol.* **127**, 705–710.

Knauf, S., and Urbach, G. I. (1978). *Am. J. Obstet. Gynecol.* **131**, 780–787.

Knauf, S., and Urbach, G. I. (1981). *Cancer Res.* **41**, 1351–1357.

Knutson, C. A. (1975). *Carbohydr. Res.* **43**, 225–231.

Kobata, A. (1979). *Analyt. Biochem.* **100**, 1–14.

Kohn, P., Winzler, R. J., and Hoffman, R. C. (1962). *J. Biol. Chem.* **237**, 304–308.

Koide, N., Muramatsu, T., and Kobata, A. (1979). *J. Biochem.* **85**, 149–155.

Kornfeld, R. (1978). *Biochemistry* **17**, 1415–1423.

Krakower, J. M., and Aaronson, S. A. (1978). *Nature (London)* **273**, 463–464.

Krakower, J. M., Tronick, S. R., Gallagher, R. E., Gallo, R. C., and Aaronson, S. A. (1978). *Int. J. Cancer* **22**, 715–720.

Krusius, T., Finne, J., and Rauvala, H. (1976). *FEBS Lett.* **71**, 117–120.

Kuo, T. J., Rosai, J., and Tillack, T. W. (1973). *Int. J. Cancer* **12**, 532–542.

Kurth, R. (1976). *Biomembranes* **8,** 167–233.

Kurth, R., and Bauer, H. (1975). *Biochim. Biophys. Acta.* **417,** 1–23.

Kurth, R., and Mikschy, U. (1978). *Proc. Natl. Acad. Sci. U.S.A.* **75,** 5692–5696.

Kurth, R., Teich, N. M., Weiss, R., and Oliver, N. T. D. (1977). *Proc. Natl. Acad. Sci. U.S.A.* **74,** 1237–1241.

Kurth, R., Fenyo, E. M., Klein, E., and Essex, M. (1979). *Nature (London)* **279,** 197–201.

Laine, R. A., Esselman, W. J., and Sweeley, C. C. (1972). *In* "Methods in Enzymology" (V. Ginsburg, ed.), Vol. 28, pp. 159–167. Academic Press, New York.

Lang, W. E., Jones, P. A., and Benedict, W. F. (1975). *J. Natl. Cancer Inst.* **54,** 173–179.

Langley, O. K., and Ambrose, E. J. (1967). *Biochem. J.* **102,** 367–372.

Ledbetter, J., and Nowinski, R. C. (1977). *J. Virol.* **23,** 315–322.

Lee, T. C., and Scocca, J. R. (1972). *J. Biol. Chem.* **247,** 5753–5758.

Lehnhardt, W. F., and Winzler, R. J. (1968). *J. Chromatogr.* **34,** 471–479.

Lemieux, R. U., Baker, D. A., Weinstein, W. M., and Switzer, C. M. (1981). *Biochemistry* **20,** 199–205.

Leonard, E. J., Richardson, A. K., Hardy, A. S., and Rapp, H. J. (1975). *J. Natl. Cancer Inst.* **55,** 73–78.

Leung, J. P., and Edgington, T. S. (1980). *Cancer Res.* **40,** 316–321.

Leung, J. P., Plow, E. F., Nakamura, R. M., and Edgington, T. S. (1978). *J. Immunol.* **121,** 1287–1296.

Leong, S. P. L., Sutherland, C. M., and Krementz, E. T. (1977a). *Cancer Res.* **37,** 293–298

Leong, S. P. L., Sutherland, C. M., and Krementz, E. T. (1977b). *Cancer Res.* **37,** 4035–4042.

Levine, D. W., Wong, J. S., Wang, D. I. C., and Thilly, W. G. (1977). *Somatic Cell Genet.* **3,** 149–155.

Li, E., and Kornfeld, S. (1979). *J. Biol. Chem.* **254,** 1600–1605.

Li, E., Gibson, R., and Kornfeld, S. (1980). *Arch. Biochem. Biophys.* **199,** 393–399.

Li, S.-C., Mazzotta, M. Y., Chien, S.-F., and Li, Y.-T. (1975). *J. Biol. Chem.* **250,** 6786–6791.

Li, Y.-T., and Li, S.-C. (1977). *In* "The Glycoconjugates" (M. I. Horowitz and W. Pigman, eds.), Vol. I, pp. 51–67. Academic Press, New York.

Liao, T.-H., Gallop, P. M., and Blumenfeld, O. O. (1973). *J. Biol. Chem.* **248,** 8247–8253.

Lin, L.-H., and Davidson, E. A. (1981). *Cancer* (Submitted).

Lindberg, B. (1972). *In* "Methods in Enzymology" (V. Ginsbrug, ed.), Vol. 28, pp. 178–195. Academic Press, New York.

Linker, A., and Hovingh, P. (1972). *In* "Methods in Enzymology" (V. Ginsburg, ed.), Vol. 28, pp. 902–911. Academic Press, New York.

Lisowska, E. (1969). *Eur. J. Biochem.* **10,** 574–579.

Lisowska, E., and Wasniowska, K. (1978). *Eur. J. Biochem.* **88,** 247–252.

Littauer, U. Z., Giovanni, M. Y., and Glick, M. C. (1980). *J. Biol. Chem.* **255,** 5448–5453.

Lloyd, K. O., Travassos, L. R., and Takahashi, T. (1979). *J. Natl. Cancer Inst.* **63,** 623–634.

Lotan, R., and Nicolson, G. L. (1979). *Biochim. Biophys. Acta* **559,** 329–376.

Lotan, R., Beattie, G., Hubbell, W., and Nicolson, G. L. (1977). *Biochemistry* **16,** 1787–1794.

Luborsky, S. W., Chang, C., Pancake, S. J., and Mora, P. T. (1976). *Proc. Natl. Acad. Sci. U.S.A.* **71,** 990–996.

Luft, J. H. (1971). *Anat. Rec.* **171,** 347–368 and 369–416.

Luft, J. H. (1976). *Int. Rev. Cytol.* **45,** 291–382.

McKibbin, J. M. (1978). *J. Lipid Res.* **19,** 131–147.

Maddy, A. H. (1966) *Biochim. Biophys. Acta* **117**, 193–200.
Maddy, A. H., and Dunn, M. J. (1976). *In* "Biochemical Analysis of Membranes" (A. H. Maddy, ed.), pp. 177–196. Wiley, New York.
Mallucci, L. (1971). *Nature (London)* **233**, 241–244.
Mann, D. L. (1972). *Transplantation* **14**, 398–401.
Marchesi, V. T., and Andrews, E. P. (1971). *Science*, **174**, 1247–1248.
Marchesi, V. T., Tillack, T. W., Jackson, R. L., Segrest, J. P., and Scott, R. E. (1972). *Proc. Natl. Acad. Sci. U.S.A.* **69**, 1445–1449.
Marshall, R. D. (1974). *Biochem. Soc. Symp.* **40**, 17–26.
Marshall, R. D., and Neuberger, A. (1970). *Adv. Carbohydr. Chem.* **25**, 407–478.
Marshall, R. D., and Neuberger, A. (1972a) *In* "Glycoproteins" (A. Gottschalk, ed.), Part A, pp. 322–380. Elsevier, Amsterdam.
Marshall, R. D., and Neuberger, A. (1972b). *In* "Glycoproteins" (A. Gottschalk, ed.), Part A, pp. 224–299. Elsevier, Amsterdam.
Martinez-Palomo, A. (1970). *Int. Rev. Cytol.* **29**, 29–75.
Martinez-Palomo, A., Wicker, R., and Bernhard, W. (1972). *Int. J. Cancer* **9**, 676–684.
Mathews, R. A., Johnson, T. C., and Hudson, J. E. (1976). *Biochem. J.* **154**, 57–64.
Meezan, E., Wu, H. C., Black, P. H., and Robbins, P. W. (1969). *Biochemistry* **8**, 2518–2524.
Merz, D. C., Good, R. A., and Litman, G. W. (1972). *Biochem. Biophys. Res. Commun.* **49**, 84–91.
Mesa-Tejada, R., Keydar, I., Ramanarayanan, M., Ohno, T., Fenoglio, C., and Spiegelmann, S. (1978). *Proc. Natl. Acad. Sci. U.S.A.* **75**, 1529–1533.
Meyer, K. (1971). *In* "The Enzymes" (P. D. Boyer, ed.), Vol. 5, pp. 307–320. Academic Press, New York.
Miller, S. C., Hay, E. D., and Codington, J. F. (1977). *J. Cell Biol.* **72**, 511–529.
Mitchell, K. F., Fuhrer, J. P., Steplewski, Z., and Koprowski, H. (1980). *Proc. Natl. Acad. Sci. U.S.A.* **77**, 7287–7291.
Momoi, M., Kennett, R. H., and Glick, M. C. (1980). *J. Biol. Chem.* **255**, 11914–11921.
Montagnier, L., and Torpier, G. (1976). *Bull. Cancer (Paris)* **63**(1), 123–134.
Montreuil, J. (1975). *Pure Appl. Chem.* **42**, 431–477.
Montreuil, J. (1980). *Adv. Carbohydr. Chem. Biochem.* **37**, 157–223.
Montreuil, J., and Vliegenthart, J. F. G. (1979). *In* "Glycoconjugate Research" (J. D. Gregory and R. W. Jeanloz, eds.), Vol. 1, pp. 35–78. Academic Press, New York.
Mort, A. J., and Lamport, D. T. A. (1977). *Analyt. Biochem.* **82**, 289–309.
Mosesson, M. W., and Umfleet, R. A. (1970). *J. Biol. Chem.* **245**, 5728–5736.
Mosesson, M. W., Chem, A. B., and Huseby, R. M. (1975). *Biochim. Biophys. Acta* **386**, 509–524.
Mosher, D. F. (1975). *J. Biol. Chem.* **250**, 6614–6621.
Muramatsu, T. (1978). *In* "Methods in Enzymology" (V. Ginsburg, ed.), Vol. 50, pp. 555–559. Academic Press, New York.
Muramatsu, T., Atkinson, P. H., Nathenson, S. G., and Ceccarini, C. (1973). *J. Mol. Biol.* **80**, 781–799.
Muramatsu, T., Gachelin, G., Nicholas, J. F., Condamine, H., Jakob, A., and Jacob, F. (1978). *Proc. Natl. Acad. Sci. U.S.A.* **75**, 2315–2319.
Muramatsu, T., Muramatsu, H., Kasai, M., Habu, S., and Okumura, K. (1980). *Biochem. Biophys. Res. Commun.* **96**, 1547–1553.
Murray, M. J., and Kabat, D. (1979). *J. Biol. Chem.* **254**, 1340–1348.
Nachbar, M. S., Oppenheim, J. D., and Aull, F. (1976). *Biochim. Biophys. Acta* **419**, 512–529.

CELL SURFACE GLYCOPROTEIN MARKERS 101

Nakada, H., and Yamashina, I. (1978). J. Biochem. (Tokyo) 83, 79–83.
Nakada, H., Funakoshi, I., and Yamashina, I. (1975). J. Biochem. (Tokyo) 78, 863–872.
Nakada, H., Funakoshi, I., and Yamashina, I. (1977). J. Biochem. (Tokyo) 79, 280–284.
Nakagawa, H., Yamada, T., Chien, J.-L., Gardas, A., Kitamikado, M., Li, S.-C., and Li, Y.-T. (1980). J. Biol. Chem. 255, 5955–5959.
Nakajo, S., Nakaya, K. J., and Nakamura, Y. (1979). Biochim. Biophys. Acta 579, 88–94.
Narasimhan, S., Wilson, J. R., Martin, E., and Schachter, H. (1979). Can. J. Biochem. 57, 83–96.
Natori, T., Law, L. W., and Appella, E. (1977). Cancer Res. 37, 3406–3413.
Natori, T., Law, L. W., and Appella, E. (1978). Cancer Res. 38, 359–364.
Natowicz, M., and Baenziger, J. U. (1980). Anal. Biochem. 105, 159–164.
Neuberger, A., Gottschalk, A., Marshall, R. D., and Spiro, R. G. (1972). In "Glycoproteins" (A. Gottscalk, ed.), Part A, pp. 450–490. Elsevier, Amsterdam.
Neville, Jr., D. M. (1976). In "Biochemical Analysis of Membranes" (A. H. Maddy, ed.), pp. 27–54. Wiley, New York.
Nicolson, G. L. (1974). Int. Rev. Cytol. 39, 89–190.
Nicolson, G. L. (1976). Biochim. Biophys. Acta 458, 1–72.
Nicolson, G. L., and Singer, S. J. (1971). Proc. Natl. Acad. Sci. U.S.A. 68, 942–945.
Nicolson, G. L., and Singer, S. J. (1974). J. Cell Biol. 60, 236–248.
Nicolson, G. L., Birdwell, C. R., Brunson, K. W., Robbins, J. C., Beattie, G., and Fidler, I. J. (1977). In "Cell and Tissue Interaction" (J. W. Lash and M. M. Burger, eds.), pp. 225–241. Raven, New York.
Nilsson, K., Andersson, L. C., Gahmberg, C. G., and Wigzel, H. (1977). Int. J. Cancer 20, 708–716.
Ogata, S.-I., Muramatsu, T., and Kobata, A. (1975). J. Biochem. (Tokyo) 78, 687–696.
Ogata, S.-I., Muramatsu, T., and Kobata, A. (1976). Nature (London) 259, 580–582.
Ogata, S.-I., Ueda, R., and Lloyd, K. O. (1981). Proc. Natl. Acad. Sci. U.S.A. 78, 770–774.
Ohkubo, Y., Funakoshi, F., and Yamashina, I. (1981). J. Biochem. 89, 161–167.
Okada, Y., and Spiro, R. G. (1980). J. Biol. Chem. 255, 8865–8872.
Onodera, K., and Sheinin, R. (1970). J. Cell Sci. 7, 337–355.
Onodera, K., Yamaguchi, N., Kuchmo, T., and Aoi, Y. (1976). Proc. Natl. Acad. Sci. U.S.A. 73, 4090–4094.
Painter, T. J. (1965). In "Methods in Carbohydrate Chemistry" (R. L. Whistler, ed.), Vol. 5, pp. 280–285. Academic Press, New York.
Parry, G., and Hawkes, S. P. (1978). Proc. Natl. Acad. Sci. U.S.A. 75, 3703–3707.
Paulson, J. C., Prieels, J.-P., Glasgow, L. R., and Hill, R. L. (1978). J. Biol. Chem. 253, 5617–5624.
Pazur, J. H., Dreher, K. L., and Forsberg, L. S. (1978). J. Biol. Chem. 253, 1832–1837.
Perdue, J. F. (1974). In "Methods in Enzymology" (S. Fleischer and L. Packer, eds.), Vol. 31, pp. 162–168. Academic Press, New York.
Phillips, D. R., and Morrison, M. (1971). Biochemistry 10, 1766–1771.
Phillips, E. R., and Perdue, J. F. (1977). Int. J. Cancer 20, 798–804.
Phillips, E. R., and Perdue, J. F. (1978). Cancer Res. 38, 1281–1285.
Prat, M., and Comiglio, P. M. (1976). Immunochemistry 13, 97–102.
Prat, M., Landolfo, S., and Comiglio, P. M. (1975). FEBS Lett. 51, 351–354.
Prehm, P., and Scheid, A. (1978). J. Chromatogr. 166, 461–467.
Pritchard, D. G., and Niedermeier, N. (1978). J. Chromatogr. 152, 487–494.
Quissel, D. O., Changus, J. E., Yonan, T., and Pitot, H. C. (1977). Analyt. Biochem. 79, 240–256.
Rambourg, A., Neutra, M., and Lebland, C. P. (1966). Anat. Res. 154, 41–72.

Rapin, A. M. C., and Burger, M. M. (1974). *Adv. Cancer Res.* **20**, 1–91.

Rasilo, M.-L. (1980). *Can. J. Biochem.* **58**, 281–286.

Raz, A., Bucana, C., McLellan, W., and Fidler, I. J. (1980a). *Nature (London)* **284**, 363–364.

Raz, A., McLellan, W. L., Hart, I. R., Bucana, C. D., Hoyer, L. C. Sela, B.-A., Dragsten, P., and Fidler, I. J. (1980b). *Cancer Res.* **40**, 1645–1651.

Reading, C. L., Penhoet, E. E., and Ballou, C. E. (1978). *J. Biol. Chem.* **253**, 5600–5612.

Reisfeld, R. A., Pellegrino, H. A., and Kahan, B. D. (1971). *Science* **172**, 1134–1136.

Reynolds, J. A., and Tanford, C. (1970). *J. Biol. Chem.* **245**, 5161–5165.

Rieber, M., Bacalao, J. and Alonso, G. (1975). *Cancer Res.* **35**, 2104–2108.

Rifkin, D. B., Compans, R. W., and Reich, E. (1972). *J. Biol. Chem.* **247**, 6432–6437.

Rifkin, D. B., Loeb, J. N., Model, J., and Reich, E. (1974). *J. Exp. Med.* **139**, 1317–1328.

Robinson, J. M., Smith, D. F., Davis, E. M., Gilliam, E. B., Capetillo, S. C., and Walborg, Jr., E. F. (1976). *Biochem. Biophys. Res. Commun.* **72**, 81–88.

Roll, D. E., and Conrad, H. E. (1977). *Analyt. Biochem.* **77**, 397–412.

Rosenberg, S. A., and Guidotti, G. (1969). *J. Biol. Chem.* **244**, 5118–5124.

Rosenthal, K. L., Tomkins, W. A. F., and Rawls, W. E. (1980). *Cancer Res.* **40**, 4744–4750.

Rous, P. (1911). *JAMA* **56**, 198–203.

Ruoslahti, E., and Vaheri, A. (1974). *Nature (London)* **248**, 789–791.

Sadler, J. E., Paulson, J. C., and Hill, R. L. (1979). *J. Biol. Chem.* **254**, 2112–2119.

Saito, M., Toyoshima, S., and Osawa, T. (1977). *J. Biochem. (Tokyo)* **81**, 1203–1208.

Sakiyama, H., and Burge, B. W. (1972). *Biochemistry* **11**, 1366–1376.

Sanford, B. H. (1967). *Transplantation* **5**, 1272–1279.

Santer, U. V., and Glick, M. C. (1979). *Biochemistry* **18**, 2533–2540.

Santer, U. V., and Glick, M. C. (1980). *Biochem. Biophys. Res. Commun.* **96**, 219–226.

Schleicher, J. B. (1973). *In* "Tissue Culture: Methods and Applications" (P. F. Kruse and M. K. Patterson, eds), pp. 333–338. Academic Press, New York.

Schlom, J., Wunderlich, D., and Teramoto, Y. A. (1980) *Proc. Natl. Acad. Sci. U.S.A.* **77**, 6841–6845.

Schmidt-Ullrich, R., Knuffermann, H., and Wallach, D. F. H. (1973). *Biochim. Biophys. Acta* **307**, 353–365.

Segrest, J. P., Wilkinson, T. M., and Sheng, L. (1979). *Biochim. Biophys. Acta* **554**, 533–537.

Sheinin, R., and Onodera, K. (1972). *Biochim. Biophys. Acta* **274**, 49–63.

Sherblom, A. P., and Carraway, K. L. (1980). *J. Biol. Chem.* **255**, 12051–12059.

Sherblom, A. P., Buck, R. L., and Carraway, K. L. (1980). *J. Biol. Chem.* **255**, 783–790.

Shimada, A., and Nathenson, S. G. (1969). *Biochemistry* **8**, 4048–4062.

Shin, B. C., and Carraway, K. L. (1973). *Biochim. Biophys. Acta* **330**, 254–268.

Silverberg, M., and Marchesi, V. T. (1978). *J. Biol. Chem.* **253**, 95–98.

Simmons, R. L., and Rios, A. (1971). *Science* **174**, 591–593.

Simmons, R. L., and Rios, A. (1973). *J. Immunol.* **111**, 1820–1825.

Simpson, D. L., Hranisavljevic, J., and Davidson, E. A. (1972). *Biochemistry* **11**, 1849–1855.

Slayter, H. S., and Codington, J. F. (1973). *J. Biol. Chem.* **248**, 3405–3410.

Sloneker, J. H. (1972). *In* "Methods Carbohydrate Chemistry" (R. L. Whistler and J. N. BeMiller, eds.), Vol. 6, pp. 20–24.

Smart, J. E., and Hogg, N. (1976). Nature (*London*) **261**, 314–316.

Smets, L. A., VanBeek, W. P., and van Rooy, H. (1976). *Int. J. Cancer* **18**, 462–468.

Smith, D. F., and Ginsburg, V. (1980). *J. Biol. Chem.* **255**, 55–59.

Smith, D. F., Neri, G., and Walborg, Jr., E. F. (1973). *Biochemistry* **12**, 2111–2118.

Snyder, H. W., and Fleissner, E. (1980). *Proc. Natl. Acad. Sci. U.S.A.* **77**, 1622–1626.

Spiro, R. G. (1966a). *In* "Methods in Enzymology" (E. F. Neufeld and V. Ginsburg, eds.), Vol. 8, pp. 3–26. Academic Press, New York.

Spiro, R. G. (1966b). *In* "Methods in Enzymology" (E. F. Neufeld and V. Ginsburg, eds.), Vol. 8, pp. 26–52. Academic Press, New York.

Spiro, R. G. (1970). *Annu. Rev. Biochem.* **39**, 599–638.

Spiro, R. G. (1972). *In* "Methods in Enzymology" (V. Ginsburg, ed.), Vol. 28, pp. 3–43. Academic Press, New York.

Spiro, R. G. (1973). *Adv. Protein Chem.* **27**, 349–467.

Spiro, R. G., and Bhoyroo, V. D. (1974). *J. Biol. Chem.* **249**, 5704–5717.

Springer, G. F., and Desai P. R. (1975) *Carbohydr. Res.* **40**, 183–192.

Springer, G. F., Desai, P. R., and Scanlon, E. F. (1976). *Cancer* **37**, 169–172.

Steck, T. L., and Wallach, D. F. H. (1970). In "Methods in Cancer Research" (H. Busch ed.), Vol. 5, pp. 93–153. Academic Press, New York.

St. Groth, S. F, de, and Scheidegger, D. (1980). *J. Immunol. Methods* **35**, 1–21.

Strecker, G., Pierce-Gretel, A., Fournet, B., Spik, G., and Montreuil, J. (1981). *Analyt. Biochem.* **111**, 17–26.

Strnad, B. C., Schuster, T., Klen, R., and Neubauer, R. H. (1981). *Biochem. Biophys. Res. Commun.* **98**, 1121–1127.

Struck, D. K., and Lennarz, W. J. (1980). *In* "The Biochemistry of Glycoproteins and Proteoglycans (W. J. Lennarz, ed.), pp. 35–83. Plenum, New York.

Suzuki, S. (1972). *In* "Methods in Enzymology" (V. Ginsburg, ed.), Vol. 28, pp. 911–917. Academic Press, New York.

Tai, T., Yamashita, K., Ogata-Arakawa, M., Koide, N., Muramatsu, T., Iwashita, S., Inoue, Y., and Kobata, A. (1975). *J. Biol. Chem.* **250**, 8569–8575.

Takahashi, T., and Nishibe, H. (1978). *J. Biochem.* (*Tokyo*) **84**, 1467–1473.

Takahashi, T., and Nishibe, H. (1981). *Biochim. Biophys. Acta* **657**, 457–467.

Takasaki, S., and Kobata, A. (1974). *J. Biochem.* (*Tokyo*) **76**, 783–789.

Takasaki, S., and Kobata, A. (1976). *J. Biol. Chem.* **251**, 3603–3609.

Takasaki, S., Ikehira, H., and Kobata, A. (1980). *Biochem. Biophys. Res. Commun.* **92**, 735–742.

Tanner, M. J. A., and Gray, W. R. (1971). *Biochem. J.* **125**, 1109–1117.

Tarentino, A. L., Trimble, R. B., and Maley, F. (1978). *In* "Methods in Enzymology" (V. Ginsburg, ed.), Vol. 50, pp. 574–580. Academic Press, New York.

Teramoto, Y. A., Kute, D., and Schlom, S. (1977). *Proc. Natl. Acad. Sci. U.S.A.* **74**, 3564–3568.

Thom, D., Powell, A. J., Lloyd, C. W., and Rees, D. A. (1977). *Biochem. J.* **168**, 187–194.

Thomas, D. B., and Winzler, R. J. (1969). *J. Biol. Chem.* **244**, 5943–5946.

Tikhomirov, M. M., Khorlin, A. Ya., Voelter, W., and Bauer, H. (1978). *J. Chromatogr.* **167**, 197–203.

Troy, F. A., Fueyo, E. M., and Klein, G. (1977). *Proc. Natl. Acad. Sci. U.S.A.* **74**, 5270–5274.

Tsao, D., and Kim, Y. S. (1975). *J. Biol. Chem.* **253**, 2271–2278.

Tuszynski, G. P., Baker, S. R., Fuhrer, J. P., Buck, C. A., and Warren, L. (1978). *J. Biol. Chem.* **253**, 6092–6099.

Umemoto, J., Bhavanandan, V. P., and Davidson, E. A. (1977). *J. Biol. Chem.* **252**, 8609–8614.

Umemoto, J., Bhavanandan, V. P., and Davidson, E. A. (1981). *Biochim. Biophys. Acta,* in press.

Unkeless, J. C., Tobia, A., Ossowski, T., Quigley, J. P., Rifkin, D. P., and Reich, E. (1973). *J. Exp. Med.* **137**, 85–111.

Vaheri, A., and Ruoslahti, E. (1975). *J. Exp. Med.* **142**, 530–538.

Van den Eijnden, D. H., Codington, J. F., and Jeanloz, R. W. (1976). *Carbohydr. Res.* **52**, 209–213.

Van den Eijnden, D. H., Evans, N. A., Codington, J. F., Reinhold, V. N., Silber, C., and Jeanloz, R. W. (1979). *J. Biol. Chem.* **254**, 12153–12159.

Van Nest, G. A., and Grimes, W. J. (1977). *Biochemistry* **16**, 2902–2908.

Vischer, P., and Reuter, W. (1978). *Eur. J. Biochem.* **84**, 363–368.

Viza, D., and Phillips, J. (1975). *Int. J. Cancer* **16**, 312–317.

Vorbrodt, A., and Koprowski, H. (1969). *J. Natl. Cancer Inst.* **43**, 1241–1248.

Walborg, Jr., E. F., Lantz, R. S., and Wray, V. P. (1969). *Cancer Res.* **29**, 2034–2038.

Wallach, D. F. H. (1968). *Proc. Natl. Acad. Sci. U.S.A.* **61**, 868–874.

Warren, L. (1959). *J. Biol. Chem.* **234**, 1961–1975.

Warren, L. (1974). *In* "Methods in Enzymology" (S. Fleischer and L. Packer, eds.), Vol. 31, pp. 156–162. Academic Press, New York.

Warren, L., Glick, M. C., and Nass, M. K. (1966). *J. Cell. Physiol.* **68**, 269–287.

Warren, L., Critchley, D., and MacPherson, I. (1972a). *Nature (London)* **235**, 275–277.

Warren, L., Fuhrer, J. P., and Buck, C. A. (1972b). *Proc. Natl. Acad. Sci. U.S.A.* **69**, 1838–1842.

Warren, L., Fuhrer, J. F., Tuszynski, G. P., and Buck, C. A. (1974). *Biochem. Soc. Symp.* **40**, 147–157.

Warren, L., Zeidman, I., and Buck, C. A. (1975). *Cancer Res.* **35**, 2186–2190.

Warren, L., Buck, C. A., and Tuszynski, G. P. (1978). *Biochim. Biophys. Acta* **516**, 97–127.

Watanabe, K., Hakomori, S.-I., Powell, M. E., and Yokoto, M. (1980). *Biochem. Biophys. Res. Commun.* **92**, 638–646.

Weiss, L., Fisher, B., and Fisher, E. R. (1974). *Cancer* **34**, 680–683.

Wells, G. B., and Lester, R. L. (1979). *Analyt. Biochem.* **97**, 184–190.

Wennogle, L. P., and Berg, H. C. (1978). *J. Mol. Biol.* **124**, 689–699.

Wise, K. S., Allerton, S. E., Trump, G., Powars, D., and Beierle, J. W. (1975). *Int. J. Cancer* **16**, 199–210.

Wolfrom, M. L., and Franks, N. E. (1965). *In* "Methods in Carbohydrate Chemistry" (R. L. Whistler, ed.). Vol. 5, pp. 276–280. Academic Press, New York.

Woodbury, R. G., Brown, J. P., Yeh, M.-Y., Hellstrom, I., and Hellstrom, K. E. (1980). *Proc. Natl. Acad. Sci. U.S.A.* **77**, 2183–2187.

Wu, H. C., Meezan, E., Black, P. H., and Robbins, P. W. (1969). *Biochemistry* **8**, 2509–2517.

Yamada, K. M., and Weston, J. A. (1974). *Proc. Natl. Acad. Sci. U.S.A.* **71**, 3492–3496.

Yamada, K. M., and Pouyssegur, J. (1978). *Biochimie* **60**, 1221–1233.

Yamada, T., and Yamada, M. (1973). *Nature (London)* **244**, 297–299.

Yamashita, K., Ichishima, E., Arai, M., and Kobata, A., (1980). *Biochem. Biophys. Res. Commun.* **96**, 1335–1342.

Yang, J., Tang, R., and Nandi, S. (1977). *Biochem. Biophys. Res. Commun.* **76**, 1044–1050.

Yeh, M.-Y., Hellstrom, I., Brown, J. P., Warner, G. A., Hansen, J. A., and Hellstrom, K. E. (1979). *Proc. Natl. Acad. Sci. U.S.A.* **76**, 2927–2931.

Yogeeswaran, G., Stein, B. S., and Sebastian, H. (1978). *Cancer Res.* **38**, 1336–1344.

Yoshima, H., Furthmayr, H., and Kobata, A. (1980). *J. Biol. Chem.* **255**, 9713–9718.

Yosizawa, Z., Sato, T., and Schmid, K. (1966). *Biochim. Biophys. Acta* **121**, 417–420.

Yurchenco, P. D., Ceccarini, C., and Atkinson, P. H. (1978). *In* "Methods in Enzymology" (V. Ginsburg, ed.), Vol. 50, pp. 175–204. Academic Press, New York.

Zechel, K. (1977). *Analyt. Biochem.* **83**, 240–251.
Zopf, D. A., Ginsburg, A., and Ginsburg, V. (1975). *J. Immunol.* **115**, 1525–1529.
Zopf, D. A., Tsai, C.-M. and Ginsburg, V. (1978). *Arch. Biochem. Biophys.* **185**, 61–71.
Zwaal, R. F. A. and van Deenen, L. L. M. (1968). *Biochim. Biophys. Acta* **163**, 44–49.

ANTIGEN MARKERS OF TUMOR CELLS AND NUCLEI

CHAPTER III

NUCLEOLAR ANTIGENS OF HUMAN TUMORS

HARRIS BUSCH, ROSE K. BUSCH, PUI-KWONG CHAN, DAVID KELSEY, AND KEI TAKAHASHI

I. Introduction

The nucleolar antigens have recently become of increased interest because of the possibility that they may reflect unique functions in human
cancer cells and because of their potential immunodiagnostic use. This
chapter presents a general review of the approaches taken toward the
evaluation, identification, isolation, and functional analysis of the nucleolar antigens of human cancer cells.

II. Nucleolar Antigens

Two general types of antinucleolar antibodies are of interest, namely,
the autoantibodies formed in various disease states and the antibodies induced by immunization of experimental animals with whole nucleoli or
specific nucleolar fractions (Tan, 1979; H. Busch *et al.*, 1979). Antinucleolar
antibodies along with a variety of other antinuclear antibodies arise in
human autoimmune diseases, such as Sjogren's syndrome, lupus erythe-
matosus, mixed connective disease, and other autoimmune states including rheumatoid arthritis. These antibodies are directed against a variety of
macromolecules including DNA, histones, nonhistone proteins, RNA,
and other nuclear elements. There are many mysterious features of these
autoimmune diseases including the number and types of antibodies elicited, their specificity and binding constants, and their potential destruc-
tive effects which are not well understood, either in terms of pathology or
relation to the disease.

In the experimentally produced antibodies directed against specific nucleolar products, the complexities of the antibodies produced increases
with the duration of the immunization program as well as the complexity
of the antigens. In two instances, involving tumors, i.e., with the Novikoff rat hepatoma and human HeLa and Namalwa tumors, specific nu-

cleolar antigens have been purified and have been found to be proteins (at least in part) (Chan *et al.*, 1980). These purified protein immunogens probably differ from the DNA–protein complexes utilized by Hnilica and his associates (Hnilica *et al.*, 1978) in their studies on DNP–specific antigens of a variety of tissues and tumors.

The initial goal of our experimental studies on nucleolar antigens was to define conditions that might permit an analysis of very minute amounts of proteins important to nucleolar functions, some of which could be "promoters" for rDNA. Surprisingly, the results obtained with these studies became of particular interest for possible differentiation of human cancer cells and other cells; this point will be discussed below in more detail.

A. EXPERIMENTAL PRODUCTION OF ANTINUCLEOLAR ANTIBODIES

To determine whether nucleoli or their subfractions could induce immunological responses in rabbits, nucleoli were prepared by standard procedures developed in earlier studies in this laboratory (Busch and Smetana, 1970) and injected into rabbits in Freund's adjuvant (Busch *et al.*, 1974). The sites of injection were initially subcutaneous and intramuscular but in later studies injection into footpads was found to be particularly useful. The initial testing for the immunological response was by the direct immunofluorescence assays of Hilgers *et al.* (1972). Ouchterlony gel analysis and immunoelectrophoresis were employed to determine whether precipitating antibodies were produced (Busch and Busch, 1977) In the initial studies (Busch *et al.*, 1974), complement fixation was used but this procedure was not utilized in the later more definitive studies.

B. TISSUES EMPLOYED AND IMMUNOFLUORESCENT MICROSCOPY

In the initial studies, nucleoli from the Novikoff hepatoma cells and normal rat liver cells were employed as the immunogens. In both cases, the rabbits produced remarkably specific antisera which either specifically reacted with the nucleoli and exhibited only comparatively minor extranucleolar reactions (Busch *et al.*, 1974). When these antisera were not absorbed with other tissues, cross reactions were found so that the antiliver nucleolar antisera produced indirect immunofluorescence in the Novikoff hepatoma cells and the antihepatoma nucleolar antisera also produced immunofluorescence in the liver cells (Fig. 1). In addition to these cross reactions, these antisera also produced positive immunofluorescence in the normal kidney and in Walker tumor cells (Fig. 2).

Complement fixation studies indicated that as with most self-antigens

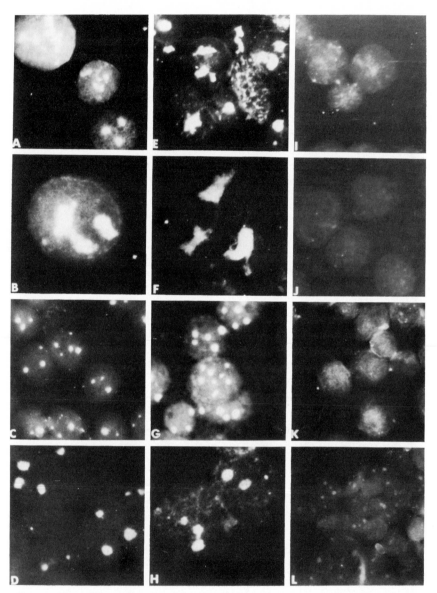

Fig. 1. Photomicrographs of nuclei analyzed with antisera or normal sera by the indirect immunofluorescent technique. Tumor antinucleolar antisera were incubated with Novikoff hepatoma nuclei (A, × 1800; B, × 4500) and liver nuclei (C, × 1800; D, × 4500). Liver antinucleolar antisera were incubated with Novikoff hepatoma nuclei (E, × 1800: F, × 4500) and liver nuclei (G, × 1800; H, × 4500). Normal rabbit sera were incubated with Novikoff hepatoma nuclei (I, × 1800) and liver nuclei (J, × 1800). Tumor antinucleolar antiserum absorbed with Novikoff tumor nucleoli was incubated with Novikoff nuclei (K, × 1800), and liver antinucleolar antiserum absorbed with liver nucleoli was incubated with liver nuclei (L, × 1800). (From Busch *et al.*, 1974.)

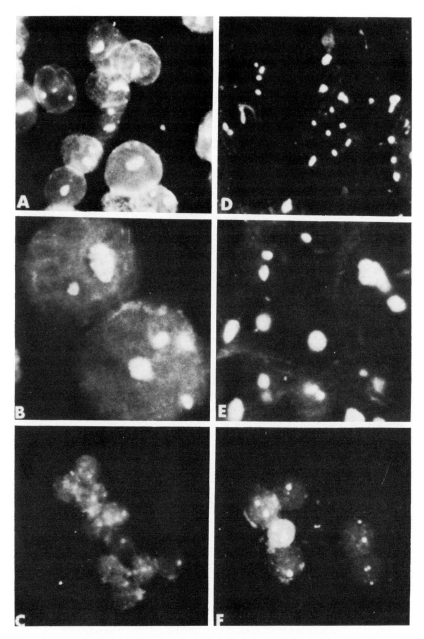

Fig. 2. Photomicrographs of nuclei analyzed with antisera by the indirect immuno-fluorescent technique. Novikoff hepatoma antinucleolar antisera were incubated with Walker nuclei (A, × 1800; B, × 4500) and kidney nuclei (C, × 1800). Liver nucleolar antisera were incubated with Walker nuclei (D, × 1800; E, × 4500) and kidney nuclei (F, × 1800). (From Busch et al., 1974.)

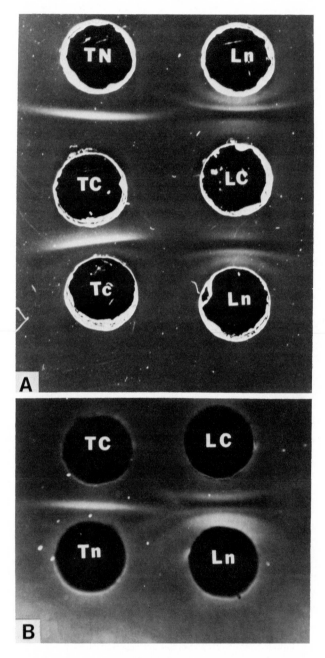

FIG. 3. (A) Immunodiffusion plate which contains a 0.6 *M* NaCl extract of tumor nuclear chromatin TCAg in the left center well and liver chromatin LCAg in the right center well (300–400 gm) as antigens. The TCAg formed precipitin bands with tumor nuclear (TNAb)

the titers of the antisera were not high, i.e., activity was noted up to dilutions of 1:160. Initial absorption studies indicated that there was little loss of complement fixation activity following absorption of liver antinucleolar antiserum with the tumor proteins but there was a greater loss following treatment of tumor antisera with the liver proteins. Generally, the titers for complement fixation were not remarkably reduced by single absorptions. In further studies, absorbed antisera were used.

C. Tumor Specificity

Ouchterlony gel analysis was used to evaluate the similarity and difference in the immunoprecipitin bands formed between the tumor and liver nucleolar antigens and their corresponding antibodies (Busch and Busch, 1977). This study was initially designed to determine whether there were antigenic differences in proteins of various fractions extracted from the nucleoli of these cells with different extractants. However, a striking finding obtained was that there were nucleolar antigens in the Novikoff tumor (Fig. 3) that were not present in the liver and vice versa. When the liver nucleolar antigens were reacted with the antiliver antibodies, three immunoprecipitin bands were formed. When the antitumor nucleolar antibodies were reacted with the tumor nucleolar antigens, a single, dense immunoprecipitin band was formed. Both findings were striking. No evidence was obtained for cross reactivity of these tumor and liver antigens.

It seemed likely that if the immunizations were continued for a longer period, more antibodies would be formed. This result was demonstrated by immunoelectrophoresis (Fig. 4) which showed that up to 14 antigens were detectable in nucleoli of Novikoff hepatoma ascites cells (Davis *et al.*, 1978). The antisera to normal liver nucleoli detected 10 of the 14 antigens detected by the anti-Novikoff hepatoma nucleolar antiserum. Moreover, in analysis of fetal tissues, particularly fetal liver, it was found that there were antigens common to the tumor and fetal liver that were not present in the adult liver. This finding supported the earlier result of Yeoman *et al.* (1976) that there are fetal nuclear antigens in tumors that are

---

and tumor chromatin (TcAb) antibodies. The LCAg antigen formed at least three precipitin bands with the liver nucleolar (LnAn) antibodies. The antibody wells contained 33 μl. (B) Immunodiffusion plate which contains 0.6 *M* NaCl extracts of tumor nuclear chromatin TCAg in the top left well and liver nuclear chromatin LNAg in the top right well (300–400 μg). The tumor chromatin antigen formed a precipitin band with the tumor nucleolar antiserum (TnAb). The LCAg antigen formed at least three precipitin bands with the liver nucleolar antibodies (LnAb). The antibody wells contain 33 μl. (From Busch and Busch, 1977.)

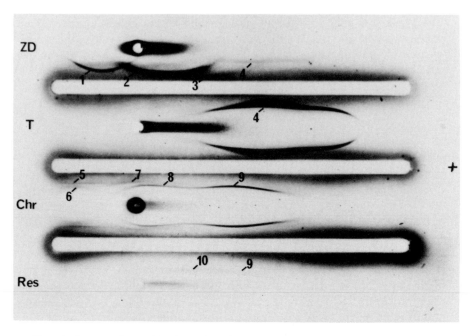

FIG. 4. Immunoelectrophoretic profile of tumor nucleolar antigens. The Zubay–Doty (ZD), low-ionic-strength Tris (T), 0.6 M NaCl/5 M urea extract (Res) of Novikoff hepatoma nucleoli were analyzed by immunoelectrophoresis. The immunoelectrophoresis slide was presoaked in running buffer for 2 hours. ZD (20 μg) and 40 μg of the other antigens were placed in the antigen wells. After electrophoresis at 100 V for 30 minutes, 50 μl of antitumor nucleolar immunoglobulin at 80 mg protein per ml was placed in the antiserum troughs, and the precipitin arcs that formed in 24 hours were stained with Coomassie Brilliant Blue. (From Davis et al., 1978.)

not present in normal adult tissues. Results of this type for cytoplasmic enzymes, serum proteins, and a variety of "oncofetal" and "oncoembryonic" antigens have been reported on in great detail in other systems (Fishman and Busch, 1979).

D. ADSORPTION OF THE ANTIBODIES

Although the results of immunoelectrophoresis provided some evidence for distinctive antigens in the Novikoff hepatoma and normal and fetal liver, an impressive distinction occurred after absorption of the antisera with extracts of nucleoli and nuclei of both tissues. As indicated in Fig. 5, bright nucleolar fluorescence was observed in the Novikoff hepatoma cells after absorption of the antiserum with normal liver nuclear products. However, the absorbed antiserum did not produce nucleolar fluorescence in the normal liver nucleoli. The corresponding result was obtained with antisera to normal liver nucleoli, i.e., when the antisera had been absorbed with Novikoff hepatoma nuclear products to the point that no nucleolar fluorescence was evident, they still produced immunofluorescence in the normal liver nucleoli (Davis *et al.*, 1979).

Taken together, all these studies with antinucleolar antisera whether by immunoprecipitin band analysis, analysis of immunoelectrophoresis patterns, or evaluation of the results of absorption by immunofluorescence indicated that antigens in the nucleoli of Novikoff hepatomas differed from those of normal liver nucleoli and vice versa.

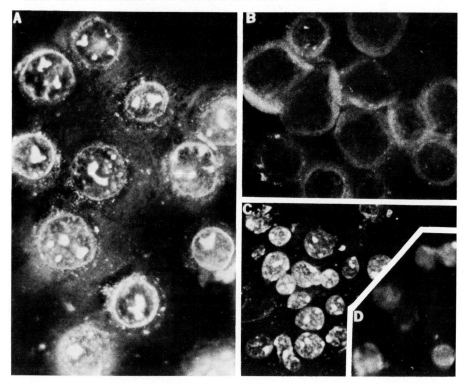

FIG. 5. Photomicrographs of cells tested with preabsorbed antinucleolar antisera by indirect immunofluorescent technique. Preabsorbed antitumor nucleolar antiserum was incubated with Novikoff hepatoma cells (A) or with normal liver cells (D). Preabsorbed antiliver nucleolar antiserum was incubated with Novikoff hepatoma cells (B) or with normal liver cells (C). All photomicrographs, × 1800. (From Davis *et al.*, 1978.)

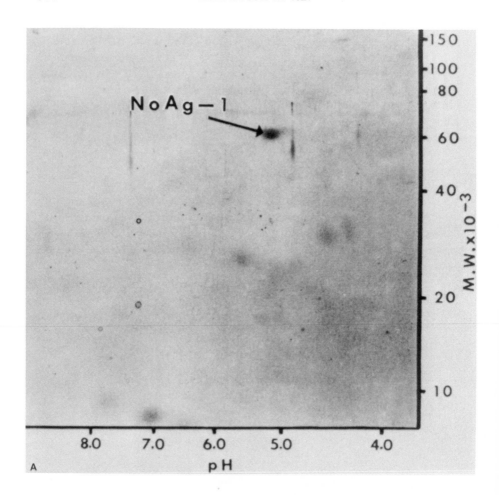

FIG. 6. (A) Two-dimensional gel electrophoresis of NoAg-1, the tumor antigen. NoAg-1 (10 μg) was added to lyophilized sample buffer [9 M urea/2% ampholines (3/10 Bio-lyte)/2 M dithiothreitol] and subjected to two-dimensional electrophoresis (Marashi et al., 1979). (B) Rocket immunoelectrophoresis of NoAg-1 from the SDS–polyacrylamide slab gel. A 1-cm² area containing the single NoAg-1 spot from SDS–polyacrylamide slab gel was placed on a blank agarose gel and electrophoresed into antibody-containing agarose gel containing anti-nucleolar antiserum (1.0 mg/ml). A strip of agarose gel containing 1.5% Triton X-100 was placed between the blank and antibody containing agarose gel to trap SDS and release NoAg-1 (Marashi et al., 1979.)

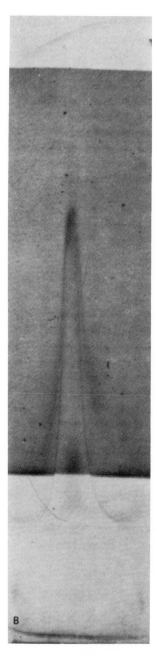

FIG. 6B.

E. What Are These Tumor Nucleolar Antigens?

To advance the studies on these antigens, it was essential to purify one of the antigens to homogeneity. For this purpose, the nucleoli were isolated from the Novikoff hepatoma and subjected to a series of extractions generally employed for chromatin (Rothblum *et al.*, 1977). In the first of these steps, the nucleoli were extracted with an approximately isotonic extractant (0.075 *M* NaCl/0.025 *M* EDTA/pH 8) designed to remove divalent ions important to the maintenance of the nucleolar ultrastructure. The nucleoli were then exposed to buffers of very low ionic strength (0.01 *M* Tris–HCl/pH 7.8) designed to permit the chromatin to swell and to release nuclear particles entrapped in the chromatin. In addition, a number of nucleolar components such as RNA polymerases and kinases are apparently soluble in this low ionic strength buffer but are not soluble in isotonic buffers. In subsequent extraction procedures, a variety of salt solutions of higher ionic strengths, e.g., 0.35, 0.6, and 1.0 *M* NaCl were successively used as extractants. Finally the nucleoli were extracted with 3 *M* NaCl/7 *M* urea. Although this last solution does not completely solubilize all the nucleolar elements, the residue fraction was very small (Rothblum *et al.*, 1977; Marashi *et al.*, 1979).

In the studies on the major antigens of the Novikoff rat hepatoma nucleoli, it was found that the majority of the antigen (more than 50%) was not extracted with either the isotonic buffer or the low ionic strength buffers employed but rather with the 0.6 *M* NaCl extract which followed these initial extraction steps (Marashi *et al.*, 1979). The antibodies to these antigens were used for the preparation of affinity columns for binding the antigen. Further purification of the antigen was accomplished by elution with putrescine at pH 11. Because there were small contaminants in some of the samples, hydroxylapatite chromatography was used for final purification. Under these conditions, a Coomassie Blue stained gel (Fig. 6A) showed that only a single protein was present which had a molecular weight of approximately 60,000 an an isoelectric point of approximately 5.0 (Marashi *et al.*, 1979).

This result represented the first purification of a specific nucleolar antigen from a tumor. To prove that the antigen was indeed in this spot, it was excised from the two-dimensional gel and "rocket" electrophoresis was done. A distinctive "rocket" (Fig. 6B) was produced which demonstrated the presence of the antigen in this sample (Marashi *et al.*, 1979). In view of these potentially important results with human tumor nucleoli, it will be of interest to determine what if any similarities existed between the 60,000 MW antigen of the Novikoff hepatoma cells and the 68,000 MW antigen of the human tumors (Chan *et al.*, 1981) which is discussed below.

Their overall similarities in positioning of the spot on two-dimensional gel electrophoresis suggest that they may have some similarities, despite the apparent difference in antigenic determinants.

F. Liver Nucleolar Antigens

The antigens in normal liver nucleoli differ from those of Novikoff hepatoma nucleoli. Abelev *et al.* (1979) had reported earlier that there are liver-specific antigens but none has been characterized. In the nucleus of rat liver, a protein (MW 20,000) was found that was reported to be liver-specific. In studies of R. K. Busch *et al.*, (1979) on the liver nuclear antigens, three nucleolar antigens were found in the liver; two of these were not present in the Novikoff hepatoma (Fig. 7).

One liver antigen-1 (Ln-1) was not found in any tissue other than liver; but in kidney, an antigen was present that formed an overlapping band. However, this antigen did not exhibit identity to the liver antigen. Of the total antigen Ln-1, 99% was present in the cytosol and only 1% was found in the nucleus. Of this, approximately 10% was in the chromatin from which it was extracted with 0.6 M NaCl.

When purified by absorption on affinity columns and eluted with 0.2 M Tris–HCl/0.05 M NaCl/pH 11, the antigens contained three RNA bands. These bands were all rich in guanylic and cytidylic acids and had approximate molecular weights of 200,000 (ca. 600 nucleotides). These antigens could then fall into the category of small nuclear ribonucleoprotein particles (snRNPs). The functions of the RNA or the snRNPs are not defined.

The antigen Ln-2 was found in several tissues, including spleen, Novikoff hepatoma, normal liver, and regenerating liver. However, it was not found in kidney or rat serum. Antigen Ln-3, like antigen Ln-1, was found in the normal and regenerating rat liver but it was not present in the other tissues studied. Further characterization of these antigens, their associated RNA species and definition of their nucleolar and cellular functions will certainly be of much interest in the future.

G. mRNA for Nucleolar Antigens

To determine whether the polysomes and the mRNA for synthesis of the nucleolar antigens were unique to the tumors, the antibodies to the Novikoff hepatoma nucleolar proteins were first purified by absorption with liver nucleolar proteins (Davis *et al.*, 1978). They were then subjected to affinity chromatography on Sepharose-4B columns containing normal rat liver proteins to remove the antibodies that were nonspecifi-

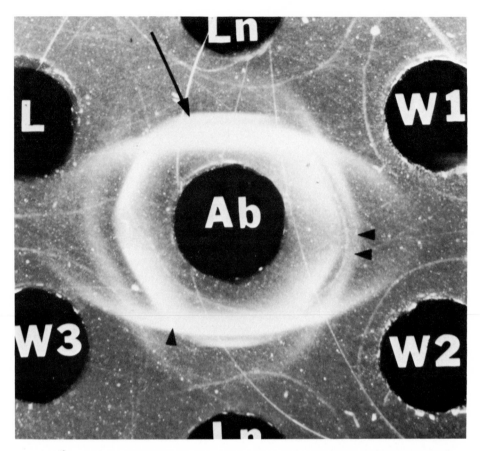

FIG. 7. Immunodiffusion plate with Ig from antiserum to liver nucleoli in the center well. The following antigens were in the outer wells: (Ln) the 0.15 M NaCl extract of liver nucleoli; the supernatants from the three consecutive 0.15 M NaCl extracts of liver pressate designated (w1), (w2), and (w3); the 0.15 M NaCl extract (1 hour) of the "washed" liver pressate (L). The following immunprecipitin bands formed between the nucleolar antibodies (Ab) and the antigens: Ln-1 (arrow) with antigens w1, w2, w3, L, and Ln; Ln-2 (arrowhead) with antigen Ln; and Ln-3 (double arrowheads) with antigens w1, w2, w3, and L. Extraction of liver pressate with 0.15 M NaCl readily solubilized antigens Ln-1 and Ln-3. (From R. K. Busch *et al.*, 1979.)

cally absorbed to such proteins. The IgG which did not bind to the liver Sepharose column after 12 hours of incubation at 4°C was then applied to a column containing Novikoff hepatoma nucleolar proteins. The IgG which did not bind was discarded and the bound IgG was eluted with 1 M NaCl/3 M urea/0.2 M Tris–HCl/pH 7.5 and dialyzed. These IgG fractions (which constituted only 1–2% of the total IgG) were then labeled with [125]I.

The first finding obtained (Fig. 8) was that the antibodies bound readily with a sharply defined plateau to the polysomes of the Novikoff hepatoma cells but not at all to the polysomes of the normal liver cells (Reiners *et al.*, 1980). Binding of the labeled antibodies to the regenerating liver polysomes was about one-third that of the Novikoff hepatoma. Competition studies (Fig. 9) showed that the tumor nucleolar and nuclear extracts effectively competed with the antibody binding to the polysomes but the normal liver nuclear and nucleolar extracts did not. These studies demonstrated a high order of specificity of the interactions of the antinucleolar antibody and IgG fractions with the tumor polysomes and the tumor products from nucleoli and nuclei (Reiners *et al.*, 1980).

The binding of the antibody to the polysomes was dependent upon Mg^{2+} and was inhibited almost completely by puromycin but only partially by RNase indicating that the interactions were protein–protein interactions rather than protein–RNA interactions. Some cross reactivity occurred with the fetal liver nuclear extracts which supports the idea that

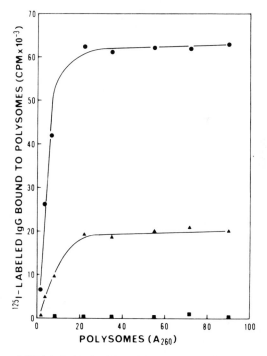

FIG. 8. Titration of ^{125}I-labeled IgG with variable amounts of polysomes. Iodinated absorbed affinity chromatography-purified antitumor nucleolar IgG (2.5×10^5 cpm) was incubated with tumor (●), regenerating liver (▲), and normal liver (■) polysomes. Over the range of polysomes titered, 5800 to 6600 cpm were precipitated in the absence of Mg^{2+} and were subtracted from the values for sedimented polysome–IgG complexes. (From Reiners *et al.*, 1980.)

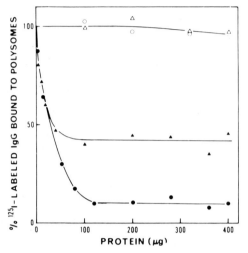

FIG. 9. Competition by nuclear and nucleolar extracts with tumor polysomes for ^{125}I-labeled antitumor IgG. Competition by extracts with 20 A_{260} units of tumor polysomes for iodinated absorbed affinity chromatography-purified antitumor nucleolar IgG (2.5 × 10^5 cpm) was performed. ●, Tumor nuclear extract; ▲, nucleolar 0.075 M NaCl/0.025 M EDTA extract; ○, normal rat liver extract; △, nucleolar 0.075 M NaCl/0.025 M EDTA extract. One hundred percent precipitation is represented by 71,000 cpm. Data are uncorrected for the 6500 cpm (9% maximum) sedimented in the absence of Mg^{2+}. (From Reiners *et al.*, 1980.)

some of the antigens are "oncofetal" or "oncoembryonic" as noted in earlier studies of Yeoman *et al.* (1976) and Davis *et al.* (1978).

H. NUCLEOLAR ANTIGENS IN HUMAN TUMORS

Although the studies on the nucleolar antigens of the rodent tumors and nontumor tissues indicated that there might be important differences in these nucleolar proteins, initial attempts to extend these studies to human neoplasms met with the problem that human tumor nucleoli did not exhibit bright fluorescence when treated with antibodies to rat tumor nucleoli. After preliminary studies showed that these antibodies did not

FIG. 10. Bright nucleolar fluorescence in a series of squamous cell carcinomas and adenocarcinomas. The antibody concentration was 0.3 to 0.5 mg/ml. (a) Squamous cell carcinoma, skin. × 160. (b) Squamous cell carcinoma, lung. × 400. (c) Squamous cell carcinoma, metastatic to muscle. × 630. (d) Squamous cell carcinoma, esophagus. × 400. (e) Squamous cell carcinoma, metastatic to muscle. × 400. (f) Higher power squamous cell carcinoma, lung. × 630. (g) Adenocarcinoma, prostate. × 160. (h) Adenocarcinoma, lung. × 400. (i) Adenocarcinoma, lung (high power). × 630. Arrows, positive fluorescent nucleoli; arrowheads, negative region in adjacent tissue. (From H. Busch *et al.*, 1979.)

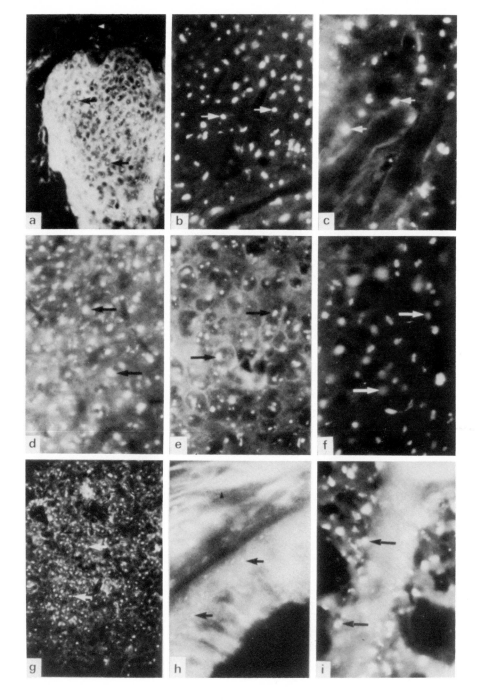

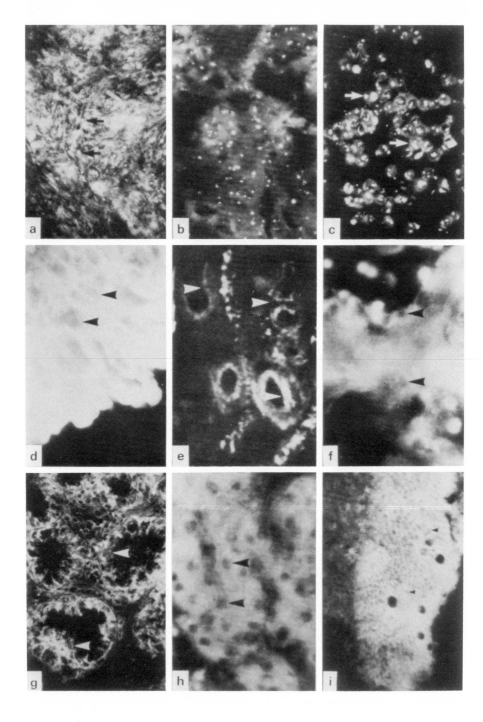

produce corresponding immunoreactivity with nucleolar antigens of human tumor specimens, nucleolar preparations and nuclear Tris extracts (0.01 M Tris–HCl/pH 8.0) of human HeLa cells were used as immunogens. Happily, the immunized rabbits developed antihuman tumor nucleolar antibodies and more definitive studies on human tumor nucleolar antigens were done (Davis *et al.*, 1979; H. Busch *et al.*, 1979).

As shown in Figs. 10 and 11, a broad array of human malignant tumors contains nucleolar antigens recognizable by bright nucleolar fluorescence (H. Busch *et al.*, 1979). These tumors include (Table I) carcinomas of many types, a variety of sarcomas, and many hematological neoplasms. To discriminate the nucleolar fluorescence of the tumors from that found in other tissues, such as placenta, it was clear that extensive absorption of nontumor antibodies from the antisera, Ig, or IgG fractions was necessary. First, because the HeLa cells initially used were grown in fetal calf serum, fetal calf serum was an essential absorbent. Second, since most human normal tissues were not widely available for isolation, a source of nuclei or nuclear products was necessary. Inasmuch as placentas are discarded and are a good source of nuclei, they were utilized as a source of nuclear extracts for absorption (Davis *et al.*, 1979; H. Busch *et al.*, 1979). In addition, normal human serum contains some minor cross reactive elements so that absorption was done with serum proteins or whole serum.

Although it would be highly desirable to have a precipitating antibody of the type found with the anti-Novikoff hepatoma antibodies, such precipitins have not yet been found with human tissues despite the use of multiple rabbits, sheep, and goats. It appears that the antigenic determinants of human nucleolar antigens differ from those of the rodent but as yet, no specific information is available on either the amino acid or other determinants in either of these types of antigens.

I. Antibodies to Other Tumors

For comparative purposes, two malignant tumors other than HeLa cells were used as sources of the antigen. The Namalwa cell line is a derivative of a Burkitt tumor provided to us by the National Cancer Institute and the

---

Fig. 11. Bright nucleolar immunofluorescence in a number of tumors and lack of nucleolar fluorescence in a number of nontumorous tissues. (a) Brain, glioblastoma. × 160. (b) Adenocarcinoma of stomach, liver metastasis. × 400. (c) HeLa cells, S3, culture, × 400. (d) Bronchial epithelium, newborn. × 400. (e) Bronchial glands × 400. (f) Thyroid adenoma, × 630. (g) Intestinal crypts. × 400. (h) Adenoma, parathyroid. (i) Gastric epithelium (hyperplastic) × 160. Arrows, positive fluorescent nucleoli, arrowheads, negative nucleus or negative regions in cells. (From H. Busch *et al.*, 1979.)

TABLE I

BRIGHT NUCLEOLAR FLUORESCENCE IN HUMAN MALIGNANT TUMOR SPECIMENS

I. Carcinomas
  1. Lung
    Adenocarcinoma (3)
    Oat cell (4)
    Squamous cell (22)
  2. Gastrointestinal
    Oral cavity (8)
    Pharynx (4)
    Esophagus, squamous cell (5)
    Stomach, adenocarcinoma (5)
      Metastasis: liver
      Metastasis: liver node
    Colon, adenocarcinoma (9)
      Metastasis: liver (2)
    Transplantable carcinoma
    (GW-39)
    Liver, primary carcinoma (3)
    Pancreas (4)
  3. Genitourinary
    Kidney (4)
    Prostate, adenocarcinoma (22)
    Bladder (4)
  4. CNS
    Glioblastoma (1)
    Astrocytoma (5)
  5. Endocrine
    Breast (3)
    Cervix (4)
    Parathyroid (1)
    Thyroid (5)
  6. Skin
    Basal cell (8)
    Eccrine gland (1)
    Squamous cell (7)
      Metastasis: lymph node
    Melanoma, malignant (4)
      Cerebral metastasis (1)
    Sweat gland (3)

II. Sarcomas
  1. Chondrosarcoma (1)
  2. Fibrosarcoma (4)
  3. Giant cell tumor (1)
  4. Granulocytic myoblastoma (2)
  5. Leimyosarcoma (4)
  6. Lymphoma (10)
  7. Meningiosarcoma (1)
  8. Myoblastoma (2)
  9. Osteogenic (6)
  10. Pulmonary blastoma (1)
  11. Reticulum cell sarcoma (1)
  12. Synovial sarcoma (1)

III. Hematological neoplasms
  1. Acute lymphocytic leukemia (2)
  2. Acute myelocytic leukemia (7)
  3. Acute monocytic leukemia (2)
  4. Chronic myelocytic leukemia (5)
  5. Hodkins disease (9)
  6. Leukemia: CLL (12), hairy cell (1)
  7. Mycosis fungoides
  8. Plasmacytomas (7)

Frederick Cancer Research Center through the generosity of Drs. V. De-Vita, J. Douros, and Mr. Fred Klein. A human prostate carcinoma grown in tissue culture was used by Dr. F. Gyorkey and Mrs. P. Gyorkey. Both of these tumors contain nucleolar antigens as demonstrated by production of antinucleolar antibodies with similar titers and specificities in rabbits. With the prostatic carcinoma, a nucleolar preparation was used for immunization and a Tris extract of nuclei of the Namalwa cells was used as the immunogen. The similarity of the results obtained suggested that there were common antigens in these cells and the HeLa cells.

J. ARE THE TUMOR NUCLEOLAR ANTIGENS PRESENT IN NONTUMOR TISSUES?

It is a logical question to ask whether antigens of the types found reflect a neoplastic process or a normal process involved in growth, cell division or other normal physiological effect. Our theory of carcinogenesis (Busch, 1976) pointed out that cancer is probably the resultant of misapplication of normal gene readouts as a dysplastic phenomenon involving fetal genes rather than a process which involves "totally new" events, such as integration of a viral genome or other gene aberration. Accordingly, a search has been made for the antigens in a variety of normal, growing, and fetal tissues. As noted in Table II, the nucleolar antigens were not found in a broad array of nontumor tissues which presumably have exhibited slow growth or none at all.

An important question was whether the nucleolar antigens were present in normal growing nontumor tissues. In studies on bone marrow, skin Malpigian layers, and intestinal epithelium, the nucleolar antigens were not found. In studies on bone marrow of patients with leukemias, the neoplastic cells contained the antigens but their nontumor counterparts in the same maturation series did not contain the antigens (Smetana et al., 1979). As controls for the nontumor tissues, studies were made on cells of patients with acute infectious mononucleosis and lymphoid hyperplasia but neither exhibited bright nucleolar fluorescence under the circumstances of these studies. These results, like those indicated above, suggested that immunological analysis of whole cells, cell suspensions, or cell sections for the nucleolar antigen could be useful for immunodiagnosis of malignant disease.

In extending the studies to various types of tissues, fetal tissues were studied, partly because in earlier studies nucleolar fetal antigens were found to be expressed in the Novikoff hepatoma (Davis et al., 1978; Yeoman et al., 1976) and also because there may be important conclusions if

TABLE II
NEGATIVE NUCLEOLAR FLUORESCENCE IN HUMAN TISSUES

I. Normal tissue
  1. Lung
  2. Gastrointestinal
      Stomach
      Intestine
      Small, crypts of Lieberkuhn
      Large
      Liver
      Pancreas
  3. Genital urinary
      Kidney
      Bladder
      Prostate
  4. Endocrine
      Thyroid
      Breast
      Placenta
  5. Skin
II. Hematologic
  1. Bone marrow
  2. Lymph nodes
      Lymphocytes
      Hyperplastic lymph nodes
  3. Benign growing tissues
      Thyroid, goiter
      Prostate, hyperplastic
III. Inflammatory diseases
  1. Chronic ulcerative colitis
  2. Glomerulonephritis
  3. Granuloma and fibrosis of lung
  4. Liver: cirrhosis, hepatitis
  5. Lupus profundus (mammary gland and skin)
  6. Pemphigus: bullous
  7. Ulcer, gastric

the neoplastic cells contained functional fetal antigens (Busch, 1976). Initially, in more mature fetal tissues, such as 9-month fetal lung or 6-month fetal liver, no evidence was found for bright nucleolar fluorescence. However, examination of the IMR-90 and WI-38 diploid fetal fibroblast lines in tissue culture indicated that they exhibited brightly positive nucleolar fluorescence (H. Busch *et al.*, 1979). Such studies, along with evidence to be presented in the section on staining of gels, indicated that the nucleolar antigens in the malignant tumors might reflect activation of the fetal genes which could be important in the overall neoplastic process (H. Busch *et al.*, 1979; Busch, 1976).

K. Breast Cancer

Because of the need for a "preliminary" evaluation of the possible diagnostic use of the fluorescence assay for the human tumor antigens, it was important to find a series of a particular tumor type that would lend itself to a "blind" evaluation. It was fortunate that at the Michigan Cancer Foundation, a prospective study on human breast cancer is in progress. As part of this study, a large series of patients with breast cancer are being analyzed for relationships between the pathology of the neoplasm and the course of the disease (Busch *et al.*, 1981). Sections of normal breast tissue as well as benign and malignant tumors were analyzed for bright nucleolar fluorescence by the indirect immunofluorescence technique. These investigations were all approved by the Human Research Committee of Baylor College of Medicine and the Committee for Protection of Human Subjects of the Michigan Cancer Foundation.

The cryostat sections of the human tumors were kept at $-20°C$; they were cut at 2 μm and fixed for 12 minutes in acetone at 4°C. The tumors were evaluated histopathologically by a panel of five pathologists who provided a consensus diagnosis, designation of tumor grade, and other characteristics on the basis of H and E staining. The specimens were treated with either Ig or IgG fractions prepared from antisera absorbed with human placental nuclear extracts, fetal bovine serum, and human serum.

Before the "blind" study was initiated, known samples of breast carcinomas were examined. In 19 of 20 of these, bright nucleolar fluorescence was found to be either distributed throughout the sections or in a few instances in cell masses in particular portions of the sections. The 95% positive result for nucleolar fluorescence was similar to the first result (H. Busch *et al.*, 1979) in which 81 of 84 samples (96%) were positive in the variety of malignant tumors.

Figure 12 presents some micrographs of bright nucleolar fluorescence in the breast carcinomas. In some cases, the whole specimen consisted of cells with irregular, large brightly fluorescent nucleoli (Busch *et al.*, 1981). In others, the neoplastic cells were either in focal lesions or randomly distributed and in some, chords of tumor cells were distributed throughout the specimens. The background fluorescence ranged from negligible to moderately intense (Fig. 12).

In some sections, the neoplastic cells were confined to small areas or were not visible. In some "false negatives," the antibodies did not penetrate the cells either as a result of sample thickness, proteolysis, or "waxy deposits." In other instances, the region containing the tumor cells was lost or only at the periphery of the specimen. To avoid such problems,

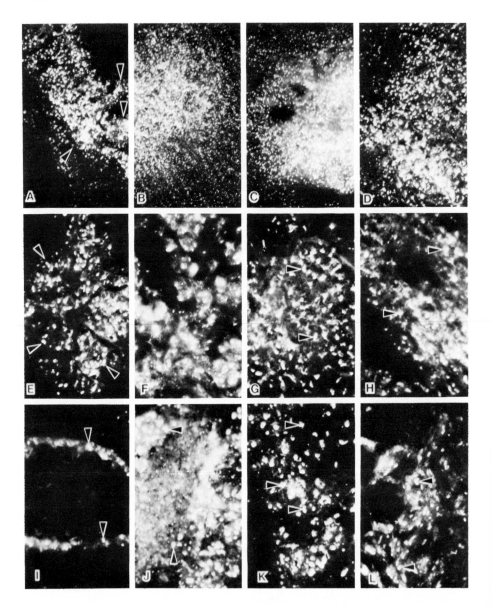

FIG. 12. (A–D) Low power (160×) views of bright nucleolar fluorescence in breast carcinomas illustrating clustering of cells, extensions from masses (A—pointers) and variable
densities within masses. (E–H) High power views of bright nucleolar fluorescence of fields
within breast carcinomas showing abortive pseudolobular formations (E,F) and nucleolar
irregularity (G,H). ×400. (I–L) Ductule in a carcinoma (I), two sizes of brightly fluorescent
nucleoli (J), large nucleoli (K), and irregular nucleoli (L). Pointers—brightly fluorescent nucleoli. ×400.

examination of several slides from a single specimen was necessary to sharply define the area of the neoplastic cells.

L. Normal Breast Tissue and Benign Tumors

In the normal breast tissue, utilizing the same antibodies that were used in the studies on the known carcinomas, there were no visible brightly fluorescent nucleoli. In some sections, there were "minispots" which were either intraluminal or in extracellular spaces. The antinucleolar antibodies apparently were nonspecifically absorbed by basement membrane elements inasmuch as fluorescent boundaries were occasionally visible around the terminal ducts either as a thin or thick limiting membrane or both (Fig. 13).

In the benign tumors, the results were very similar to those observed in the normal breast tissues. The lining membranes were larger and less regular than those observed with the normal breast tissues. In all cases, such "limiting membranes" were visible. In a few instances, fluorescent "spots" were observable in the benign tumors, usually in small confined areas but occasionally in larger areas. Whether the antibodies bound to some relatively nonspecific but "sticky" substance such as procollagen, keratin, vimentin or other nucleolus unrelated macromolecule which has common antigenic determinants to those of the nucleolar antigens is not yet defined. Further studies are needed to improve the specificity of the antibody preparation either by purification to monospecificity or by utilizing monoclonal preparations for monospecific antibodies.

In a few benign breast tumors, nucleolar fluorescence was apparent. These nucleoli were smaller and fewer in number than in the malignant tumors. Although such nucleolar fluorescence was found in only a few benign tumors, it led to an investigation of the sizes of the nucleoli in these benign lesions. Tables III and IV show that it was possible to distinguish sharply between benign and malignant lesions on the basis of overall nucleolar diameters, but it was not possible to specify for any one cell whether it is malignant or not simply by observing the nucleolar size or fluorescence. It is not known whether the antigen in the benign tumors is the same that is found in the malignant tumors or whether another molecular species accounts for the positive nucleolar fluorescence in a few benign tumors.

M. "Blind" Study

In this study, 80 breast samples were evaluated. Of these, 55 were carcinomas and 25 were either normal breast or benign tumor specimens

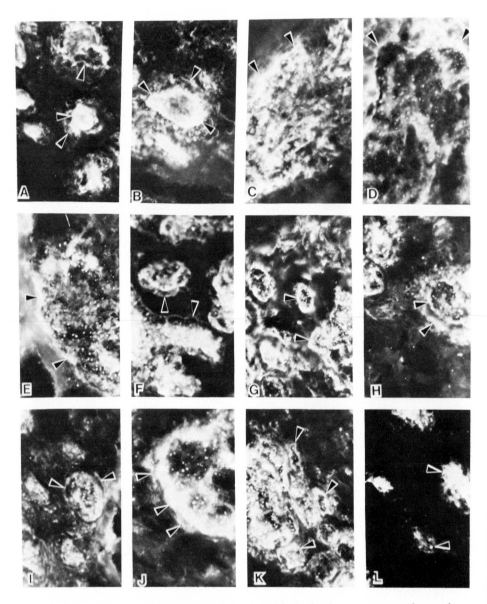

FIG. 13. Varying types of fluorescence observed in benign breast tumors and normal breast tissues. (A,B) Normal breast tissue. Central nonfluorescent areas are surrounded by a dense fluorescent "boundary" (pointers) around which there are light fluorescent elements (pointers). (A) × 160; (B) × 400. (C) Adenosis. Pointers show dense outer "boundary." Within the structures are "microspherules" and semiparallel "fibrillar" elements. × 160.

TABLE III

MAXIMUM NUCLEOLAR DIAMETERS IN A SERIES OF HUMAN BREAST CARCINOMAS

Sample	1 Less than 2.5 μm	2 Greater than 2.5 μm	3 Ratio 2/1
589-1	15	11	0.68
588	6	17	2.8
78	3	13	4.3
79	14	30	2.1
76	10	34	3.4
70	7	20	2.8
75	7	26	3.7
598	30	42	1.4
596	21	44	2.1
589-2	36	24	0.66
4	33	34	1.0
5	27	59	2.2
7	10	34	3.4
8	17	33	1.9
9	15	33	2.2
10	29	42	1.5
		Mean	2.3

(Busch *et al.*, 1981). Although this series of samples contained a preponderance of carcinomas, it was designed to determine whether one could distinguish tissues other than carcinomas in a series of breast samples. In further studies now in progress, additional benign tumors and other breast diseases are being evaluated.

The code for this study was kept in Detroit and the samples were evaluated in Houston. The results were reported in 4 series containing 13–29 samples per group. In the initial review of the samples, some were readily interpreted as positive for the nucleolar antigen and others were clearly

---

(D) Fibrocystic disease. Pointers show dense boundaries surrounding inner areas containing "microspherules." × 160. (E) Sclerosing adenosis. Pointers show dense boundaries surrounding inner areas containing "microspherules." × 160. (F) Adenosis. Area containing "microspherules" surrounded by thin boundaries (pointers). × 160. (G) Fibrocystic disease. Dense "boundary" layer (pointers) surrounding areas containing microspherules. × 160. (H) Normal breast tissue. Dense and less dense "boundaries" (pointers) surrounding areas containing "microspherules." × 160. (I) Sclerosing adenosis. Note boundary layers (pointers) surrounding areas containing microspherules. × 160. (J) Sclerosing adenosis. Dense and less dense "boundaries" (pointers) surrounding areas containing "microspherules." × 400. (K) Normal breast tissue. Large number of structures containing "microspherules" surrounded by "boundary elements. × 400. (L) Normal breast tissue. Fluorescent structures (pointers) seen in normal breast tissue specimens. × 400.

TABLE IV

MAXIMUM NUCLEOLAR DIAMETERS IN A SERIES OF BENIGN BREAST TUMORS

Sample	1 Less than 2.5 μm	2 Greater than 2.5 μm	3 Ratio 2/1
Fibrocystic disease			
65	45	1	0.05
(2 others)	—	—	0
Cystic disease			
55	95	6	0.06
(7 others)	0	0	0
Adenosis			
49–42	65	13	0.2
63	38	2	0.05
Mazoplasia			
38	9	1	0.10
2	0	0	0
Sclerosing adenosis			
73-1	39	4	0.11
73-2	61	7	0.11
		Mean benign tumors	0.036
Normal breast tissue			
42	40	2	0.05
(9 others)	0	0	0
		Mean	0.005

Ratio 3—carcinomas/normal breast	460
Ratio 3—carcinomas/benign tumors	66.7

negative. In the first group (Table V), the most readily interpreted, the 14 samples reported as positive were correctly identified as carcinomas and the 6 reported as negative were all correct except for 1 sample, a benign tumor that contained some fluorescent nucleoli.

In the next series, 29 samples, all those reported as negative were normal or benign tumors. Of the 18 carcinomas, one was a false negative. Accordingly, in the first two series, the overall correct percentage of 95% was equal to that originally reported for the larger known series of different tumor types and the series of known breast carcinomas.

It was quite surprising that in the third series of samples (Table V) which contained 16 carcinomas and 2 benign tumors, the reported results were all correct. This was a result in part of increased experience and in part of other criteria such as limiting membranes and limiting structures

TABLE V
RESULTS OF EVALUATION OF BRIGHT NUCLEOLAR FLUORESCENCE IN UNKNOWN
SPECIMENS (BLIND STUDY) OF BENIGN AND MALIGNANT BREAST SPECIMENS[a]

Specimens studied in order of difficulty	Positive	Negative	Percentage correct
I. Less difficult			
A. Generalized fluorescence or absence of fluorescence	14	6(1)	95
B. Less generalized fluorescence or unusual structures (Fig. 2)	18(1)	11	96
C. More localized fluorescence or more unusual structures	16	2	100
	48(1)	19(1)	97
II. More Difficult			
Limited fluorescence or limited visualization of cells; questionable regions	7(2)	6(1)	77
Overall correct			94%

[a] Numbers in parentheses are errors, i.e., after positive = malignant tumor reported as negative, and after negative = a benign tumor reported as positive.

notable in the normal tissues and benign lesions aided in the conclusions.

Major problems emerged in evaluation of the last group (13 samples) which contained fewer malignant cells and two benign tumors which exhibited nucleolar fluorescence. In this series, only 77% of the specimens were correctly diagnosed. In two of the malignant tumors, nucleolar fluorescence was not observed. In the overall series, 52 of 55 of the carcinomas were correctly identified and the overall percentage was 94.6% correct. This result correlated well with the initial studies. However, in the series of benign lesions, 2 of 27 were incorrectly diagnosed so the overall correct percentage was only 92%.

Among the technical problems encountered in these studies were high background fluorescence in some samples and failure to develop satisfactory fluorescence in others. In the "blind study," the H and E stained sections were unavailable but they were provided in the later review. Among the reasons for the errors in diagnosis of the malignant tumors were the failure of the antibodies to penetrate the samples as shown by fluorescence along the borders, excessive thickness of the samples, and necrosis of the specimen. These problems were similar to those noted in earlier studies on the broad range of malignant tumors (H. Busch et al., 1979).

These studies indicated that important improvements were necessary, both to substantiate and expand these results and more importantly to improve their specificity. Inasmuch as the antibodies were not shown to be completely specific for nucleolar antigens in carcinomas, it seems essential that the antigens be purified and that monospecific antibodies be provided. Second, it is necessary to evaluate the benign tumors which exhibited nucleolar fluorescence to determine whether they contain the same or different antigens and whether the nucleolar fluorescence has any prognostic significance.

III. Characterization of the Nucleolar Antigens

A. WHAT ARE THE NUCLEOLAR ANTIGENS?

Because of the necessity for more complete information on the numbers and types of antigens, studies were undertaken to chemically characterize the nucleolar antigens in these human tumors. Although it would be highly desirable and ultimately possible to isolate and purify the antigens from a variety of tumors, it was first necessary to develop techniques for their purification from a satisfactory source. The initial attempts at characterization were made with nucleolar products from HeLa cells but unfortunately there is no satisfactory commercial source and the cell masses required are extremely expensive.

It was most fortunate that during this period, the Frederick Cancer Researh Laboratories were in the process of large scale production of interferon from Namalwa cells, a Burkitt tumor line. Through the cooperation of Drs. Vincent DeVita, John Douros, and Fred Klein, quantities of such cells from 100 to 250 gm were made available. Although not completely satisfactory from the point of view that the nuclear preparations from these frozen cells were less elegant than those from fresh cells, these cells were a satisfactory source of the nucleolar antigens for purification and for further characterization (Chan et al., 1980).

B. ISOELECTRIC FOCUSING OF THE NUCLEOLAR ANTIGENS

The studies on the nucleolar antigens of the Novikoff hepatoma showed that multiple antigenic determinants and multiple antigens might exist in the human tumor nucleoli. To initiate studies on these human antigens (recognizing that some methods might preclude identification of a number of other antigens) isoelectric focusing of the antigens was undertaken (Chan et al., 1980). For this purpose, the proteins were incorporated into the gels so that antigens would not be lost by loading on either the basic or acidic side and second, 8 M urea was added to the ampholine solution to enhance the resolution of the bands. However, it seemed likely that the urea and the ampholines might react with or modify some of the antigens and make them unrecognizable.

For visualization of the antigens, the gels were washed three times with isotonic saline, immersed in acetone briefly to shrink the gel, and then the gels were soaked in the antitumor nucleolar antibodies (antiserum, Ig fraction, or IgG fraction). Excess antiserum was then removed from the gel by washing six times with the buffered saline solution and the fluorescein or peroxidase-conjugated goat-antirabbit antibody was added to the preparation. With this procedure, it was possible to visualize the antigen in the gel either by fluorescence or by the peroxidase staining methods (Fig. 14).

C. IDENTIFICATION OF THE pl 6.3 AND 6.1 ANTIGENS

In the isoelectric focusing gels, two antigens were identified both by fluorescence and peroxidase staining methods. The major antigen focused at pl 6.3 and the minor band focused at pl 6.1. Later studies showed these antigens had molecular weights (Fig. 15) of approximately 68,000 and 61,000, respectively, and accordingly they were referred to as HuAg 68/6.3 and 61/6.1 (MW + 10^{-3}/pl) (Chan *et al.*, 1981). These antigens were not detected with preimmune serum and were not found in the normal liver cells, nuclei, or nucleolar proteins focused on corresponding gels (Fig. 16), in this group of studies.

In addition to these two bands which were regularly observed in such preparations, weakly immunostained bands were occasionally observed at pl 6.6, 5.5, 5.7, and 5.9. However, they were also observed following incubation with preimmune serum.

Another set of bands which were nonspecifically bound to either the first or second antibody was the basic side of the gels. These bands were also observed with preimmune serum and they were generally present and also were in both normal human liver samples and HeLa and Namalwa samples. These bands may be of importance in nonspecific nucleolar staining reactions which have been a problem in some diagnostic studies. They may also be tissue specific but this has not been shown yet.

It was important to run the gels for short periods in view of the possibility that some antigens might migrate rapidly off the acidic or basic sides. However, no reproducible antigens were found other than the HuAg 68/6.3 and HuAg 61/6.1 even when the gels were run for very short periods. No additional antigens were demonstrable when higher concentra-

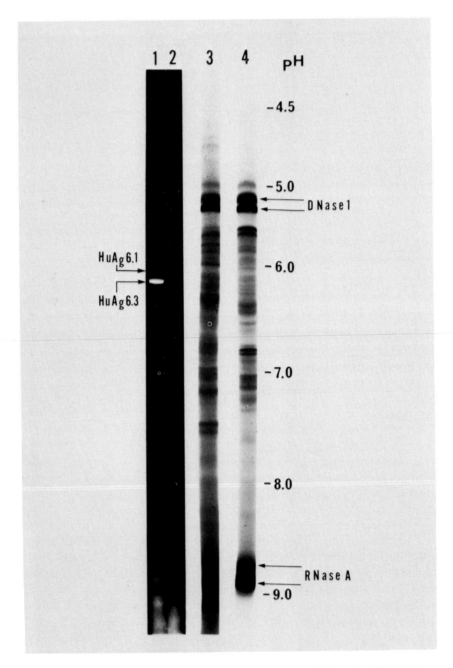

FIG. 14. Identification of the human tumor nucleolar antigens HuAg 6.3 and HuAg 6.1 on 4% polyacrylamide IF gels. The HeLa nucleoli were treated with DNase and RNase, and the

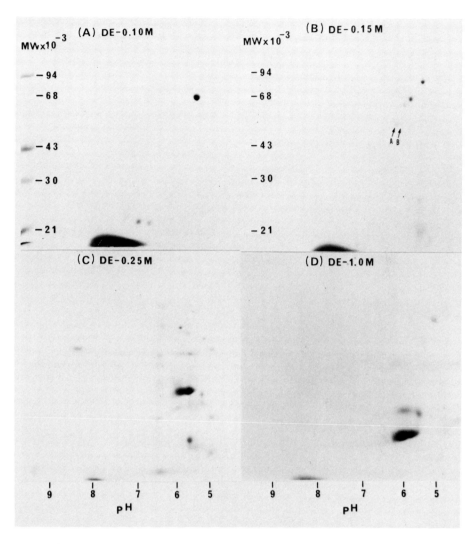

FIG. 15. Two-dimensional gel electrophoresis of the DEAE fractions. The proteins of the DEAE fractions (Fig. 18) were fractionated first on IF gels and then by 12% sodium dodecyl sulfate–polyacrylamide slab gel electrophoresis. (A) De-0.1 M; (B) DE-0.15 M. The Coomassie Blue-stained spots which comigrate with HuAg 6.3 (Arrow A) and HuAg 6.1 (Arrow B) are indicated. (C) DE-0.25 M; (D) DE-1 M. (From Chan et al., 1980.)

proteins were then analyzed by IF. The gels were reacted with immune or preimmune serum and then with fluorescein-conjugated goat anti-rabbit IgG. Photographs were made with a green filter under the long-wavelength UV lamp. Lane 1, Coomassie Blue-stained HeLa nucleolar proteins; Lane 2, Coomassie Blue-stained human liver nucleolar proteins; Lane 3, tumor proteins with immune serum; Lane 4, tumor proteins with preimmune serum. (From Chan et al., 1980.)

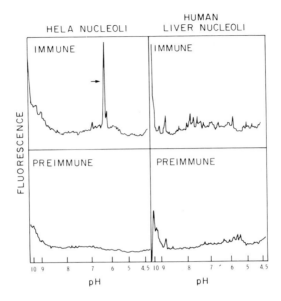

Fig. 16. Fluorometric tracing of IF gels of nucleolar proteins of HeLa cells and human liver. The nucleolar proteins of HeLa and human liver were analyzed on IF gels and immunostained with fluorescein-conjugated goat anti-rabbit IgG. The p*I* 6.3 antigen band (arrow) is present in the HeLa nucleolar proteins. A corresponding fluorescent band was not found in human liver nucleolar proteins. (From Chan *et al.*, 1980.)

tions of antibodies or proteins were used or when loading was done on the acidic or basic ends of the gels. Of course, none of these results eliminates the possibility that antigens are present that are denatured or are altered by the ampholines or the urea (Chan *et al.*, 1980).

From the point of view of localization of the HuAg 68/6.3 and HuAg 61/6.1, it is notable that they were not present in the "nuclear sap" (75 mM NaCl/25 mM EDTA/0.1 mM PMSF/pH 8 extracts) of HeLa cells nuclei nor in the cytosol fraction of these cells. They were found in the whole nucleolar protein extracts and in the 10 mM Tris extracts of nuclei after the nuclear sap was extracted with 75 mM NaCl/25 mM EDTA.

D. Densitometric Scanning of the Fluorescent Antigens

Figure 16 shows that in the isoelectric focusing gel of the nucleolar proteins of the HeLa cells, there was a fluorescent peak at p*I* 6.3 when the gel was treated with immune serum but not with the preimmune serum. Corresponding analysis of the nucleolar proteins of the normal liver did not show the presence of a corresponding antigen. Staining of the same gels with the Coomassie Blue staining indicated that there were 36 protein bands which on two-dimensional gels separated into more than 60 peptides (Fig. 14).

Similar studies on Namalwa nuclear Tris extracts demonstrated the presence of the same major and minor antigens (Fig. 17). Because of the interest in whether fetal cells contain these antigens, a similar analysis was made of IMR-90 fetal human fibroblasts. Both nucleolar antigens with

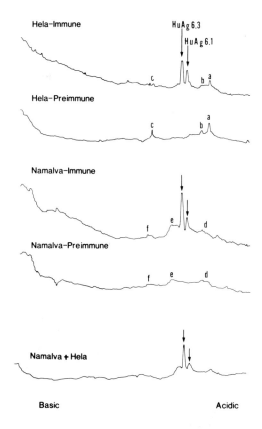

FIG. 17. Identification of the nucleolar antigens HuAg 6.3 and 6.1 in the Namalwa cells. The Tris extract of the Namalwa nuclei was analyzed on IF gels. The gels were immunostained with peroxidase-conjugated goat anti-rabbit IgG and scanned with an absorption wavelength of 475 nm. It is noted that the HuAg 6.3 and the HuAg 6.1 of the HeLa sample comigrated with those of the Namalwa sample. Several weakly immunostained bands (a,b,c in the HeLa sample and d,e,f in the Namalwa sample) and the heavily stained bands at the basic side of the IF gel were found in both immune and preimmune gels. These bands were not consistently found in different experiments. (From Chan et al., 1980.)

p*I* values of 6.3 and 6.1 were demonstrable in these cells. These results provide further support for the presence of oncofetal or "oncoembryonic" antigens in human malignant tumors. The question of what period in fetal life contains the "time window" at which these antigens are normally produced remains to be defined.

E. PURIFICATION OF THE HUMAN TUMOR NUCLEOLAR ANTIGENS

For characterization of these proteins, it was first necessary to develop a satisfactory purification procedure with preservation of antigenicity and production of a homogeneous product. Initially, ammonium sulfate fractionation was used. At a concentration of 40% ammonium sulfate, none of the antigen was precipitated and accordingly the 40% sediment was discarded.

The 40–100% fraction contained the antigen and after sedimentation, it was chromatographed on a DEAE-cellulose column. As shown in Fig. 18, a stepwise NaCl gradient was used to selectively elute the antigens at a concentration 0.15 M NaCl. This resulted in approximately a 10-fold purification inasmuch as 10% of the protein and most of the antigen was eluted in this fraction. Analysis of the proteins in this fraction by isoelectric fo-

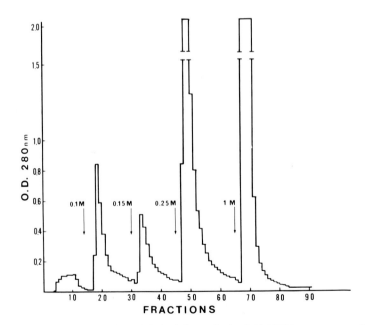

FIG. 18. Interrupted gradient elution of the nucleolar 0.01 M Tris extract proteins from DEAE cellulose. The gels for these fractions are shown in Figure 15.

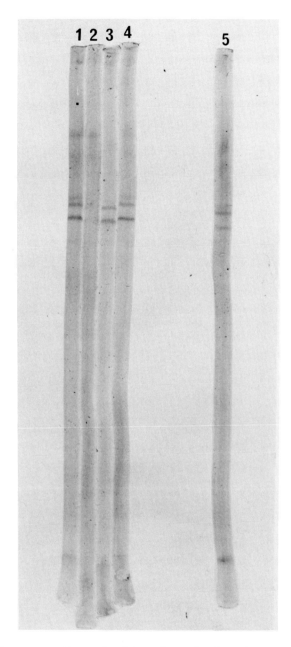

FIG. 19. Immunoperoxidase stain of the antigen using the antiserum preabsorbed with DE-0.15 M fractioned by IF gels and subsequently immunoperoxidase-stained using the antisera preabsorbed with various DEAE fractions (Fig. 18). Lane 1, antiserum preabsorbed with DE-0.1 M; Lane 2, antiserum preabsorbed with DE-0.15 M; Lane 3, antiserum preabsorbed with DE-0.25 M; Lane 4, antiserum preabsorbed with DE-1 M; Lane 5, control antiserum. (From Chan et al., 1981.)

cusing gels indicated that only this fraction reproducibly contained the HuAg 6.3 and HuAg 6.1 antigens. A Coomassie Blue-stained band which corresponds to this fraction was identified; this band was shown to be concentrated in the 0.15 M NaCl fraction but not in the other fractions.

To test whether the antigens in these fractions could absorb the Ig fraction or the antiserum, the antibodies were initially treated with the NaCl eluted fractions and then used for the double-antibody immunostaining of the gels. Only the antibody fraction absorbed with the 0.15 M NaCl eluate did not stain the antigen bands indicating that the antigens in this fraction had bound the anti-HuAg antibodies (Fig. 19).

F. Two-Dimensional Electrophoresis of the Antigens

Initially, the two antigens were detected on isoelectric focusing gels; they were subjected to a second dimensional analysis on 12% sodium dodecyl sulfate (SDS) gels. Inasmuch as only two faint spots were visible on the two-dimensional gel in the 6.3 and 6.1 region, these faint spots were suggested to be the Coomassie Blue-stained antigens (Fig. 15). Their molecular weights compared to known standards were approximately 68,000 and 61,000. In further studies, these spots corresponded to the ^{125}I-labeled antigens which were purified from the labeled proteins in the 0.15 M NaCl eluates (Figs. 20 and 21).

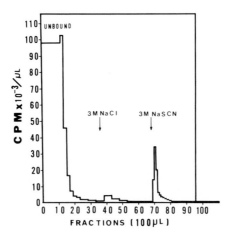

Fig. 20. Partial purification of the HuAg on the anti-0.15 M NaCl extract antibody affinity column. The HuAg were eluted with 3 M NaSCN after a 3 M NaCl wash. (From Chan *et al.*, 1981.)

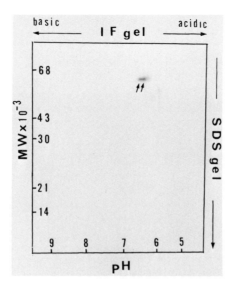

Fig. 21. Two-dimensional gel electrophoresis of purified nucleolar antigens (HuAg) from human tumors as in Fig. 20; note the dense doublet at p*I* 6.3 and the single spot at p*I* 6.1. (From Chan *et al.*, 1981.)

G. Affinity Gel Purification of the Antigens

In the previous studies on the nucleolar antigen of Novikoff hepatoma (Marashi *et al.*, 1979) affinity columns containing the antibodies were successfully used for its purification. A similar procedure was successfully employed with the Ig fraction of the antibodies to tumor nucleoli (Figs. 20 and 21). Only small amounts of the antigens were in the flow-through fraction; the fraction eluted with 3 *M* NaSCN contained highly purified antigens. To further improve the separation of the ^{125}I-labeled antigens from the nonspecifically binding proteins, the 0.15 *M* NaCl eluate was bound first to an affinity gel containing preimmune serum. The unbound fraction was then bound to the affinity gel containing the immune serum. Only two major spots were detected on the two-dimensional gel of the 3 *M* NaSCN eluate, namely, the 68/6.3 and 61/6.1 antigens (Fig. 19).

H. Separation of the Antigens into Individual Components

To further purify these antigens, preparative isoelectric focusing gels were used. With these, "single spot" antigens were purified as shown in Fig. 22. The fact that the two spots of HuAg 68/6.3 remained together sug-

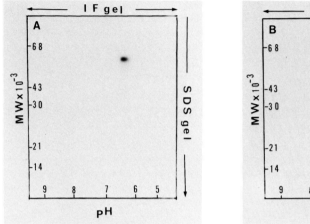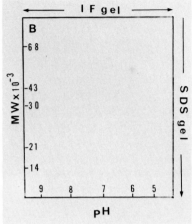

Fɪɢ. 22. Two-dimensional gel electrophoresis showing "single spot" purification of human tumor nucleolar antigens by preparative ısoelectric focusing gels. The dense p*I* 6.3 doublet is shown on (A) and the p*I* 6.1 antigen is shown on (B). (From Chan *et al.*, 1981.)

TABLE VI
Aᴍɪɴᴏ Aᴄɪᴅ Cᴏᴍᴘᴏsɪᴛɪᴏɴ ᴏғ Hᴜᴍᴀɴ
Tᴜᴍᴏʀ Nᴜᴄʟᴇᴏʟᴀʀ Aɴᴛɪɢᴇɴ 68/6.3

Amino acid	Mole %
Lysine	5.4
Histidine	2.1
Ammonia	—
Arginine	3.3
Aspartic acid	9.3
Threonine	5.7
Serine	9.1
Glutamic acid	11.6
Proline	5.3
Glycine	15.0
Alanine	8.6
Cystine	—
Valine	6.6
Methionine	1.4
Isoleucine	3.6
Leucine	7.3
Tyrosine	2.5
Phenylalanine	3.1
A/B	1.9

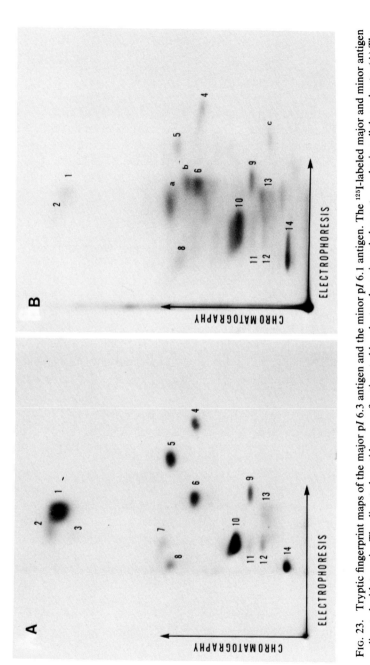

Fig. 23. Tryptic fingerprint maps of the major p*I* 6.3 antigen and the minor p*I* 6.1 antigen. The ^{125}I-labeled major and minor antigen was digested with trypsin. The digested peptides were fractionated by electrophoresis and chromatography in cellulose sheets. (A) The major p*I* 6.3 antigen. Fourteen ^{125}I-labeled peptides were identified. (B) The minor p*I* 6.1 antigen in which 12 peptides (except that peptide 3 and 7 were missing) were found identical to those obtained from the major antigen.

gests they are minor modifications of the same protein; their very similar tryptic peptide maps supported this suggestion.

I. Amino Acid Composition of the Antigen

Table VI presents the amino acid composition of the affinity purified human tumor nucleolar antigen. The amino acids in highest contents were glycine, 15%; glutamic acid, 11.6%; and serine, 9%. The ratio of the sum of the acidic to the sum of basic amino acids was 2.

J. Maps of the Tryptic Digests of the pI 6.3 and 6.1 Antigens

The major and the minor antigen (three proteins) were separately digested with trypsin. The digests were fractionated by electrophoresis and chromatography on cellulose sheets. As shown in Fig. 23A, 14 ^{125}I-labeled peptides were obtained from the trypsin digest of the major antigen. A very similar peptide map was obtained from the pI 6.1 antigen (Fig. 23B) in which 12 peptides (except that peptides 3 and 7 were missing) were identical to those obtained from the pI 6.3 antigen. These results indicate that the major pI 6.3 antigen and the minor pI 6.1 antigen are related and the pI 6.1 antigen is possibly a degradation product of the pI 6.3 antigen.

IV. Assay of the Nucleolar Antigens

A. Quantitative Analysis of the Nucleolar Antigens

In further investigations on the nature of these tumor-associated antigens, a quantitative assay was needed in addition to fluorescence microscopy and immunostaining of polyacrylamide gels. Enzyme immunoassays have recently become a useful tool for both research and clinical serodiagnosis (see review by O'Beirne and Cooper, 1979).

Nuclei from HeLa or Namalwa cells were prepared by hypotonic shock/detergent lysis as described earlier (H. Busch et al., 1979; Chan et al., 1980; Davis et al., 1979; Smetana et al., 1979). The cells were swollen on ice in 10 mM Tris–HCl/10 mM NaCl/1.5 mM MgCl$_2$/pH 7.4 (RBS) for 10 minutes, centrifuged, and resuspended in RSB containing 0.5% Nonidet P-40 (Shell Chemical Co.). The cells were homogenized in a Teflon-glass homogenizer and the crude nuclei collected by centrifugation. The crude nuclei were further purified by homogenization in 0.25 M sucrose/10 mM

MgCl$_2$ followed by centrifugation through a cushion of 0.88 M sucrose/0.5 mM MgCl$_2$.

The nuclei from liver or placenta were prepared by passing the tissues through a grinder and washing the ground tissue in 130 mM NaCl/5 mM KCl/0.8 mM MgCl$_2$. The washed tissue was homogenized in 10 volumes (w/v) of 2.2 M sucrose/10 mM MgCl$_2$ using a Teflon-glass homogenizer, filtered through cheesecloth, and centrifuged at 17,000 g for 90 minutes. The pelleted nuclei were then washed once in 0.88 M sucrose/10 mM MgCl$_2$.

B. Preparation of Nuclear Extracts and Solid-Phase Absorbents

Purified nuclei were homogenized in 75 mM NaCl/25 mM EDTA/1 mM PMSF/pH 8.0 using a Dounce homogenizer. After a 15-minute incubation on ice, the nuclei were centrifuged at 12,000 g for 10 minutes; the extraction was repeated, and the two supernatants were combined (NaCl/EDTA extract). The nuclei and resulting chromatin were then extracted three times with 10 mM Tris–HCl/1 mM PMSF/pH 8.0 (Tris extract) for 15, 30, and 15 minutes.

C. Enzyme Immunoassay (EIA)

Nuclear extracts were diluted in PBS and 50 μl was added to the wells of polystyrene microtiter plates (Dynatech, Alexandria, VA) and incubated at 4°C overnight. The solutions were removed by aspiration and the remaining protein binding sites were blocked by the addition of PBS/Tween/BSA for 2 hours at room temperature. The plates were washed with PBS/0.5% Tween 20 (PBS/Tween) and 50 μl of IgG solution (40 μg/ml in PBS/Tween/BSA) was added to each well; incubation was done for 2 hours at room temperature. This solution was removed by aspiration and the plates were washed with PBS/Tween. Alkaline phosphatase conjugated goat anti-rabbit IgG (diluted 1:1000 in PBS/Tween) was added (50 μl/well) and the plates were incubated for 1 hour at room temperature. After removal of this solution, the plates were washed again with PBS/Tween and 200 μl of 1 mg/ml p-nitrophenylphosphate (Boehringer Mannheim) in 0.05 M NaCO$_3$/1 mM MgCl$_2$/pH 9.8 was added to each well. After a 30-minute incubation at room temperature, color development was stopped by the addition of 50 μl of 4 N NaOH. The color intensity in each well was measured at 405 nm using an ELIA reader (Fischer Scientific).

D. Quantitation of the Antigen

When various amounts of Namalwa Tris extracts were assayed by enzyme immunoassay (EIA), a linear response was obtained over a protein range of 100 to 500 ng. Figure 24 shows the average result of five assays performed over a period of 2 months using unabsorbed IgG. In each assay the data were fit by linear regression analysis to a straight line with a correlation coefficient of >0.98. In addition to detecting antigens in the extract of tumor nuclei, the unabsorbed antibodies also reacted significantly with extracts from placental nuclei and, to a lesser extent, with extracts from normal liver nuclei (Fig. 25). Because of the variability of the EIA with <100 ng of protein, the lines in Fig. 2 are shown only in the linear range of 100–500 ng. Increasing the amount of protein beyond 500 ng resulted in a marked reduction in the slope of the response.

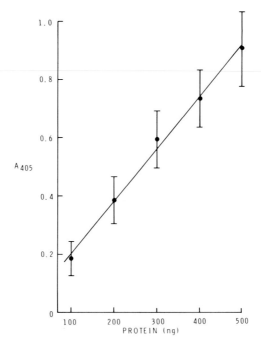

Fig. 24.   EIA of Namalwa Tris extract. Assays were performed using unabsorbed IgG. Microtiter wells initially contained 100–500 ng protein from Namalwa Tris extract. The values for normal rabbit IgG were subtracted from each point. The results are plotted as the average (± SD) of five separate assays. The correlation coefficients for the straight lines in each assay were between 0.980 and 0.997.

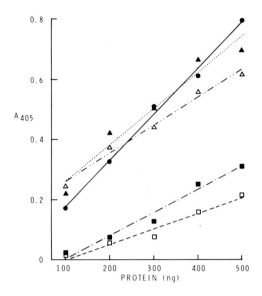

Fɪɢ. 25.   EIA of nuclear extracts using unabsorbed IgG. Various nuclear extracts were assayed using unabsorbed IgG. Microtiter wells initially contained 100–500 ng protein from Namalwa Tris extract (●——●), placental NaCl/EDTA extract (▲——▲), placental Tris extract (△——△), liver NaCl/EDTA (■——■), or liver Tris extract (□----□). Values for normal rabbit IgG were subtracted from each point.

Liver and placental nuclear extracts were concentrated by ultrafiltration (M_r cutoff = 10,000), dialyzed against 0.1 M NaHCO$_3$/0.5 M NaCl/pH 8.0, and coupled to CNBr-activated Sepharose 4B (Pharmacia, Piscataway, NJ). Approximately 8 mg of protein was added per ml of activated gel and the mixture was rotated overnight at 4°C. The coupling efficiency was approximately 90–95%. Unreacted coupling sites were blocked by treatment with 1 M ethanolamine/0.5 M NaCl/pH 8.0 overnight, and the Sepharose was washed three times each with alternating washes of 1 M NaCl/0.1 M sodium acetate (pH 4) and 1 M NaCl/0.1 sodium borate (pH 8). The coupled Sepharose was stored at 4°C as a 50% suspension in 10 mM Na$_2$HPO$_4$/150 mM NaCl/pH 7.4 (PBS) with 0.02% NaN$_3$. Protein concentrations were determined by the method of Bradford (1976) using a protein assay kit from Bio Rad Laboratories (Richmond, CA).

E. Improved Analysis by Absorptions of Antibodies

Absorption of the IgG was performed by both column and batch methods. In the column method, an absorption mixture containing 200 μl each of Sepharose coupled with liver NaCl/EDTA, liver Tris, and placental NaCl/EDTA extracts, and 400 μl of placental–Tris coupled Sepharose was centrifuged for 2 minutes at 12,800 g; the supernatant was removed, and the pellet was resuspended in 0.5 ml of 10 mM Na$_2$HPO$_4$/1 M NaCl/pH 7.4. To this suspension was added 0.5 ml of IgG (1 mg/ml) and the mixture was rotated overnight at 4°C. The mixture was then placed in a 1-ml syringe and the flowthrough fraction was collected. The column was washed with 0.1 ml of 10 mM Na$_2$HPO$_4$/1 M NaCl/pH 7.4. In the batch method, the IgG was diluted to a concentration of 40 μg/ml in PBS/0.05% Tween 20/0.5% BSA (PBS/Tween/BSA) which also contained the absorbents. These samples were mixed overnight. The solid phase was pelleted by centrifugation for 2 minutes at 12,800 g, and the supernatant was used directly in the EIA.

The contaminating antibodies directed against antigens present in normal cells were also absorbed with extracts from normal cell nuclei which were covalently coupled to Sepharose 4B. Sepharose coupled to the NaCl/EDTA extract from human liver nuclei was used to assay the liver NaCl/EDTA and Tris extracts by EIA. The effect of increasing amounts of absorbent on the EIA activity is shown in Fig. 25. Approximately 80% of the EIA activity toward the liver NaCl/EDTA extract was removed by absorbing the IgG (30 μg) with 50 μl of the liver NaCl EDTA containing Sepharose suspension. Figure 25 also shows that this absorption also significantly reduced the EIA activity toward the the liver Tris extract. However, the reduction in activity (compared to unabsorbed IgG) to the Tris extract was somewhat less than the reduction in the NaCl/EDTA activity (Fig. 25). This result indicates that many of the antigens are in both extracts but some in the Tris extract may not be present in the NaCl/EDTA extract. In a similar experiment, IgG absorbed with combined liver extract Sepharose absorbents had a high EIA activity to the Tris extract from placental nuclei.

Inasmuch as any one extract seemed to be insufficient for complete absorption, IgG was absorbed by the column method using a mixture of Sepharose-coupled extracts. After two rounds of column absorption, the IgG was absorbed once more by the batch method using 200 μl of this mixture. These absorptions greatly reduced the binding activity of the IgG for the normal tissue nuclear extracts (Fig. 26), but binding to the tumor extract was not markedly affected. The slopes of the best-fit straight line for each set of points showed the activity toward the normal nuclear ex-

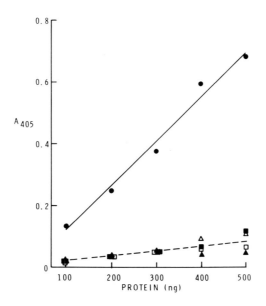

FIG. 26. EIA of nuclear extracts using absorbed IgG. IgG was absorbed three times as described in the text. See legend to Fig. 25 for details. Absorption of liver NaCl/EDTA antibodies. Five hundred nanograms protein liver NaCl/EDTA (●——●) and liver Tris (○----○) extracts were assayed using IgG which has been absorbed with various amounts of liver NaCl/EDTA-bound Sepharose. The results are expressed as percentage of activity remaining compared to unabsorbed IgG. The IEA was performed as above except that peroxidase-conjugated goat anti-rabbit IgG was used as a second antibody. The substrate was 0.015% 2,2′azino-di-(3-ethylbenzthiazoline sulfonate) (Levy and Sober, 1960) and 0.015% H_2O_2 in 0.1 M citrate/pH 4.0. The reaction was stopped with 1 M NaF and the absorbence measured at 417 nm.

tracts was reduced by an average of 82% by the absorptions, compared with only a 6% reduction in activity toward the tumor extract.

Coupling of the antigen to CNBr-Sepharose 4B was done as described by Bustin and Kupfer (1976). The RNP antigens (30–60 mg) were dialyzed against 0.5 M NaCl/0.1 M NaHCO$_3$/pH 8.0 overnight before coupling to CNBr-Sepharose 4B gels. The antigen-coupled Sepharose 4B was incubated with 40–70 mg antibodies (rabbit IgG to HeLa nucleoli) by end-over-end rotation at room temperature for 2 hours and then at 4°C overnight. The unbound IgG was removed and the gel was washed with PBS/0.05% Tween 20 until the absorbance at 280 nm of the flow-through fraction was less than 0.01. The bound IgG (2–3 mg) was eluted with 3 M NaSCN. The antibodies were purified by using the same affinity gel. Approximately 0.6–0.9 mg IgG was finally obtained.

F. Immunoabsorption

Immunoabsorption was carried out with Sepharose 4B coupled with liver nuclear extract (Kelsey *et al.*, 1981). The 100 μl of the affinity purified antibodies (24 μg), 400 μl of the gel (50% suspension in PBS) was added and incubated at 4°C overnight. After low-speed centrifugation to remove the Sepharose 4B bound complexes, the absorbed antibodies were used for further studies.

Figure 27 shows the purification of the antibodies by affinity chromatography. In a typical experiment, 96% of the total IgG was in the flow-through fraction and 4% of the total was in the bound fraction. The titer of the purified antibodies was measured by the ELISA procedure. The antibodies were diluted with PBS/Tween 20/BSA (1:5 to 1:200) and tested against the Namalwa RNP antigens (0.7 μg/well). To compare the titer of antibodies, the 0.2 O.D. level at 417 nm was used; this value was twice

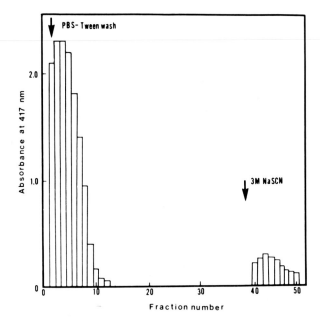

Fig. 27. Affinity chromatography of antinucleolar antibodies on Sepharose bound RNP extract. The RNP antigens (30–60 mg) were coupled to CNBr-Sepharose 4B (3–6 gm). After the affinity gel was incubated with IgG (40–70 mg), it was transferred to a sintered glass funnel and the unbound IgG was removed. The initial wash with PBS/0.05% Tween 20 was continued until the absorbance at 280 nm was less than 0.01. The bound IgG was eluted with 3 *M* NaSCN.

that of the preimmune IgG at the highest concentration (0.6 μg/well) used (Field *et al.*, 1980). The specific activity of the antibodies was calculated assuming that 1 O.D. in the ELISA assay equals 1 unit of the antibody activity at the indicated antigen concentration. As shown in Fig. 28, the purified antibodies had a titer of 50 (1:50 dilution; 60 ng antibodies). The specific activity was about 8 times that of the original IgG. Much of the activity (73% of the total) was in the flow-through fraction which indicates that either the antigen content of the gel was low or the equilibration was incomplete.

When the antibodies were repurified on the same affinity gels, about 75% of the IgG was found in the flow-through fractions, while 25% was again found in the bound fractions. The ELISA assay indicated that the IgG in the flow-through fractions had virtually no antigen-binding activity. The titer of the IgG in the bound fractions (Fig. 28) was 138 (1:138 dilution, 20 ng antibodies). A 23-fold purification of the antibodies was obtained by these two affinity chromatography steps.

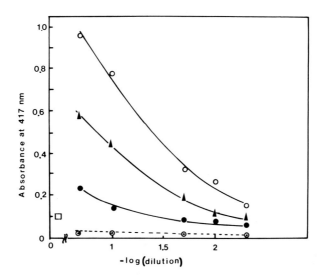

FIG. 28. Titration of antibodies by ELISA procedure. Antibodies (0.6 μg/well) from different fractions after the first and the second run of affinity chromatography were diluted with PBS/Tween 20/BSA [1:5 to 1:200 dilutions as expressed by $-$ log (dilutions)] and reacted to 0.7 μg of RNP antigens/well. (O———O), Bound IgG of the second affinity chromatography; (▲———▲), bound IgG of the first affinity chromatography; (O-----O), unbound IgG of the second affinity chromatography; (●-----●), original IgG; (□), represents the preimmune IgG level.

G. Specificity of Antibodies

To test the specificity of the purified antibodies, human liver and placenta nuclear RNP antigens were bound to microtiter wells for the ELISA assay. As shown in Fig. 29, the titer of the antibodies toward Namalwa antigens at 0.2 O.D. was 138 (1:38 dilution), while the titer toward placental and liver was 8 (1:8 dilution). Therefore, the antibodies had a 17-fold greater reactivity with the Namalwa antigens than with placenta or liver samples.

H. Effects of Immunoabsorption of the Purified Antibodies

The binding of the purified antibodies pretreated with liver-Sepharose 4B to Namalwa, liver, and placental antigens was determined by the ELISA assay. Figure 30 shows that at the highest antigen concentration 0.7 µg/well) used, the activity of the absorbed antibodies was decreased about 17% for the tumor (O.D.), but its activity was decreased more for liver and placenta, 36 and 51%, respectively. The titer was calculated from the experiments in Fig. 29 as about 115 (Namalwa), 5 (liver), and 4 (placenta). This indicates the absorbed antibodies had much a higher

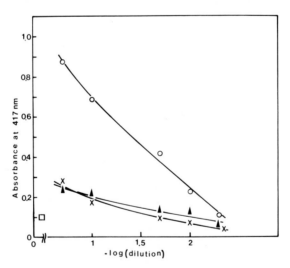

FIG. 29. Specificity of affinity purified antibodies by ELISA procedure. The antibodies purified twice on affinity gels (0.6 µg/well) were diluted with PBS/Tween 20/BSA (1:5 to 1:200 dilutions) and reacted to 0.7 µg antigens/well. (O———O), Namalwa RNP antigens; (▲———▲), normal human liver antigens extracted with 10 mM Tris–HCl/pH 8.0; (×———×), normal placenta antigens extracted with 10 mM Tris–HCl/pH 8.0; (□), represents the preimmune IgG level.

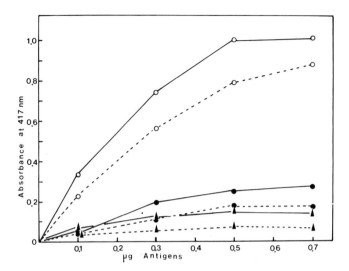

FIG. 30. Effect of liver-Sepharose on the purified antibodies by ELISA procedure. Affinity purified antibodies before and after immunoabsorption on Sepharose coupled liver Tris extract were reacted to extracts from Namalwa (O——O), human liver (●——●), and placenta (▲——▲). The solid lines represent results with unabsorbed antibodies, the broken lines represent results with absorbed antibodies.

specificity for tumor, 23-fold greater than for liver and 29-fold greater than for placenta.

V. Nuclear Localization of the Antigen

To aid in the localization of the antigen and provide further information on its relationship to nuclear RNP particles, immunoelectron microscopic analysis of the antigen was initiated with the specific immunoperoxidase–antiperoxidase (PAP) reaction and antibody preparations against HeLa or cell nucleoli (Busch *et al.*, 1980; Davis *et al.*, 1979; Sternberger, 1979).

A. Fixation of the Human Nucleolar Antigen

Various fixatives were evaluated to determine the optimal preservation of the antigen which was evaluated in smears by the indirect immunofluorescence described previously (Busch *et al.*, 1980; Davis *et al.*, 1979).

Table VII lists the fixatives evaluated on a relative scale when compared to the standard fixation in acetone. The satisfactory preservation of the nucleolar antigenic activity as well as relatively reasonable ultrastruc-

TABLE VII

SENSITIVITY OF HeLa NUCLEOLAR ANTIGEN TO VARIOUS FIXATION CONDITIONS

Fixative	Concentration	Time	Fluorescence
Acetone	100%	10 minutes	+++
Ethanol	100%	10 minutes	+++
Formaldehyde	0.5%	1 hour	++
in 0.1 M Na-			
cacodylate	1	1 hour	++
0.1 M sucrose		Overnight	++
	2	1 hour	−
	3	1 hour	−
	4	1 hour	−
Glutaraldehyde			
in 0.1 M Na-			
cacodylate	0.075	1 hour	−
0.1 M sucrose	0.1	1 hour	−
	0.2	1 hour	−
	0.5	1 hour	−
	1	1 hour	−
	2	1 hour	−
Glutaraldehyde	0.075	1 hour	−
followed by NaBH₄	0.1	1 hour	−
	0.2	1 hour	−
	0.5	1 hour	−
Acetone followed by			
glutaraldehyde (0.2%)		10 minutes and 1 hour	−
Formaldehyde followed			
by OsO₄ (2%)		1 hour and 1 hour	−

ture to permit its localization in the nucleus was obtained with freshly prepared 1% paraformaldehyde in sodium cacodylate buffer (pH 7.4) for 1 hour to overnight. The stock solution of 10% paraformaldehyde (Polysciences, Inc., Warrington, PA) was prepared by dissolving an appropriate amount of paraformaldehyde in deonized glass distilled water at 60°C. After 5 minutes of constant stirring, 100 μl of 1 N NaOH was added to completely solubilized the paraformaldehyde. The final working solutions were made in 0.1 sodium cacodylate buffer (pH 7.4) containing 0.1 sucrose.

B. POSTEMBEDDING IMMUNE LOCALIZATION OF THE ANTIGEN (STERNBERGER, 1979)

The paraformaldehyde (1%) fixed HeLa cells were processed through dehydration in ethanol and infiltration with Epon-Araldite (Mollenhauer, 1964) by routine procedures. The ultrathin sections were deposited on

300-mesh gold or nickel grids, and etched with sodium hydroxide or 10% hydrogen peroxide. SEM was used to evaluate the effects of the various etching procedures on the surfaces of the fine sections that were deposited on the grids. Following the etching procedures, the sections were rinsed with the etching vehicle solution and air-dried. The grids were then coated with approximately 100 Å of gold in a DSM-1 sputtering module (Denton vacuum) at 175 mTorr pressure, at 10 mA current. The coated grids were examined with ASID-TEM-SCAN 100CS electron microscope operated at 40 kV. The etching with 10% H_2O_2 (Moriarty and Halmi, 1972) for 10 minutes provided satisfactory results although no visible effects were noted with the scanning electron microscope. In contrast, the etching with sodium hydroxide (H. Busch *et al.*, 1979) (calibrated in ethanol or 0.5 *N* solution in 50% ethanol), completely or partially dissolving the polymerized epoxy resins as seen by scanning microscopy, produced a loss of the nucleolar antigenic activity.

The etched sections were washed three times in separate beakers containing distilled water. Without allowing these sections to air-dry, they were incubated with normal goat serum (1:100) dilution for 3 minutes (the "blocking reaction"). Without further washing of the section, the grids were incubated at 4°C for 24 hours with rabbit antibodies to the human tumor nucleolar antigen (Busch *et al.*, 1980; Chan *et al.*, 1980; Davis *et al.*, 1979) at the dilution of 1:100 followed by a wash in 0.05 *M* phosphate buffer, pH 6.8 containing 1% normal goat serum. The control sections were incubated with preimmune rabbit IgG.

The sections were incubated again for the blocking reaction with normal goat serum for 3 minutes followed by an incubation with goat anti-rabbit IgG (Cappel Labs, Cochranville, PA) at a dilution of 1:100 for 3 minutes. The grids were washed in 0.05 *M* phosphate buffer, pH 6.8 and floated on top of a peroxidase antiperoxidase (PAP) rabbit IgG complex (Miles Yeda, Rehovot, Israel) solution for 3 minutes diluted in phosphate buffer. Following a wash in 0.05 *M* phosphate buffer/pH 6.3, the grids were incubated in reaction mixture containing 0.0125% diaminobenzidine tetrahydrochloride (DAB) (Sigman, St. Louis, MO)/0.0025% hydrogen peroxide/0.05 *M* Tris, pH 7.6 with constant gentle stirring to prevent DAB flakes from being deposited on the fine sections. After 3 minutes, the grids were washed in water and transferred to a solution of osmium tetroxide (EMS Inc.) for 10 minutes. The grids were then air-dried and examined with either a Philips 200 EM or JEOL 100-CS at 60 or 80 kV without any additional electron staining.

Nucleoli of HeLa cells were characterized by the presence of variably distinct nucleolonemas (Fig. 31); their ultrastructural organization did not differ from the previous descriptions. The nucleolonemas contained mainly dense fibrillar and granular components (Fig. 32). The etching of

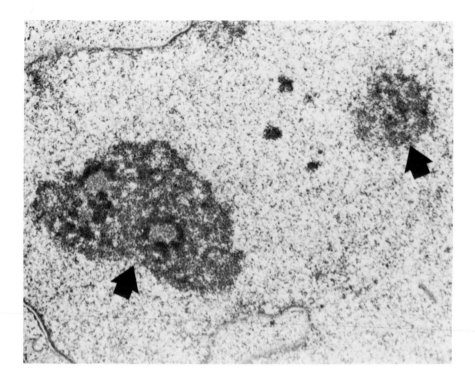

Fɪɢ. 31. Nucleoli (arrows) of a HeLa cell fixed in paraformaldehyde and osmium tet-
raoxide, stained with uranyl acetate and lead citrate. They are characterized by the presence
of nucleolonemas of varying density.

sections before the immune PAP reaction apparently altered the morphology of both cytoplasmic and nuclear components but the basic organization of nuclear and nucleolar structures was preserved (Figs. 33 and 34).
    When the investigated cells were incubated with anti-HeLa nuclear an-
tibodies, the highest positive immune PAP–diaminobenzidine reactions
were observed in nucleoli as shown by their high density at low magnifications (Fig. 33). In nucleoli, the nucleolonemas had the highest density
(Figs. 33 and 34); the nucleolar antigen was concentrated in these structures which contain nucleolar RNP components (Busch and Smetana,
1970). The densest positive immune reactions were noted in some nucleolonemas (Fig. 34) which contain dense fibrillar RNP components (Busch
and Smetana, 1970). Other nucleolar components and nuclear structures
appeared to be less dense or did not react in the specific immune PAP–
diaminobenzidine reaction. Moreover, a few small dense areas were
noted in the nucleus and the chromatin associated with the nuclear mem-

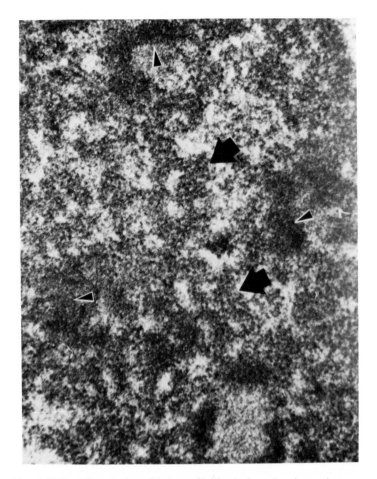

FIG. 32. A HeLa cell nucleolus with dense fibrillar (pointers) and granular components (arrows). The same fixation and staining as in Fig. 1. × 48,000.

brane (Fig. 33). However, the density of these structures might be also due to the staining with the osmium tetroxide used in the procedure as postfixation (Sternberger, 1979).

C. LOCALIZATION OF THE HUMAN TUMOR NUCLEOLAR ANTIGEN(S) IN NUCLEOLI OF HeLa CELLS TREATED WITH ADRIAMYCIN

As in other cells (Merski *et al.*, 1976), adriamycin produced in HeLa cells marked changes in the nucleolar structural organization (Figs. 35 and 36). Nucleoli with nucleolonemas segregated to rounded and compact nucleolar structures (Fig. 35) with a relatively uniform distribution of dense

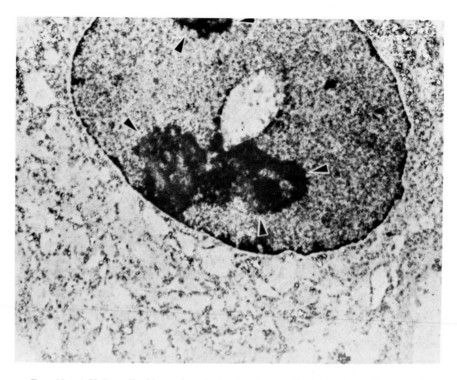

Fig. 33. A HeLa cell with an altered ultrastructure produced by the etching procedure with H_2O_2. Nucleoli (pointers) had a very high density after the specific immune PAP–diaminobenzidine reaction.× 18,500.

fibrillar RNA components in segregated areas (Fig. 36). After etching the sections and incubation with antinucleolar antibodies followed by the PAP–diaminobenzidine reaction, the cell ultrastructure was altered but the products of the specific immunoreaction were densest in nucleoli (Figs. 37 and 38). The distribution of the nucleolar antigen(s) after treatment of HeLa cells with adriamycin was mainly in the areas containing the dense nucleolar RNP components.

With shorter treatment of specimens (previously incubated with antibodies to nucleoli) with diaminobenzidine in the PAP–diaminobenzidine reaction, distinct PAP complexes were seen at high magnifications in the nucleolus (Fig. 39) but their localization to fibrillar or granular RNP components was not well defined. The size of these PAP complexes was about 20–30 nm and was therefore similar to that in the literature (Moriarty *et al.*, 1972; Sternberger, 1979). Few PAP complexes were also noted in the extranucleolar regions of the nucleus (Fig. 39).

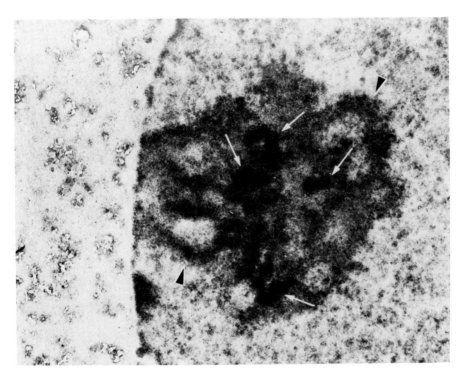

Fig. 34. Higher magnification of a nucleolus of a HeLa cell. Nucleolonemas (pointers and arrows) are characterized by a high density after the specific immune PAP–diaminobenzidine reaction. The cytoplasmic structure was altered by etching with H_2O_2. × 30,000.

D. The Control of the Specificity of the Immune PAP Reaction

Incubation of the specimens with rabbit preimmune IgG (Busch *et al.*, 1979, 1980) did not produce specific accumulation of the products of the PAP–diaminobenzidene reaction in nuceloli in HeLa cells. They were unstained or stained only slightly like other cell components (Figs. 40 and 41).

E. Evidence That the Nucleolar Antigen Is Associated with Nuclear Miniparticles

During the course of the studies on purification of the nuclear antigens, improved sources of the antigen were sought. During a brief sabbatical in this laboratory, M. Fukushima noted that the extracellular concentration

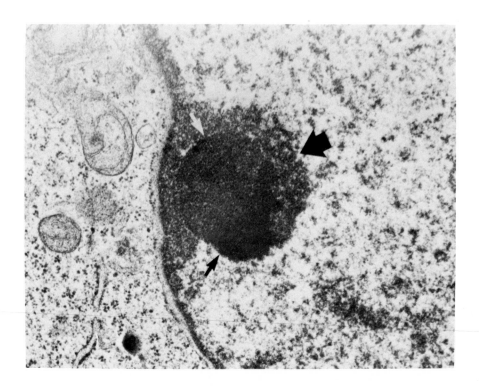

Fig. 35. A HeLa cell treated with adriamycin (fixation and staining were done as for Fig. 31). The nucleolus is compact with segregated fibrillar (black thin arrow) and granular (white arrow) components. The perinucleolar chromatin—thick arrow. × 25,000.

of the antigen was higher by comparsion with the intracellular concentration. After this finding was confirmed, F. Harmon carried out a series of purification studies including exclusion chromatography on Sephacel G-200 which indicated that the antigen was mainly a particle which has an approximate MW of 600,000.

Sucrose density gradients revealed that the particle sedimented in one or two bands with approximate sedimentation coefficients of 14 S and 21 S. This particle is also found in the nucleoli of HeLa cells but not in the nucleoli of normal liver cells (Fig. 42A and B). These preliminary studies are of interest because they support prior studies which showed that approximately 60–70% of the antigen was in a particle.

Electron microscopy showed that this particle has a "donut" shape at 150,000 × (Fig. 43A); the appearance of the particle at higher magnification is indicated in Fig. 43B and C. These "donut-shaped" particles may

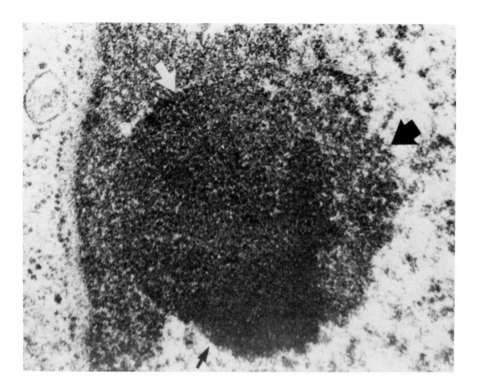

FIG. 36. The same nucleolus as in Fig. 35 at a higher magnification. Note the uniform distribution of nucleolar dense RNP fibrillar (black thin arrow) and granular (white arrow) components in segregated areas. The perinucleolar chromatin—black thick arrow. × 68,000.

or may not be similar to those observed by different workers. They bear a relationship to the "miniparticle" reported by Narayan and Rounds (1973), but they differ in that the particle they described was sensitive to DNase and not RNase. These particles are destroyed by RNase. Donut-shaped particles of similar size have been found in preparations of bacterial RNase polymerase and in preparations of complement reactive proteins (CPR). There has also been a report that *Herpes* virion may contain such small particles in their surface structure. At present, chemical information that would permit discrimination of these various potential structures is being obtained. In the higher magnification of 1×10^6 and 3.5×10^6 (Fig. 43C and D) it is clear that these particles are composed of 7 or 8 subunits which surround an oval center. A number of the subunits have a small central core. Further studies are in progress on the composition and structure of the subelements of these novel nucleolar particles.

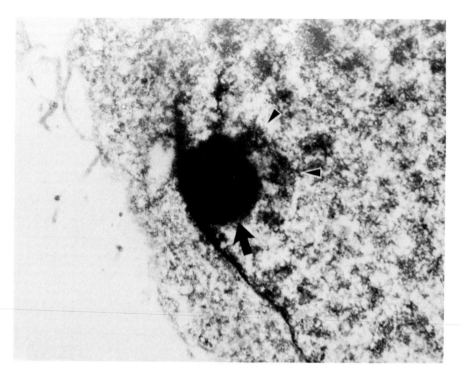

FIG. 37. A highly dense and compact nucleolus in a HeLa cell treated with adriamycin and stained with specific immune PAP–diaminobenzidine reaction. The nucleolus (thick arrow) has the highest density in comparison with other cell structures. The contrast of the nucleolus was slightly reduced by printing to increase the visibility of other cell components. The perinucleolar chromatin—pointers. × 20,000

VI. Discussion

A. POSSIBLE FUNCTIONS OF THE NUCLEOLAR ANTIGEN

Although there is no specific information yet on the precise role of the nucleolar 68/6.3 antigen, its localization has been analyzed both by light and electron microscopy. The present evidence shows it is present in the various soluble and formed elements of the nucleolus and it is concentrated in the "fibrillar" elements (approximately 70% of the antigen is in RNP particles) of the fundamental nucleolonemal structure of the nucleolus. Its localization is quite similar to the "silver staining protein C23" of rat tumor nucleoli, although evidence has not been obtained that the antigen is a silver staining or an NOR protein. However, this is one possibility that needs further examination.

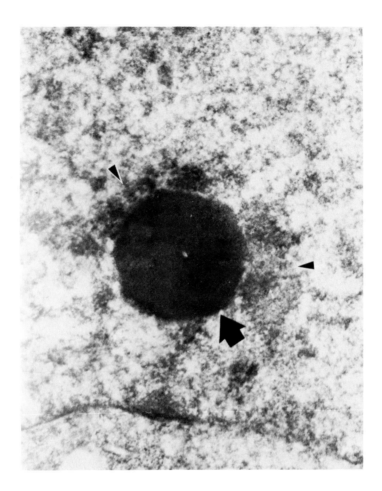

Fig. 38. A compact nucleolus (arrow) of a HeLa cell treated with adriamycin after staining with the specific immune PAP–diaminobenzidine reaction. The density of the nucleolus is higher than that of other cell structures although the contrast of the electron micrograph was reduced by printing. The high density of the nucleolus did not permit localization of the reaction products to segregated dense fibrillar or granular components. The perinucleolar chromatin—pointers. × 33,000.

Another nucleolar element that is distributed in a similar fashion is the U3 RNP particle. Although the function of the U3 RNA of the nucleolus is not defined, it may serve a role similar to the "splicing" function of the U1 RNA and possible other small nuclear RNAs. The U3 RNA is in a small RNP particle which is intimately associated with the large 60 S and 80 S subunit elements of the nucleolar preribosomal RNP particles. Inasmuch as the antigen is concentrated in the particulate elements of the nu-

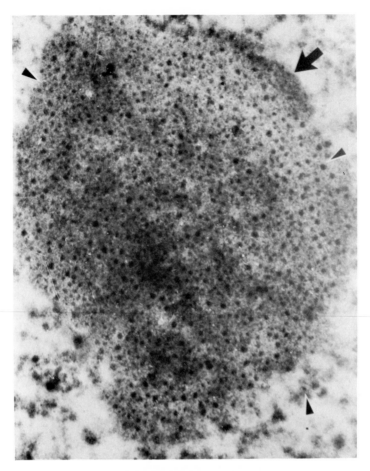

Fig. 39. A compact nucleolus of a HeLa cell treated with adriamycin. The time of the specific immune PAP reaction with diaminobenzidine was reduced to demonstrate the products of this reaction (pointers) in the nucleolus (large arrow). The size of the reaction products is about 20–30 nm and their precise localization to dense nucleolar RNP components is not possible. × 14,000.

cleolus, one possibility being explored is that it constitutes a structural element of these small particles.

At intriguing recent problem is the finding, by ELISA analysis for the antigen, of a particle which is approximately 100 Å in diameter and has a "donut" or "ring-shaped" appearance. This particle was found in large amounts in saline extracts of Namalwa cells and in corresponding extracts of HeLa cells. It represents a possible contaminant of these cells, although it seems unlikely that such a contaminant would exist in two cell

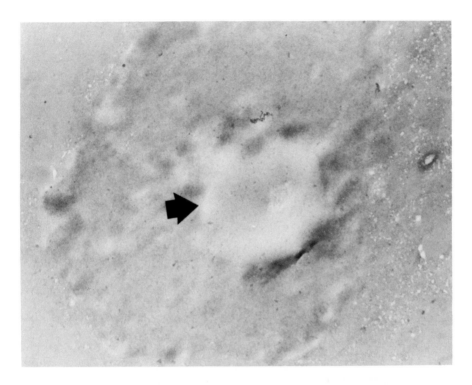

Fig. 40. A compact nucleolus (arrow) of a HeLa cell treated with adriamycin. In the immune PAP reaction the antinucleolar antibodies were replaced by preimmune rabbit IgG as the control. The nucleolus does not show any positive reaction. × 14,000.

lines of such diverse origin (a Burkitt lymphoma and a uterine carcinoma). Whether the antigen is on its surface is not yet clear.

This type of "miniparticle" was found earlier by Narayan and Rounds (1973) who observed them in tissue culture fluids of KB, HeLa, and CMP (a human adenocarcinoma). The particles were reported to contain approximately 5% DNA and 10% RNA. Whether they are U3 RNP particles, unique molecular elements, some rhino or other virus is not known.

Recently evidence has been adduced that nuclei of human cancer cells contain a novel DNA polymerase, Cm (Lowenstein et al., 1980) which differs from the normal DNA polymerases of human cells. Inasmuch as the antigen might serve a special role in the replication of rDNA, it is conceivable that it is either the same DNA polymerase or possibly an rDNA polymerase. Studies on this point will be done.

Another possibility that requires study is that the antigen may reflect the presence of unusual or "fetal" subunits of RNA polymerase I. It is

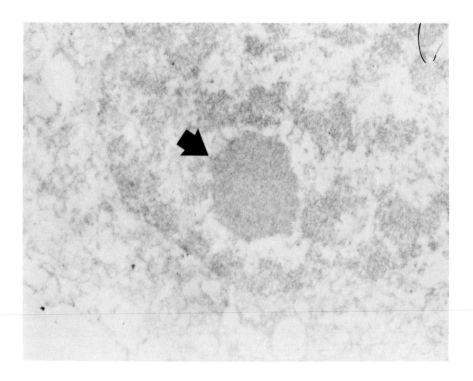

FIG. 41. A HeLa cell treated with adriamycin after the PAP–diaminobenzidine reaction in which the antinucleolar antibodies were replaced by the preimmune rabbit IgG as the control. The contrast was increased by printing and the nucleolus did not show a higher density in comparison with other cell components. × 16,000.

well known that RNA polymerase I is a multisubunit enzyme and little is known about it in human tissues. The antigen is present in such small amounts that it is likely to serve as an enzymatic function. In the nucleolus, a major function is synthesis of rRNA but one cannot rule out a role in any of the many synthetic, modification, or other functions that characterize the nucleolus. The "particles" may be a multiheaded enzyme.

B. IS THE ANTIGEN AN ACCELERATOR OR GENE CONTROL ELEMENT?

The almost ubiquitous presence of the antigen in human cancers certainly requires an explanation both in terms of function and why this element should be present. If it were transmitted epigenetically, as the data

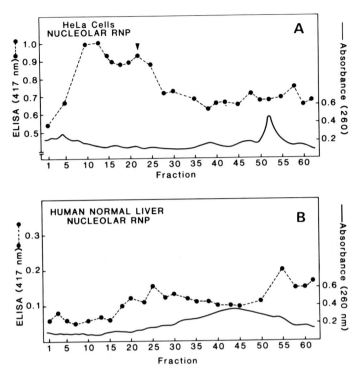

FIG. 42. Sucrose density gradients of nucleolar RNP particles. The maximum ELISA activities in the nucleoli of HeLa cells (A) corresponds with the peak (arrowhead) containing the particle shown in Fig. 43. A corresponding peak was not found in normal liver nucleoli (B).

on the HeLa cells indicate (H. Busch *et al.*, 1979), it might serve to "bypass" the usual gene controls on G_1 entry. It might also serve to activate genes either directly or through feedback mechanisms that were normally not functional or were normally blocked and yet were essential for growth and cell division. It is clear that there is a "circus movement" of sorts in cancer cells which is insensitive to extrinsic or intrinsic controls. Accordingly, some system is activated in cancer cells to produce this antigen which is a common product of the activated genes of cancer cells. This system may be intimately related to the cancer process or it may be involved in some essential function for the growth of these cells.

C. Relation of the Nucleolar Antigens to the "src Gene" Product

When the nucleolar antigen was shown to have a molecular weight of approximately 68,000 and a p*I* of 6.3, it became of interest to compare it

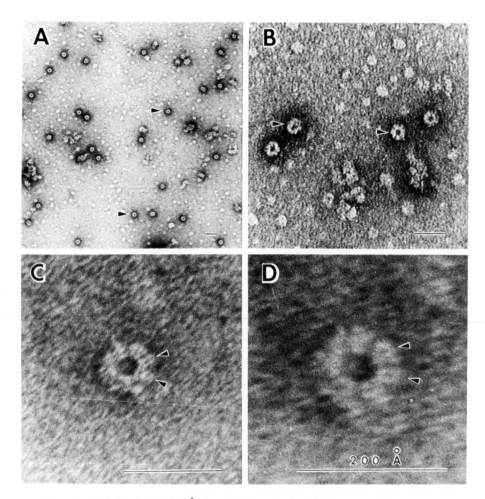

Fig. 43. "Miniparticles" (100 Å) found in the nucleoli of HeLa and Namalwa cells and in the medium. These particles contain a center dark area which gives them a "donut" appearance (A and B). At higher magnifications, 7 or 8 subunits are visible (C and D). Several of these subunits contain a dark center (D). These particles are rich in the antigen(s); their concentration is 10 or more times greater than in the nuclear Tris extract of HeLa cells. (A) × 150,000; (B) × 500,000; (C) × 1,600,000; (D) × 2,500,000. (Courtesy of Drs. N. Domae and F. Harmon.)

with other reported proteins of similar molecular weights and isoelectric points. As noted earlier (Marashi *et al.*, 1979), the antigen in Novikoff hepatoma nucleoli had a very similar molecular weight. Its lower p*I* of 5.1 probably reflects differences in amino acid content or modification which also may account for the differences in immunological properties by comparison to the human tumor nucleolar antigens.

A protein of much interest was the "src gene" product which has been studied in detail by Erickson's group (Erickson *et al.*, 1980; Collett *et al.*, 1978a,b). This protein has a similar molecular weight and p*I*, but it differs in cellular localization inasmuch as it is a membrane protein (Krueger *et al.*, 1980a,b). It is primarily localized to the nuclear envelope and jutanuclear reticular membrane structure in rat cells (Krueger *et al.*, 1980a) and on the plasma membrane of Rous sarcoma virus-transformed chicken fibroblasts. Kreuger *et al.* (1980a) proposed that the "pp60src" is a membrane protein that associates with cellular membranes by hydrophobic interactions. Collett and Erickson (1978) found the "src gene" product was a protein kinase but in our studies, the human tumor nucleolar antigens were not found to be phosphorylated or to exhibit properties of kinases.

To compare the structures of the nucleolar antigens with the "src

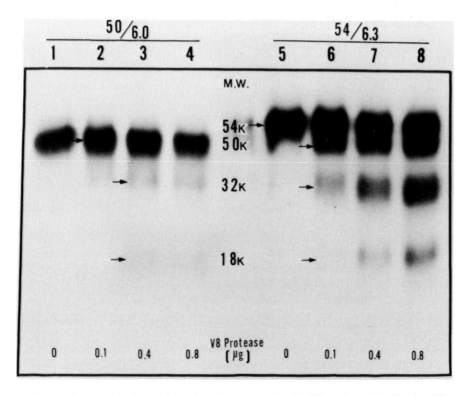

Fig. 44. Fractionation of the antigen fragments after the V8 protease digestion by 12% SDS–polyacrylamide gel electrophoresis. (1–4) The minor antigen. (5–8) The major antigen. (1 and 5) No enzyme added. (2 and 5) 100 ng enzyme. (3 and 7) 400 ng enzyme. (4 and 8) 800 ng enzyme.

gene'' product, the ^{125}I-labeled antigens were subjected to partial proteolysis with *Staphylococcal* V8 protease and chymotrypsin. Under the conditions employed, a number of cleavage products were detected (Fig. 44)
but these did not parallel those reported for the src gene product (Collett
et al., 1978). Although the products of protein 68/6.3 and 61/6.1 probably
were similar, they did not have identical cleavage patterns. Whether they
are similar in some structural respects remains to be determined.

Occasionally an autoimmune antiserum is produced which recognizes
all nucleoli. Such a product either has reacted to rDNA, RNA polymerase
I, U3-RNP, or common structural or processing proteins in human nucleoli. Inasmuch as we have been successful in immunizing rabbits to the
common nucleolar phosphoproteins C23 and B23 (110/5.1; 40/5.1) it is not
surprising that many types of determinants were identified by rabbit immune systems. To distinguish the nucleolar antigens 68/6.3 and 61/6.1
from other proteins, exhaustive absorptions are necessary and the best
results have been obtained with affinity absorption methods.

The immunological absorption techniques vary in their efficacy and in
their ability to remove conflicting reactants. One would like to have a
monospecific antibody for each of the antigens that would not recognize
other proteins. In these studies, this goal has not yet been achieved. Accordingly, there are problems of background, problems of ''false posi-
tives,'' false negatives, etc. Quite consistently, 95% of the tumors analyzed have developed bright nucleolar fluorescence but the problems of
differentiation of benign tumors and other disease states from malignant
tumors have not been adequately approached.

D. Malignant and Benign Tumors

It is interesting that the nucleolar antigen is found in 95% of the malignant tumor samples studied and in few, if any, of the benign tumors studies. One of the interesting questions with respect to growth is whether the
antigen is specifically in malignant tumors or whether it appears in the benign tumors. This has been a difficult question, not because it has been
found in benign tumors, but because some of the early studies in the fluorescence method lacked the present level of sophistication. In the course
of those studies, false positivies appeared in normal liver nucleoli and in
kidney nucleoli in some specimens. The false positive analysis was undertaken because four samples of benign breast tumors (sample numbers 24,
55, 58, and 73) were reported as positive in the ''blind study.''

As an approach to this study of the samples, the specimens were pretreated in a number of ways. When treated with preimmune serum followed by unlabeled second antibody as a preliminary step to bind the

"nonspecific" sites or with antibody that had been preabsorbed in a number of ways including with normal liver nucleoli, improved results with benign tumors have been more satisfactory (3 of 3) correct and some early samples were found to be negative. Further studies on benign tumors and other nontumor tissues are in progress.

Inasmuch as the antigen was mainly absent from nontumor cells and benign tumors, it may be related to rapid growth as discussed earlier (H. Busch *et al.*, 1979) in connection with the WI-38 and IMR-90 fetal lung fibroblast lines. It was suggested that a possible loss of the usual nucleolar matrix elements may make the antigen visible in such tissues and its detection in normal cells may be "blocked." Scheer and his associates (1980) have reported the presence of a "matrix" protein (145/6.3) in *Xenopus* nucleoli which may be responsible for the nucleolar configuration. It is possible that tumors may either not synthesize this protein or may substitute for the antigen in some way not yet clear.

ACKNOWLEDGMENTS

The original research in this report was supported by the Public Health Service–Nucleolar Antigen Grant CA27-27534, Michael E. DeBakey Fund, Pauline Sterne Wolff Memorial Foundation, William Stamps Farish Foundation, the Bristol-Myers Fund, and the Sally Laird Hitchcock Fund.

REFERENCES

Abelev, G. I., Engelhardt, N. V., and Elgort, D. A. (1979). *In* "Methods in Cancer Research" (H. Busch, ed.), Vol. XVIII, pp. 2–38. Academic Press, New York.
Bradford, M. (1976). *Anal. Biochem.* **72**, 248–254.
Busch, H. (1976). *Cancer Res.* **36**, 4291–4294.
Busch, H., and Smetana, K. (1970). "The Nucleolus." Academic Press, New York.
Busch, H., Gyorkey, F., Busch, R. K., Davis, F. M., and Smetana, K. (1979). *Cancer Res.* **39**, 3024–3030.
Busch, H., Busch, R. K., Chan, P. K., Daskal, Y., Gyorkey, F., Gyorkey, P., Kobayashi, M., Smetana, K., and Sudhakar, S. (1980). *Transplant. Proc.* **12**, 99–102.
Busch, H., Busch, R. K., Chan, P. K., Isenberg, W., Weigand, R., Russo, J., and Furmanski, P. (1981). *Clin. Immunol. Immunopathol.* **18**, 155–167.
Busch, R. K., and Busch, H. (1977). *Tumori* **63**, 347–357.
Busch, R. K., Daskal, I., Spohn, W. H., Kellermayer, M., and Busch, H. (1974). *Cancer Res.* **34**, 2362–2367.
Busch, R. K., Reddy, R. C., Henning, D. H., and Busch, H. (1979). *Proc. Soc. Exp. Biol. Med.* **160**, 185–191.
Bustin, M., and Kupfer, H. (1976). *Biochem. Biophys. Res. Commun.* **68**, 718–723.
Chan, P.-K., Feyerbend, A., Busch, R. K., and Busch, H. (1980). *Cancer Res.* **40**, 3194–3201.
Chan, P.-K., Frakes, R. L., Busch, R. K., and Busch, H. (1981). *Transplant. Proc.*, in press.
Collett, M. S., and Erikson, R. L. (1978). *Proc. Natl. Acad. Sci. U.S.A.* **75**, 2021–2024.

Collett, M. S., Brugge, J. S., and Erikson, R. L. (1978). *Cell* **15,** 1363–1369.

Davis, F. M., Busch, R. K., Yeoman, L. C., and Busch, H. (1978). *Cancer Res.* **38,** 1906–1915.

Davis, F. M., Gyorkey, F., Busch, R. K., and Busch, H. (1979). *Proc. Natl. Acad. Sci. U.S.A.* **76,** 892–896.

Erikson, R. L., Purchio, A. F., Erikson, E., Collett, M. S., and Brugge, J. S. (1980). *J. Cell Biol.* **87,** 319–325.

Field, A. K., Davies, M. E., and Tytell, A. A. (1980). *Proc. Soc. Exp. Biol. Med.* 524–529.

Fishman, W. H., and Busch, H., eds. (1979). "Methods in Cancer Research: Onco-Developmental Antigens," Vol. XVIII. Academic Press, New York.

Hilgers, J., Nowinski, R. C., Geering, G., and Hardy, W. (1972). *Cancer Res.* **32,** 98–106.

Hnilica, L., Chiu, J., Hardy, K., Furitani, H., and Briggs, R. (1978). *In* "The Cell Nucleus" (H. Busch, ed.), Vol. 5, pp. 307–334. Academic Press, New York.

Kelsey, D. E., Busch, R. K., and Busch, H. (1981). *Cancer Lett.* **12,** 295–303.

Krueger, J. G., Wang, E., and Goldberg, A. R. (1980a). *Virology* **101,** 25–40.

Krueger, J. G., Wang, E., Garber, E. A., and Goldberg, A. R. (1980b). *Proc. Natl. Acad. Sci. U.S.A.* **77,** 4142–4146.

Levy, H. B., and Sober, H. A. (1960). *Proc. Soc. Exp. Biol. Med.* **103,** 250–252.

Lowenstein, P. M., Lange, G. W., and Gerard, G. F. (1980). *Cancer Res.* **40,** 4398–4402.

Marashi, F., Davis, F. M., Busch, R. K., Savage, H. E., and Busch, H. (1979). *Cancer Res.* **39,** 59–66.

Merski, J., Daskal, Y., and Busch, H. (1976). *Cancer Res.* **36,** 1580–1584.

Mollenhauer, H. H. (1964). *Stain Technol.* **39,** 111–114.

Moriarty, G. C., and Halmi, N. S. (1972). *Z. Zellforsch.* **132,** 1–14.

Narayan, K. S., and Rounds, D. E. (1973). *Nature (London) New Biol.* **243,** 146–150.

O'Beirne, A. J., and Cooper, H. R. (1979). *J. Histochem. Cytochem.* **27,** 1148–1162.

Reiners, J. J., Jr., Davis F. M., and Busch, H. (1980). *Cancer Res.* **40,** 1367–1371.

Rothblum, L. I., Mamrack, P. M., Kunkle, H. M., Olson, M. O. J., and Busch, H. (1977). *Biochemistry* **16,** 4716–4720.

Smetana, K., Busch, R. K., Hermansky, F., and Busch, H. (1979). *Life Sci.* **25,** 227–234.

Sternberger, L. A. (1979). *In* "Immunocytochemistry." Wiley, New York.

Scheer, U. (1980). *Oxford Symp. Soc. Exp. Biol.*

Tan, E. M. (1979). *In* "The Cell Nucleus" (H. Busch, ed), Vol. 7, pp. 457–478. Academic Press, New York.

Yeoman, L. C., Jordan, J. J., Busch, R. K., Taylor, C. W., Savage, H. E., and Busch, H. (1976). *Proc. Natl. Acad. Sci. U.S.A.* **73,** 3258–3262.

CHAPTER IV

PROSTATE ANTIGEN OF HUMAN CANCER PATIENTS

M. C. WANG, M. KURIYAMA, L. D. PAPSIDERO,
R. M. LOOR, L. A. VALENZUELA,
G. P. MURPHY, AND T. M. CHU

I. Introduction

Prostate cancer is a prevalent disease for older men. The incidence of prostate cancer is second highest among all cancers in males. This malignancy is the third highest cause of cancer deaths for men (Silverberg, 1979). Prostate cancer, if detected at an early stage, is potentially curable (Schmidt and Pollen, 1979). Unfortunately, metastases have already occurred in the majority of cases when first diagnosed (Gittes and Chu, 1976). Therefore, it is of utmost importance to develop methods for early detection of prostate cancer. Equally important in controlling prostate cancer is the availability of parameters whereby the course or recurrence of the disease can be monitored effectively, so that proper and timely treatments can be executed. Ideally, such methods should possess a high degree of sensitivity and specificity for measurement of subtle biochemical changes associated specifically with prostate cancer in serum and other body fluids. In this regard, highly sensitive immunoassay proce-

179

dures, such as radioimmunoassay and enzyme-linked immunosorbent assay (ELISA), appear to be the methods of choice; not only are these procedures capable of detecting the picogram level of substances but they also are endowed with a high degree of sensitivity due to reactions between antigen and antibody. In developing immunoassay procedures for detecting prostate cancer, it is essential to search for antigenic markers that are associated with this disease. These antigens need not to be tumor-cell specific; they can be the antigens showing prostate specificity and be released into serum or other body fluids, where a quantitative change can be a specific indication for the occurrence of prostate cancer.

There are a number of previous studies in which human prostate-specific antigens are demonstrated (Ablin *et al.*, 1970; Flocks *et al.*, 1960; Moncure *et al.*, 1975; Shulman *et al.*, 1964). One of these antigens has been identified as prostatic acid phosphatase (PAP) by Ablin *et al.* (1970), Moncure *et al.* (1975), and Shulman *et al.* (1964). Various immunoassay procedures have been developed for assaying this enzyme in the serum of prostate cancer patients (Choe *et al.*, 1978, 1979; Cooper and Foti, 1974; Chu *et al.*, 1978; Foti *et al.*, 1975, 1978; Killian *et al.*, 1980; Lee *et al.*, 1978; Mahan and Doctor, 1979; McDonald *et al.*, 1978; Romas *et al.*, 1978; Vihko *et al.*, 1978, 1980). In this chapter, we shall describe a new prostate-specific antigen, distinct from PAP, which has been identified, purified, and evaluated in our laboratory to be of potential value as a diagnostic and prognostic marker in prostate cancer. Throughout this article and in our previous publications the term prostate antigen has been used to refer to this new prostate-specific antigen. It does not imply that there are no other non-PAP antigens yet to be identified that may possess specificity for prostate or prostate tumor.

II. Occurrence of Prostate Antigen (PA) in Human Prostate and Prostatic Fluid

A. IDENTIFICATION OF PA IN THE PROSTATE

A number of precipitin arcs were observed after subjecting crude extract of human prostate to immunoelectrophoresis employing antiserum produced from rabbit immunized with these extracts. Subsequent absorption of the antiserum with normal female serum, prior to immunoelectrophoresis, resulted in reduction of the precipitin arcs to two (Fig. 1). Further absorptions of the treated antiserum with normal female serum and with the extracts of other human tissues failed to abolish these two precipitins. However, if the antiserum was absorbed with crude extract of pros-

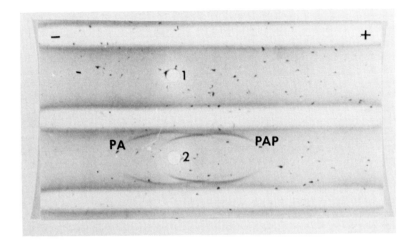

FIG. 1. Immunoelectrophoresis of the crude extract of normal prostate. Well 1, blank as control. Well 2, the extract. Troughs: normal female serum-absorbed rabbit antiserum to crude extract. Experimental conditions were as previously described (Wang *et al.*, 1979).

tate regardless of pathological origin, the reactive antibodies were neutralized and no precipitin arc was formed in immunoelectrophoresis. One of the two precipitin arcs represents PAP, as identified by its reactivity with acid phosphatase staining solution. The inference from the results of these experiments (Wang *et al.*, 1979) is that an antigen, in addition to PAP, specific to prostate is present in extracts of the prostate. This conclusion is substantiated further by experiments with the use of an antiserum, collected from rabbits immunized with a partially purified PA preparation which was devoid of PAP. This anti-PA serum reacted with the extract of prostate, but not with that of kidney, bladder, liver, intestine, pancreas, lung, breast, or spleen in double immunodiffusion (Wang *et al.*, 1979). Prostate specificity of the antiserum was confirmed by further experiments in which a more sensitive rocket immunoelectrophoresis technique (Papsidero *et al.*, 1981) was employed. The results showed that PA was detectable in all of the normal, benign, and cancerous prostate specimens examined, but not in other normal or malignant tissues (Table I).

B. IDENTIFICATION OF PA IN PROSTATIC FLUID AND SEMINAL PLASMA

To investigate if PA is a secretory product of the prostate and released into prostatic fluid, both prostatic fluid and seminal plasma were allowed

TABLE I

Specificity of PA as Examined by Rocket Immunoelectrophoresis

Tissue source	Number of specimens[a]	Number of PA positive[b]
Prostate, normal	11	11
Prostate, BPH	24	24
Prostate, carcinoma	17	17
Others (normal and cancerous)[c]	28	0

[a] Prior to testing, protein concentration of all specimens was adjusted to approximately 10 mg/ml.

[b] Sensitivity of the rocket immunoelectrophoresis employed was 0.5 μg/ml.

[c] Other tissues included liver, spleen, lung, bladder, breast, intestine, heart, pancreas, kidney, and cerebral cortex (Papsidero et al., 1981).

to diffuse against rabbit anti-PA serum in an agarose gel. As shown in Fig. 2, precipitin lines were formed indicating the presence of PA in the specimens. Fused lines seen in the figure also indicate the immunological identity among the reactive PA in prostatic fluid, seminal plasma, and that of normal, benign hypertrophic (BPH) and cancerous prostates.

Concentration of PA in seminal plasma specimens collected from different individuals was determined with radial immunodiffusion technique (Mancini et al., 1965) and found to range from 0.41 to 1.78 mg/ml with mean and standard deviation (SD) of 0.70 ± 0.38 ($n = 11$). PA content in prostatic fluid was even higher, reaching 3.6 mg/ml in some specimens examined.

C. Concentration of PA in the Prostate

It has been reported that total acid phosphatase activity, on a per gram tissue basis, was less in cancerous prostate than in normal or benign hypertrophic prostate on the average (Grayhack et al., 1977; Kircheim et al., 1964; Reif et al., 1973; Woodard, 1952). Recently, Loor et al. (1980) found that PAP activity per microgram DNA or per cell was decreased in cancerous prostate as compared with the activity in normal or benign hypertrophic prostate. These observations were of interest from the standpoint of studying carcinogenic processes of prostate malignancy, and thus prompted us to examine whether a quantitative difference in PA concentration also occurred in malignant prostatic tissues. As revealed in Table II, there is no significant difference in PA concentration, per gram tissue or per milligram DNA, among normal, BPH, and cancerous prostates.

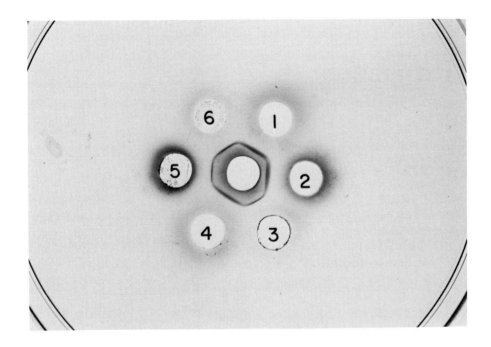

FIG. 2. Demonstration of PA in seminal plasma by double immunodiffusion. Center well, anti-PA serum. Wells 1 and 4, crude extracts of normal prostate obtained from two different individuals. Well 2, prostatic fluid. Well 3, crude extract of cancerous prostate tissue. Well 5, seminal plasma. Well 6, crude extract of BPH prostate. Protein concentration of sample in each well ranged from 10 to 20 mg/ml. Immunodiffusion was carried out as previously described (Chu *et al.*, 1977).

D. CELL LOCALIZATION OF PA IN THE PROSTATE

Papsidero *et al.* (1981) have probed the localization of PA in prostate as well as the specificity of this antigen with the immunoperoxidase staining technique of Heyderman and Neville (1977). Tissue sections were incubated with rabbit anti-PA serum and subsequently washed to remove the excess serum. The tissue sections were then incubated with peroxidase-labeled goat anti-rabbit γ-globulin, washed, and stained for peroxidase activity. Under these experimental conditions, if a tissue section contained PA, an immune complex, PA/anti-PA antibody/anti-γ-globulin peroxidase, would be formed, resulting in a positive stain. It was observed that the staining was restricted to epithelial cells comprising the prostate ductal elements (Fig. 3). Within prostatic ductal cell elements, positively

TABLE II
CONCENTRATION OF PA IN PROSTATES[a]

Pathology	Number of specimens	μg PA/gm tissue	μg PA/mg DNA[b]
Normal	7	49–304 (120 ± 89)[c]	12–85 (38.5 ± 23.8)[c]
BPH	16	33–207 (95 ± 57)	9–117 (36.8 ± 25.7)
Cancerous	9	26–353 (118 ± 123)	8–82 (33.6 ± 25.1)

[a] Concentration of PA was measured by the ELISA method (Kuriyama *et al.*, 1980).

[b] DNA was extracted from the homogenate of tissue with 10% trichloroacetic acid at 90°C and the concentration was determined by the method of Burton (1956).

[c] Range (mean ± SD given in parentheses).

stained secretory materials were evident. Specific staining was not seen for other cell components of the prostate, including the stromal and vascular elements. Furthermore, PA was not detected in the tissue sections of other organs, including breast, pancreas, colon, stomach, and liver. Using a similar immunohistochemical technique, Nadji *et al.* (1981) de-

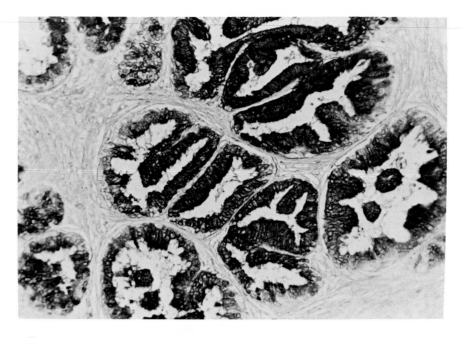

FIG. 3. Immunoperoxidase staining of formalin-fixed paraffin-embedded prostatic tissue section. The tissue section was incubated with rabbit anti-PA serum and then with peroxidase-labeled goat anti-rabbit γ-globulin as described in the text. Strong staining (dark areas) of peroxidase was found within the cytoplasm of ductal epithelial cells. No counterstain. × 200.

tected PA in the ductal epithelia of normal and hyperplasmic prostate as well as in primary and metastatic prostatic tumor. However, PA was not detected in the epithelia of periurethral glands, seminal vesicle, vas deferens, transitional epithelium, of urinary bladder and prostatic urethra or glandular lining of Von Brune's nest, or cystitis glandularis, nor was PA detected in normal or nonprostatic malignant tissues from testis, kidney, intestine, stomach, salivary gland, pancreas, liver, and breast.

III. *In Vitro* and *in Vivo* Expressions of PA by Human Prostate Tumor

To determine if malignant prostatic cells in long-term culture retain the expression of PA, cultured cells of three established lines, which originated from prostatic carcinoma metastasized to lymph node (LNCaP), lumbar vertebra (PC-3), and brain (DU-145), were extracted and analyzed with an ELISA procedure (see Section VI) for the presence of PA (Papsidero *et al.*, 1981). Results showed that LNCaP and PC-3 cells contained PA. In the spent culture fluids of LNCaP and PC-3 cells, PA was also detected. However, PA was not detected in the cultured cells originated from human fibroblast, lymphoma, carcinomas of the colon, thyroid, breast, pancreas, bladder, and skin, nor was PA detected in the spent culture fluids of these cells.

Expression of PA was also retained by DU-145 and LNCaP cells implanted in athymic nude mice. In sera of the tumor-bearing mice, PA was detected and found to have concentration of 12 to 22 ng/ml; sera of nude mice carrying human melanoma, bladder carcinoma, and pancreatic carcinoma contained no PA (Papsidero *et al.*, 1981). The extract of a LNCaP tumor and of DU-145 tumor exercised from nude mice was shown by ELISA to contain PA. Isoelectric focusing of the extract of LNCaP xenograft revealed that it contained more alkaline PA isomers (see Section IV,B) as compared with prostatic tissues collected at surgery or autopsy (unpublished observation).

IV. Purification and Characterization of PA from the Prostate and Seminal Plasma

A. PURIFICATION

Since BPH tissues and seminal plasma are more readily available than normal or cancerous prostatic tissues, we have purified PA from BPH tissues and seminal plasma.

In our original published procedure (Wang *et al.*, 1979), the crude extract of BPH tissues was first subjected to fractional precipitation with ammonium sulfate. At the salt concentration of 20 to 80% saturation, PA was almost quantitatively recovered from crude extract. The optimal salt concentration for precipitation was found between 45 and 50% saturation. In order to avoid contamination with other proteins as much as possible, the fraction between 35 and 55% saturation, which comprised approximately 60 to 70% of total PA, was collected. This preparation was subsequently applied to a DEAE-BioGel A anion exchange column, which at pH 8.0 effectively retained PA obtained from the ammonium sulfate precipitation. PA was partially separated from other proteins and dissociated from the DEAE column by NaCl at concentrations from 17 to 78 mM during concentration gradient elution (Fig. 4). Further purification of PA was achieved by means of gel filtration on Sephadex G-100 and G-75 columns, where PA was detected in the fractions corresponding to a molecular weight of 33,000. Upon rechromatography on a Sephadex G-75 column, a single symmetrical protein peak containing PA activity was obtained. However, polyacrylamide gel electrophoresis revealed heterogeneity of this preparation. Therefore, in the final step of purification, an additional preparative polyacrylamide gel electrophoresis was employed. Under our experimental conditions, PA activity emerged from the gel column from 4 to 9 hours of electrophoresis; but only those fractions collected between 8 and 9 hours of electrophoresis showed homogeneity in protein species upon analytical polyacrylamide gel electrophoresis.

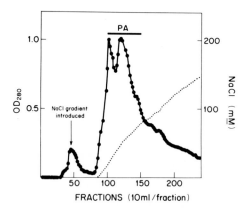

FIG. 4. Elution profile of PA from a DEAE-BioGel A column with a NaCl concentration gradient solution. Experimental details have been described elsewhere (Wang *et al.*, 1979). Horizontal bar indicates the fractions which reacted with anti-PA serum in double immunodiffusion.

Although the procedure described above yielded pure PA, the recovery was very low, often less than 0.5 mg of purified PA was obtained from 100 gm of BPH tissues. The procedure was time consuming and required painstaking preparation of a preparative gel column in a special apparatus. In addition, technical problems such as clogging of the elution channel often developed during preparative gel electrophoresis. Therefore, in order to provide purified PA for development and large scale clinical testing of immunoassay procedures, we have simplified the aforementioned purification procedure and improved the yield (Wang *et al.*, 1981b). The improved procedure is briefly described as follows. After ammonium sulfate precipitation as in the previous procedure, PA was applied to a short (2.5 × 15 cm) DEAE-BioGel A column, preequilibrated with 0.01 M Tris–HCl buffer, pH 7.7 to 8.0. After washing the column with the buffer, PA was eluted out with 80 mM NaCl and then subjected to gel fil-

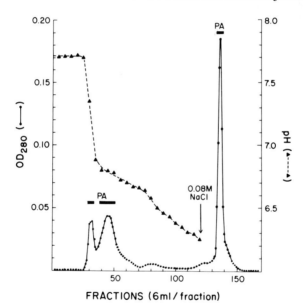

FIG. 5. Purification of PA by chromatography on DEAE-BioGel A column using pH gradient solution as eluant. Partially purified PA preparation (4.6 ml containing 10 mg total protein) from Sephadex G-100 column was applied to a 2.5 × 20 cm DEAE-BioGel A column, preequilibrated with 0.01 M Tris–HCl buffer, pH 7.7. The column was then eluted with a pH gradient solution (mixer, 300 ml 0.01 M Tris–HCl, pH 7.0; reservoir, 500 ml Tris–HCl, pH 6.0). At the end of pH gradient elution, 0.08 M NaCl in 0.01 M Tris–HCl, pH 7.7, was applied to the column. Each fraction was analyzed for PA with the double immunodiffusion technique. Horizontal bars indicate the fractions reacted with anti-PA serum in double immunodiffusion. In some experiments, no partition of PA reactivity in the first two peaks was seen (bars fused) even though two protein peaks were evident.

tration on a Sephadex G-100 column. Fractions containing PA were pooled and chromatographed on a DEAE BioGel A column (2.5 × 20 cm), using a pH gradient solution as eluant. As revealed in Fig. 5, two protein peaks, both containing PA, appeared between pH 7.5 and 6.7 and a third PA-containing peak appeared when the column was washed with 80 mM NaCl at the end of the pH gradient elution. Only the preparation obtained from the second peak showed a single protein band in polyacrylamide gel electrophoresis. Therefore, for obtaining homogeneous PA, only the second peak fractions were collected. This procedure yielded 1 to 2 mg of purified PA per 100 gm of BPH tissues. Because of the use of shorter DEAE colunmns and elimination of the Sephadex G-75 step, the time required for purification was reduced to 8 to 9 days.

PA also was purified from seminal plasma by the improved procedure described above. The yield was 1 to 2 mg per 10 ml of seminal plasma. The purified PA from seminal plasma showed immunologic and physicochemcial characteristics identical to those of PA purified from BPH tissues. Seminal plasma has become the preferred material for PA isolation as it provides some advantages. Several hours are usually required to extract PA from BPH tissue, which is omitted when seminal plasma is used. Also, it is clear from the experimental data described in Sections II,B and C that seminal plasma contains a higher PA concentration (mean: 700 μg/ml) than BPH tissues (mean: 95 μg/gm tissue or ca. 110 μg/ml tissue); thus, for example, 12 ml of pooled seminal plasma from different individuals yielded approximately the same amount of PA as 100 gm of pooled BPH tissues. Moreover, seminal plasma is more readily available than BPH tissues, and contains less contaminating proteins, such as hemoglobin, which makes the isolation of PA an easier task.

B. CHARACTERIZATION

PA was extractable from prostate specimen with 0.154 M NaCl, 0.02% disodium(ethylenediamine)tetraacetate phosphate-buffered saline, pH 6.8, 0.01% Tween 80, and 3 M KCl, but not with 1 M perchloric acid, suggesting it is not a glycoprotein high in carbohydrate content, such as carcinoembryonic antigen (Terry *et al.*, 1974).

Purified PA from BPH tissues and seminal plasma have been partially characterized (Wang *et al.*, 1979, 1981a). It is a glycoprotein containing approximately 10% (w/w) carbohydrate and having a molecular weight of 33,000 as determined by molecular sieving on a Sephadex G-75 column. Upon sodium dodecyl sulfate–polyacrylamide gel electrophoresis, it gave a single band on the gel which was located at a position of 34,000 molecular weight, indicating it contained a single polypeptide. In sucrose density gradient ultracentrifugation, a single protein band with a sedimentation coefficient of 3.1 S was detected. The isoelectric point of the purified preparation was found to be around 6.9. Using preparative isoelectric focusing and a sensitive ELISA technique (see Section VI), several isomers of PA were observed in crude extract of prostatic tissue and in seminal plasma and, therefore, pI of 6.9 should be considered as that of one particular isomer that has been purified. Proportion as well as the number of isomers in the prostate and in seminal plasma varied among specimens. Figure 6 shows an isomeric pattern as revealed in a BPH specimen. As shown, a total of five isomers with pIs ranging from 6.8 to 7.5 were detected. Treatment of the extract with neuraminidase converted isomers with pI 6.8 and to those with higher pI values (7.1 and above). These results indicated that the observed variations in the pI value reflected, at least in part, a difference in the sialic acid content. It is possible that charge microheterogeneity of PA in crude preparations may also have resulted from the association of PA to other molecules. Whether or not these isomers represent molecular species differing in their protein moiety remains to be studied.

PA is a highly immunogenic protein in animals. It is easy to produce xenoantisera in rabbits, mice, goats, and baboons. At least half of the animals immunized with purified PA or crude extract of prostate produced anti-PA antibodies. The antigenic reactivity of PA in the crude extract is stable for at least 1 week at room temperature (in the pH range of 6 to 8).

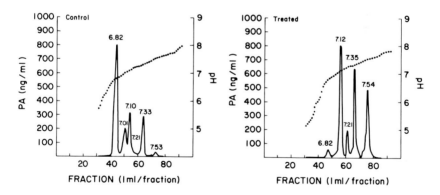

FIG. 6. Demonstration of PA isomers in a crude extract of BPH tissue by isoelectric focusing technique. Control, 2 ml of the extract (12 mg total protein) was subjected to isoelectric focusing in an LKB 8100 type 110 ml apparatus according to the LKB instruction manual. Treated, 2 ml of the same extract (as control) was treated with 0.8 mg neuraminidase (0.16 unit) in 0.1 M sodium acetate buffer, pH 5.0, for 48 hours at room temperature and then subjected to isoelectric focusing. Crude extract incubated under the same conditions but in the absence of neuraminidase gave a similar PA isomeric pattern as the control.

PA is immunologically distinct from PAP; it does not react with anti-PAP serum, nor does PAP react with anti-PA serum (Papsidero *et al.*, 1980).

V. Occurrence of PA in Serum

A. IDENTIFICATION OF PA IN SERUM BY ROCKET IMMUNOELECTROPHORESIS

As stated, one of the major objectives of our study is to develop immunodiagnostic procedures for the detection of early stage prostate cancer. It is, therefore, imperative to demonstrate the presence of PA in the sera of patients with prostate cancer. Initially, a rocket immunoelectrophoresis was used to detect PA (Papsidero *et al.*, 1980). In this preliminary study, serum samples obtained from 20 normal young adults and 20 male volunteers over the age of 55 years showed no reactivity against the antiserum; and the sera drawn from 175 patients with various advanced nonprostate cancer showed no reactivity either. However, 17 out of 219 sera from advanced prostate cancer patients showed the presence of PA.

To determine the immunological relationship between the antigen in tissue and in serum, immunological ''peak enhancement'' experiments were carried out (Papsidero *et al.*, 1980). In these experiments, samples of sera exhibiting elevated PA level and extracts of prostate specimens were subjected to rocket immunoelectrophoresis separately and after mixing. When assayed individually, each sample gave rise to a single immunoprecipitate peak on the plate. Mixtures of serum and tissue extracts also produced a single immunoprecipitation reaction and the peak height was greater than that of the individual samples. In addition to peak height enhancement, immunoprecipitation fusion occurred, showing the immunological identify of antigens from sera and prostate.

B. ISOLATION AND PARTIAL CHARACTERIZATION OF SERUM PA

After gel filtration of sera from prostate cancer patients on a Sephadex G-100 column, PA reactivity was detected at the fractions with molecular weight between 90,000 and 100,000. Since purified PA of the prostate and seminal plasma has a molecular weight of 33,000 to 34,000, the circulating protein reactive with anti-PA serum was further isolated and characterized (Papsidero *et al.*, 1980). Sera were first subjected to an affinity chromatography on a Sepharose 4B–anti-PA IgG column. The eluate was shown to contain PA activity and some normal serum components. After iodination, the preparation was incubated with rabbit antihuman whole serum to remove normal serum components. The preparation, free of normal serum components, was then incubated with rabbit anti-PA serum and with Pansorbin (*Staphylococcus aureus* containing Protein A). After centrifugation, the immunoprecipitate was dissociated with 2% sodium dodecyl sulfate, and subjected to sodium dodecyl sulfate–polyacrylamide gel electrophoresis. A major radioactive peak, located at a position corresponding to molecular weight 36,000, was detected. From these data, it was inferred that circulating PA appeared to polymerize or was associated with other proteins in the serum.

VI. Enzyme-Linked Immunosorbent Assay (ELISA) of Serum PA

The observation that some patients with prostate cancer, although small in number, had PA in their sera as examined by rocket immunoelectrophoresis had led us to the development of a more sensitive ELISA procedure (Kuriyama *et al.*, 1980).

The principle of this sandwich-type ELISA procedure for quantitation of PA is graphically illustrated in Fig. 7. The sample to be assayed for antigen is first incubated with insolubilized antibody, then centrifuged and washed to remove any unbound materials. In the second step, the washed

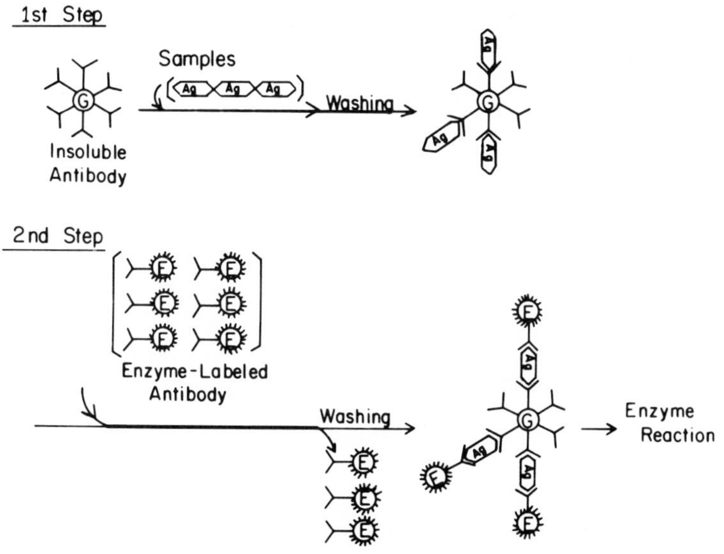

FIG. 7.   Scheme of the sandwich-type ELISA procedure for quantitation of antigen. Ag, antigen: G, insolubilized IgG antibody; E, enzyme.

solid-phase immune complex is incubated with enzyme-labeled antibody to form a sandwich immune complex, insoluble antibody/antigen/antibody enzyme, which is separated from free enzyme-labeled antibody by centrifugation and subsequent washing of the precipitated sandwich immune complex. The enzyme activity of the precipitate is then determined. Under antibody excess conditions, the amount of enzyme-labeled antibody bound and precipitated (and hence the enzyme activity associated with the sandwich immune complex) is related to the concentration of antigen in the sample. In our ELISA procedure for quantitation of PA, the insoluble antibody in the first step of the procedure is CNBr-activated Sepharose 4B–anti-PA IgG conjugate, and the enzyme-labeled antibody in the second step is peroxidase–anti-PA IgG conjugate. Preparations of these conjugates are schematically described in Figs. 8 and 9. Our ELISA procedure for PA determination is described briefly as follows:

1. The sample (100 μl) was incubated with Sepharose 4B–anti-PA IgG suspension (300 μl) for 3 hours at room temperature.

2. After centrifugation, the precipitate was washed three times with 1 ml of washing buffer (0.01 M phosphate-buffered saline, pH 7.1, containing 1% bovine serum albumin and 10 mM disodium(ethylenediamine)tetraacetate).

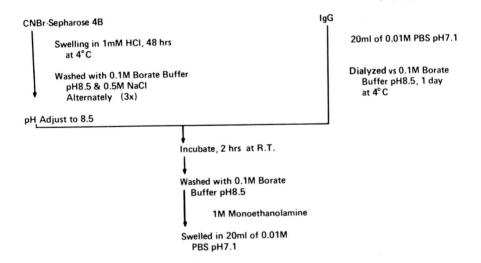

FIG. 8. Insolubilization of anti-PA IgG on Sepharose 4B beads. Anti-PA IgG (130 mg) was coupled to CNBr-activated Sepharose 4B (5 gm) according to the manufacturer's (Pharmacia) procedure with some modifications (Lee *et al.*, 1978). PBS, Phosphate-buffered saline, pH 7.1.

3. Peroxidase-labeled anti-PA IgG (100 μl) was added to the washed precipitate, and incubated at room temperature for 18 hours.

4. The incubation mixture was centrifuged and the precipitate washed three times with 1 ml of washing buffer.

5. To the precipitate 3 ml of peroxidase substrate solution (0.0083% o-dianisidine and 0.003% H_2O_2 in 0.01 M phosphate-buffered saline, pH 6.0) was added and incubated at room temperature for 90 minutes.

6. The enzyme reaction was terminated by the addition of 100 μl of 1 N HCl, followed by centrifugation.

7. Absorbance of the supernatant was read at 403 nm.

8. Percentage of peroxidase bound was calculated, taking maximal peroxidase binding at a PA concentration of 462 ng/ml as 100%.

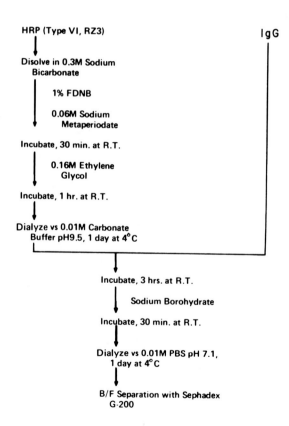

FIG. 9. Labeling of anti-PA IgG with peroxidase. The method of Nakane and Kawaoi (1974) was used to link 5 mg of horseradish peroxidase (HRP) to 5 mg of anti-PA IgG. FDNB, Fluorodinitrobenzene; R. T., room temperature; B/F, bound and free HRP or IgG.

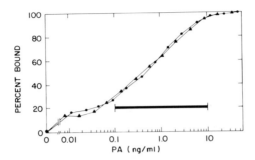

FIG. 10.. Standard calibration curve of PA as determined by ELISA procedure. Horizontal bar designates working range of the procedure. Circle, purified PA; triangle, a serum specimen of prostate cancer.

Prior to the assay, the optimal amount of IgG conjugate to be added to the incubation mixture should be determined. As shown in Fig. 10, PA concentration as low as 0.1 ng/ml can be detected with this ELISA technique.

VII. Diagnostic and Prognostic Potential of Serum PA in Prostate Cancer

To assess the possible diagnostic value of serum PA levels, Kuriyama *et al.* (1980) determined, with the ELISA procedure, the concentration of PA in the sera of normal controls, of nonprostate cancer patients, and of prostate cancer patients. Sera from 51 apparently healthy male volunteers were found to have PA levels ranging from less than 0.1 to 2.6 ng of PA/ml of serum. Taking nondetectable levels (<0.1 ng/ml, in 55% of these volunteers) as 0.1 ng/ml, the mean $\pm$ standard deviation (SD) of serum PA levels in normal male controls was calculated to be 0.47 ± 0.66 ng/ml. The circulating PA in 92 nonprostate male cancer patients was found in a range similar to that of normal controls. In half of these patients, the serum PA level was not detectable (less than 0.1 ng/ml). As expected, serum PA was not detectable in 17 normal females and 25 female cancer patients. Sera from 19 BPH patients showed a range of PA concentrations from 0.7 to 8.0 ng/ml with mean $\pm$ SD of 3.4 ± 2.05. The PA concentrations in the sera of prostate cancer patients were found to range from 0.3 to 270 ng/ml, with mean $\pm$ SD for each clinical stage as follows: stage A, 4.8 ± 4.55 ($n = 8$); stage B, 5.0 ± 4.12 ($n = 34$); stage C, 10.1 ± 15.86 ($n = 56$); and stage D, 24.2 ± 30.62 ($n = 344$). When the upper cut-off point was set at 1.79 ng/ml (mean $\pm$ 2 SD of normal controls), 68% of BPH, 63% of stage A, 79% of stage B, and 85% of stage D prostate cancer patients had an elevated level of serum PA.

Statistical analysis with the use of Student's *t* test revealed that serum

PA levels of BPH patients were significantly ($p < 0.001$) higher than those of normal individuals and nonprostate cancer patients, as were those of patients with stage A, B, C, and D prostate cancer. There was no significant difference in serum PA levels among BPH, stage A, and stage B patients. However, stage C and stage D patients exhibited significantly ($p < 0.01$ and <0.001, respectively) elevated PA levels when compared with BPH patients. Although the quantitation of serum PA concentration does not determine whether a patient had BPH or early stage prostate cancer, BPH can be differentiated from the prostate cancer by other procedure such as biopsy. Hence, abnormal levels of serum PA can be regarded as an early warning sign of prostatic abnormality, and further examination of the patient subsequently should be performed. This may lead to an increase in the detection of early stage prostate cancer. It is pertinent to mention that serum PA levels in the patients were not correlated to serum levels of PAP, a commonly used diagnostic marker of prostate cancer. In many instances, where PAP concentration in the serum was within the normal range, serum PA concentration was found to be elevated, and vice versa. Thus, simultaneous determination of serum PA and PAP levels led to a higher detection rate of these markers in prostate cancer (unpublished observations).

The prognostic value of serum PA levels has also been assessed (Kuriyama *et al.*, 1981). In 96 patients with stage D_2 prostate cancer and receiving chemotherapy, the pretreatment level of serum PA was found to relate to patients' survival. Patients ($n = 10$) who survived more than 12 months had PA level of 11.2 ± 12.7 ng/ml (mean $\pm$ SD), and those ($n = 39$) who died within 5 months exhibited PA level of 28.5 ± 31.9; levels of 13.7 ± 18.2 were found in the patients ($n = 27$) who survived 6 to 11 months. When the serum PA levels of 19 of these patients were followed for more than 6 months, it was observed that in 14 patients (74%) there was a clinicopathological correlation between PA level and the clinical course. Additionally, in another group of 32 patients who underwent curative therapies for localized prostate tumor, the serum PA levels were monitored during a period of 12 to 114 weeks (average 56 weeks). Of these patients, 5 developed metastasis during this period and all were found to exhibit increasingly elevated PA values, 0 to 68 weeks before the clinical diagnosis of the recurrence of disease.

VIII. Summary

A human PA has been identified in the prostate (normal, BPH, and cancerous) and seminal plasma as well as in human prostate carcinoma cells in culture and in nude mice. The antigen is not found in other human tissues *in vivo* and *in vitro*. Using the immunoperoxidase staining technique, this antigen has been shown to localize in ductal epithelium of the prostate. In crude extract of human prostate and in seminal plasma, PA appears to exist in several isomeric forms, one of which has been purified and found to have molecular weights of 33,000 and 34,000, contain a single polypeptide, have a p*I* of 6.9 and a sedimentation coefficient of 3.1 S, and contain approximately 10% (w/w) of carbohydrate. Purified PA is devoid of acid phosphatase activity and does not react with anti-PAP antibodies, thus it is biochemically and immunologically distinct from PAP.

Circulating PA has been demonstrated in human and nude mice bearing human prostate carcinoma. PA in human serum has molecular weight of 90,000 to 100,000 as determined by molecular sieving, but has a molecular weight of 36,000 upon sodium dodecyl sulfate–polyacrylamide gel electrophoresis. Serum PA is immunologically identical to PA of prostate. A sandwich-type ELISA procedure, capable of detecting 0.1 ng of prostate antigen/ml, has been developed and employed to assess serum level of the antigen. Results showed that circulating PA levels in BPH and in prostate cancer patients were significantly elevated as compared with those in normal males or males with nonprostate cancer. Although no quantitative difference in serum PA levels was found among BPH, stage A, and stage B prostate cancer patients, patients with stage C or stage D prostate cancer exhibited significantly elevated PA levels, quantitatively and qualitatively. Serum PA levels in prostate cancer patients were found to be of value in predicting survival time, monitoring clinical course, and predicting early recurrence of the cancer.

ACKNOWLEDGMENTS

Our work reported in this chapter was supported in part by Grant CA-15437 awarded by the National Cancer Institute through the National Prostatic Cancer Project. The authors thank Ms. J. Ogledzinski for secretarial assistance and Ms. B. Galloway for technical support.

REFERENCES

Ablin, R. J., Bronson, P., Soanes, W. A., and Witebsky, E. (1970). *J. Immunol.* **104**, 1329–1339.
Burton, K. A. (1956). *Biochem. J.* **62**, 315–323.
Choe, B. K., Pontes, E. J., Morrison, M. K., and Rose, N. R. (1978). *Arch. Androl.* **1**, 227–233.
Choe, B. K., Rose, N. R., Korol, M., and Pontes, E. J. (1979). *Proc. Soc. Exp. Biol. Med.* **162**, 396–400.
Chu, T. M., Wang, M. C., Scott, W. W., Gibbons, R. P., Johnson, D. E., Schmidt, J. D., Loening, S. A., Prout, G. R., and Murphy, G. P. (1978). *Invest. Urol.* **15**, 319–323.
Cooper, J. F., and Foti, A. (1974). *Invest. Urol.* **12**, 98–102.
Flocks, R. H., Urich, V. C., Patel, C. A., and Opitz, J. M. (1960). *J. Urol.* **84**, 134–143.

Foti, A. G., Herschman, H., and Cooper, J. F. (1975). *Cancer Res.* **35**, 2446–2452.

Foti, A. G., Cooper, J. F., and Herschman, H. (1978). *Clin. Chem.* **24**, 140–142.

Gittes, R. F., and Chu, T. M. (1976). *Semin. Oncol.* **3**, 123–130.

Grayhack, J. T., Wendel, E. F., Lee, C., and Oliver, L. (1977). *Cancer Treat. Rep.* **61**, 205–210.

Heyderman, E., and Neville, A. M. (1977). *J. Clin. Pathol.* **30**, 138–143.

Killian, C. S., Vargas, F. P., Lee, C. L., Wang, M. C., Murphy, G. P., and Chu, T. M. (1980). *Invest. Urol.* **18**, 219–224.

Kircheim, D., Gyorkey, F., Brandes, D., and Scott, W. W. (1964). *Invest. Urol.* **1**, 403–421.

Kuriyama, M., Wang, M. C., Papsidero, L. D., Killian, C. S., Shimano, T., Valenzuela, L. A., Nishiura, T., Murphy, G. P., and Chu, T. M. (1980). *Cancer Res.* **40**, 4568–4662.

Kuriyama, M., Wang, M. C., Papsidero, L. D., Killian, C. S., Inaji, H., Slack, N., Pontes, E. J., Murphy, G. P., and Chu, T. M. (1981). *Proc. Am. Assoc. Cancer Res.* **22**, 293.

Lee, C. L., Wang, M. C., Murphy, G. P., and Chu, T. M. (1978). *Cancer Res.* **38**, 2871–2878.

Loor, R. M., Wang, M. C., and Chu, T. M. (1980). *J. Cell Biol.* **87**, 283a.

McDonald, I., Rose, N. R., Pontes, E. J., and Choe, B. K. (1978). *Arch. Androl.* **1**, 235–239.

Mahan, D. E., and Doctor, B. P. (1979). *Clin. Biochem.* **12**, 10–17.

Mancini, G., Carbonara, O., and Heremans, J. F. (1965). *Immunochemistry* **2**, 235–254.

Moncure, C. W., Johnston, Jr., C. L., Koontz, Jr., W. W., and Smith, M. J. V. (1975). *Cancer Chemother. Rep.* **59**, 105–110.

Nadji, M., Tabei, S. Z., Castro, A., Chu, T. M., Murphy, G. P., Wang, M. C., and Morales, A. R. (1981). *Cancer* **48**, 1229–1232.

Nakane, P. K., and Kawaoi, A. (1974). *J. Histochem. Cytochem.* **22**, 1084–1091.

Papsidero, L. D., Wang, M. C., Valenzuela, L. A., Murphy, G. P., and Chu, T. M. (1980). *Cancer Res.* **40**, 2428–2432.

Papsidero, L. D., Kuriyama, M., Wang, M. C., Horoszewicz, J. S., Leong, S. S., Valenzuela, L. A., Murphy, G. P., and Chu, T. M. (1981). *J. Natl. Cancer Inst.* **66**, 37–41.

Reif, A. E., Schlesinger, R. M., Fish, C. A., and Robinson, C. M. (1973). *Cancer* **31**, 689–699.

Romas, N. A., Hsu, K. C., Tomashefsky, P., and Tannenbaum, M. (1978). *Urology* **12**, 79–83.

Schmidt, J. D., and Pollen, J. (1979). *In* "Prostatic Cancer" (G. P. Murphy, ed.), pp. 129–150. PSG Publ. Littleton, Massachusetts.

Shulman, S., Mamrod, L., Gonder, M. J., and Soanes, W. A. (1964). *J. Immunol.* **93**, 474–480.

Silverberg, E. (1979). *CA-A Cancer J. Clin.* **29**, 6.

Terry, W. D., Henkart, P. A., Coligan, J. E., and Todd, C. W. (1974). *Transpl. Rev.* **20**, 100–129.

Vihko, P., Sajanti, E., Jänne, O., Peltonen, L., and Vihko, R. (1978). *Clin. Chem.* **24**, 1915–1919.

Vihko, P., Kostama, A., Janne, O., Sajanti, E., and Vihko, R. (1980). *Clin. Chem.* **26**, 1544–1547.

Wang, M. C., Valenzuela, L. A., Murphy, G. P., and Chu, T. M. (1979). *Invest. Urol.* **17**, 159–163.

Wang, M. C., Kuriyama, M., Loor, R. M., Li, S. C., and Chu, T. M. (1981a). *Fed. Proc. Fed. Am. Soc. Exp. Biol.* **40**, 1564.

Wang, M. C., Valenzuela, L. A., Murphy, G. P., and Chu, T. M. (1981b). *Oncology,* in press.

Woodard, H. Q. (1952). *Cancer* **5**, 235–241.

CHAPTER V

PROSTATIC ACID PHOSPHATASE: A MARKER FOR HUMAN PROSTATIC ADENOCARCINOMA

BYUNG-KIL CHOE AND NOEL R. ROSE

I. Introduction

The prostatic acid phosphatase has served as a useful biological marker of the metastatic prostatic carcinoma for the last 4 decades (for review see Bodansky, 1972). Since Shulman and his co-workers (1964) demonstrated this enzyme to be a prostate-specific antigen, numerous immunological assay methods have been developed and these assays have given new hope for a role for this enzyme in the detection and staging of prostatic carcinoma. Since Foti *et al.* (1977) reported a radioimmunoassay for prostatic acid phosphatase that was claimed to detect intracapsular disease in a large percentage of patients, several laboratories have investigated the feasibility of mass screening of asymptomatic patients with localized prostatic carcinoma. The advantage of immunological assay seems to be the recognition of metastasis at early stage of disease. Furthermore, immunohistological investigation of bone marrow aspirates, regional lymph nodes, and other remote metastatic loci may serve as an useful auxillary diagnostic method to surgical pathologists.

From the viewpoint of basic oncology, the carcinogenesis, neoplastic progression, and the factors which determine the metastasis of prostatic cancer remain enigmas. In the past, lack of proper tissue-specific markers have made it difficult to investigate the mechanisms of tumor progression in prostatic carcinomas using the cultured or transplanted tumor as models. Although much information about the regulation of prostatic acid phosphatase biosynthesis is still lacking, the enzyme is known to be controlled by androgens since it is decreased by orchiectomy or hypophysectomy. It has been suggested that in the prostate as well as other tissues (Franks, 1980; Heatfield et al., 1980; Kastendieck and Altenähr, 1979) basal cells are progenitors of differentiated cells. Prostatic acid phosphatase may well serve as a marker for the investigation of basal cell differentiation, renewal, and malignant transformation in conjunction with other markers such as steroid receptors and prostate antigen (Wang et al., 1980).

II. Prostatic Acid Phosphatase

A. Purification

Since the discovery of acid phosphatase in human erythrocytes, several purification procedures have been reported. They were recently reviewed by Bodansky (1972). The procedure that has been adopted currently by most investigators was described by Ostrowski and his co-workers (1970). The method includes extraction and dialysis, ammonium sulfate precipitation, Sephadex G-100 filtration, and DEAE-cellulose chromatography. Final filtration through a Sephadex column yields a preparation with a specific enzyme activity of 240–300 IU/mg protein at 25°C (Derechin et al., 1971). The enzyme preparations thus purified are suitable for the enzymological and structural studies.

For the development of immunological assay methods, combinations of methods based on different principles must be employed to obtain prostatic acid phosphatase (PAP) free of impurities as judged by both immunochemical and physicochemical methods. The method currently in use in our laboratory will be described for illustrative purposes. All operations are carried out at 0–4°C. Concentration of dilute preparations is accomplished by ultrafiltration using dialysis membrane of exclusion limit, MW 10,000 under negative pressure at 4°C.

Step 1. Crude preparation: If the prostate tissue obtained from surgery or autopsy is used as the starting material, the tissue is sliced into approximately 1-mm^3 cubes and homogenized in a mixer (Sorvall-Omni) with 5 volumes of 0.1 M acetate buffer, pH 5.0. The homogenate is centrifuged at 5000 g for 30 minutes and the supernate successively centrifuged at 15,000 g for 30 minutes and at 100,000 g for 60 minutes. If pooled human seminal plasma is used as the starting material, it is simply clarified by successive centrifugations at 15,000 g and 100,000 g for the time periods described above. Particulate materials such as crystals, cell debris, membrane fragments, and ribosomes are thus eliminated.

Step 2. Ammonium sulfate fractionation: Ammonium sulfate, either as the 100% saturated solution or as fine powder, is added to the crude supernatant to obtain approximately 33% saturation. The solution was stirred gently for 1 hour in the cold room, then centrifuged at 15,000 g for 30 minutes. The supernatant, which contains the enzyme, is placed in dialysis tubings and dialyzed against 0.02 M acetate buffer, pH 4.2 overnight. If the volume of the preparation is too great, it may be reduced to approximately 5 ml by ultrafiltration. Then, the concentrated preparation should be equilibrated with 0.05 M acetate buffer, pH 4.0. If any precipitate is noticed, the solution should be centrifuged at 15,000 g for 30 minutes before ion-exchange chromatography. Globulins are partially eliminated at this step.

Step 3. Ion-exchange chromatography: The enzyme-containing fraction is absorbed on a CM-Sephadex column (2.5 × 45 cm) which was previously equilibrated with 0.05 M acetate buffer, pH 4.0, and the column is eluted with acetate buffer of increasing pH (4.0 to 5.2) and ionic strength (0.1 to 0.4 M). The pH and ionic strength gradient was generated by dropwise mixing of 0.4 M acetate buffer, pH 5.2, to a constant volume of 0.1 M acetate buffer, pH 4.0. Eluted fractions are assayed for enzyme activity and protein concentration. Fractions containing the highest enzyme activity are pooled, concentrated, and dialyzed against 20 volumes of elution buffer for the concanavalin A (Con A) affinity column. At this step of purification serum globulins (mostly IgG) and transferrins are strongly bound to the column due to their relatively high isoelectric points (pI 7.0 and 5.8) under these elution conditions. Serum albumin (pI 4.7) and PAP (pI 4.0–5.2) are weakly bound and eluted slowly by the increasing pH and ionic strength of the buffer. Haptoglobulins (pI 4.1) appear as the first eluting protein.

Step 4. Con A affinity chromatography (Van Etten and Saini, 1978): Enzyme fraction is absorbed on a Con A column and washed with elution buffer until albumin is eliminated. The bound PAP is then eluted with 0.5 M methyl-2-D-glucopyranoside in the same buffer. Concanavalin A–

Sepharose 4B matrix is available from commercial sources (e.g., Pharmacia, Uppsala, Sweden); however, it is also simple to conjugate concanavalin A to CNBr-activated Sepharose 4B in the laboratory. A small Con A column (1 to 5 ml) is made in a small syringe plugged with siliconized glass-wool and equilibrated with 0.1 M acetate buffer, pH 6.0, containing 1 M NaCl, 1 mM CaCl$_2$, 1 mM MgCl$_2$, and 1 mM MnCl$_2$. All three ions (Ca^{2+}, Mg^{2+}, and Mn^{2+}) are required for the maintenance of the tetrameric structure of concanavalin A, a protein of MW 55,000 from *Canavalia einsformis* (Jack bean), binds α-D-mannose and N-acetyl-D-glucosamine as a tetramer (Goldstein *et al.*, 1974). At this step albumin, a nonglycoprotein, is not bound to the column matrix and is eliminated by washing. PAP, a glycoprotein (Derechin *et al.*, 1971) with α-D-Man and N-acetyl glucosamine, specifically binds to the Con A and is eluted by a high concentration (0.5 M) of methyl-1-α-D-glucopyranoside which competes for binding to Con A. However, it is imperative to wash the Con A–Sepharose 4B matrix thoroughly with elution buffer prior to enzyme absorption and to investigate the leakiness of Con A protein from the matrix by spectrophotometric monitoring of the "washout" fraction at 280 nm. The bulky enzyme solution obtained at Con A chromatographic step should be concentrated to a small volume and equilibrated in 0.05 M acetate buffer, pH 5.0.

Step 5. Gel filtration: The purified enzyme is further isolated by gel filtration in a Sephacryl S-200 column (1.8 × 90 cm) previously equilibrated with 0.05 M acetate buffer, pH 5.0. The enzyme thus purified was found to be stable for over 3 months at 4°C and over a year at -25°C in the presence of 30% glycerol. Throughout the purification steps the purity of the enzyme preparation was examined by double immunodiffusion in agarose using various test antisera. γ-Globulin, serum albumin, transferrin, and haptoglobulin were the major extraneous proteins in the crude supernatant. Therefore, antisera to these proteins as well as the antiserum against "crude supernatant" were used as the test antisera.

Enzyme activity is estimated by incubating the preparation (5–10 μl) for 1 minute at room temperature with 0.1 M acetate buffer, pH 5.0, and 5 mM p-nitrophenyl phosphate as substrate, in a final volume of 0.5 ml. The reaction is started by the addition of enzyme and stopped by 2.0 ml of 0.25 N NaOH. The absorbance of the liberated p-nitrophenol is read at 410 nm. One unit of enzyme is defined as that amount that catalyzes the hydrolysis of 1 μmole of p-nitrophenyl phosphate per minute. Specific activity is expressed as units per milligram protein. The protein is estimated according to the Lowry method (Lowry *et al.*, 1951) using bovine serum albumin as the standard. Concentrations of purified enzyme solution are determined by absorbance measurement at 280 nm, assuming $E_{1\,cm}^{1\%} = 14.4$ (Derechin $et\ al.$, 1971). The enzyme thus purified is free of impurities as judged by immunochemical criteria and has a specific enzyme activity of 400–500 IU/mg protein at 37°C.

Recently, Vihko and his associates (1978) and Van Etten and Saini (1978) described a rapid and specific purification method by the use of a tartrate-affinity column. When such a specific affinity column matrix becomes available commercially, the task of PAP purification will be greatly simplified.

B. Molecular Properties

Purity of the enzyme preparations is evaluated in our laboratory according to the following criteria: (1) homogeneity and molecular weight of

TABLE I

Some Properties of Human Prostatic Acid Phosphatase[a]

Physical	
Molecular weight	102,000 at pH 7.0[b]
Sedimentation coefficient ($s_{20,w}$)	5.62[b]
Isoelectric points	4.05–5.2[c,f]
Extinction coefficient, $E_{1\,cm}^{1}$ at 280 mm	14.4[b]
Mobility on agar electrophoresis	β mobility at pH 8.6[b]
Subunit	50,000[d,f]
Chemical	
Total amino acid residues	764[b]
N-Terminal amino acid	Arginine[g,h]
N-Acetylneuraminic acid residues	6
Carbohydrate content	12.8%[b]
pH optimum	4.8–6.0[e]
Specific enzyme activity (IU/mg at 37°C)	500[e,h]
Immunochemical	
Antigenicity of polypeptide residues	Multiple, unique determinants[f]
Antigenicity of carbohydrate residues	Not demonstrated[f]
Materials cross-reacting with PAP	Not clearly identified yet[f]

[a] Adapted from Choe $et\ al.$ (1981a) with permission of the publisher.
[b] Derechin $et\ al.$ (1971).
[c] Ostrowski $et\ al.$ (1970).
[d] Luchter-Wasyl and Ostrowski (1974).
[e] Van Etten and Saini (1978).
[f] Choe $et\ al.$ (1978a,b, 1980c, 1981b).
[g] Ostrowski (1963).
[h] Choe $et\ al.$ (unpublished)

the protein in the SDS–polyacrylamide gel electrophoresis, (2) immuno-chemical homogeneity, (3) specific enzyme activity, (4) amino acid composition, and (5) N-terminal amino acid determination. For the last 20 years PAP has been studied for its physicochemical properties by Ostrowski and co-workers (Ostrowski, 1980). Some of their findings are summarized in Tables I and II.

The PAP is a glycoprotein of molecular weight approximately 100,000 with varying amounts of carbohydrate (Ostrowski et al., 1970). This heterogeneity in carbohydrate content, particularly neuraminic acid residues, gives rise to several discrete electrophoretic isozymic forms in this enzyme (Smith and Whitby, 1968; Ostrowski et al., 1970). The PAP exhibits a single homogeneous band in SDS–polyacrylamide gel electrophoresis, or SDS–8 M urea polyacrylamide gel electrophoresis and has an estimated molecular weight of 45,000 to 50,000 under reducing conditions (Fig. 1). Tryptic peptide mapping and other evidence suggested that the PAP consists of indistinguishable subunits of 50,000 (Luchter-Wasyl and Ostrowski, 1974). Arginine has been identified as the N-terminal

TABLE II

AMINO ACID COMPOSITION OF HUMAN PROSTATIC ACID PHOSPHATASE

Amino acids	Integral residues	
Aspartic acid	54[a]	50[b]
Threonine	50[a]	46[b]
Serine	54[a]	52[b]
Glutamic acid	100[a]	100[b]
Proline	50[a]	56[b]
Glycine	42[a]	40[b]
Alanine	27[a]	24[b]
Valine	34[a]	33[b]
Methionine	20[a]	16[b]
Isoleucine	27[a]	27[b]
Leucine	93[a]	100[b]
Tyrosine	43[a]	44[b]
Phenylalanine	32[a]	30[b]
Histidine	26[a]	32[b]
Lysine	45[a]	42[b]
Arginine	33[a]	32[b]
Cysteine	18[a]	18[b]
Tryptophan	18[a]	—
Total	764	742

[a] Adapted from Derechin et al. (1971) with permission of the publisher.

[b] Recalculated on the basis of PAP subunit MW 45,000 from Choe et al. (1981b) and from Choe et al. (unpublished).

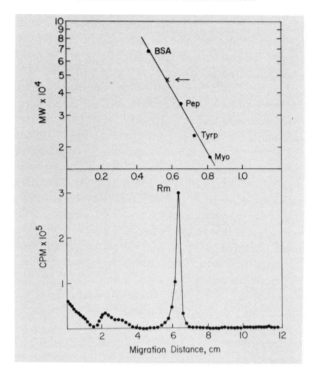

FIG. 1. Sodium dodecyl sulfate–polyacrylamide gel electrophoresis of human prostatic acid phosphatase. A mixture of ^{125}I-labeled (10 ng) and unlabeled prostatic acid phosphatase (100 ng) was immunoprecipitated with rabbit anti-PAP antibody and goat anti-rabbit IgG antibody. Tube gels were cut, and radioactivity in 2-mm gel slices was determined. Most of the ^{125}I label migrated as a single band corresponding to the molecular weight of 48,000. The mobilities of unlabeled PAP (50 μg) which is stained with Coomassie blue and that of ^{125}I-labeled PAP are identical.

amino acid of PAP and a subunit (Ostrowski, 1963; Choe, unpublished). The amino acid composition and tryptic peptide map reported by Ostrowski and co-workers (Derechin *et al.*, 1971; Luchter-Wasyl and Ostrowski, 1974) are quite reproducible (Choe *et al.*, unpublished).

III. Antibodies to Prostatic Acid Phosphatase

A. ANTIGENIC PROPERTIES OF PROSTATIC ACID PHOSPHATASE

Although antisera specific for PAP are readily prepared, little is known about the antigenic structure of the PAP molecule. PAP has been first demonstrated to be a prostate-specific marker antigen by Shulman and co-workers (1964). An immunochemical difference between lysosomal and prostatic acid phosphatases has been found by Choe *et al.* (1978a,b, 1980c). The antigenic specificity of PAP seems to reside in the protein portion of the molecule rather than in the neuraminic acid residues. Therefore, electrophoretic isozymic forms of PAP are antigenically indistinguishable (Choe *et al.*, 1978a). To date, anti-PAP antisera prepared against acid phosphatase derived from prostatic fluid, prostatic extracts, or seminal plasma in different laboratories have been immunochemically indistinguishable. Antigenic determinants of whole molecule (dimer) of PAP are conserved in subunits after the 8 M urea dissociation (Fig. 2). Cyanogen bromide cleavage of the subunits yielded several polypeptide fragments; one of the fragments seems to retain a unique antigenic determinant (Choe *et al.*, 1981b). In the hope of mapping the unique and cross-reactive antigenic determinants on a PAP molecule, several hybridoma lines secreting anti-PAP antibodies were generated in this laboratory. Some of the monoclonal antibodies distinguish PAP from lysosomal acid phosphatase (Lillehoj *et al.*, 1980). These immunochemical findings will soon provide a clearer definition of antigenic determinants in terms of peptide structure. With this structural information it will be feasible to ask pertinent questions about the biosynthesis and secretion of PAP and its regulation by androgen and estrogen in prostatic epithelial cells.

B. RABBIT ANTIBODIES TO PROSTATIC ACID PHOSPHATASE

In general, short immunization programs produce highly specific antibodies without producing antibodies against trace contaminant proteins in the enzyme preparation. Usually 250 μg to 1 mg of highly purified PAP suspended in saline or buffer is emulsified in an equal volume of complete Freund's adjuvant. Commercially available adjuvants (DIFCO, Detroit, MI or Calbiochem, LaJolla, CA) seem to be satisfactory, but home made adjuvant may be used. Single or multiple intramuscular injections of well-emulsified PAP is recommended. Subcutaneous injections of PAP emulsified in complete Freund's adjuvant often lead to sterile abscess formation, resulting in the loss of the depot. One to three months after the primary inoculation, the same dose of PAP emulsified in incomplete Freund's adjuvant is given subcutaneously in order to minimize the chance of anaphylactic shock. Test bleedings are done between 5 and 7 days after the booster injection. PAP antibody titers can be evaluated by counterimmunoelectrophoresis. If the antibody titer is high enough, rabbits are bled, 20 to 40 ml per bleeding, every third day for 3 weeks. The animals should then be rested for some weeks before being boosted and bled again.

Counterimmunoelectrophoresis for the Antibody Titration
(*Choe* et al., 1980b)

a. Materials. Prostatic acid phosphatase preparation: 100 ng/ml in electrophoresis buffer containing 1% bovine serum albumin. Anti-PAP serum: Serial dilutions in electrophoresis buffer. Gel: 2% agarose in distilled water. Electrophoresis: 0.05 M barbital buffer, pH 7.5 to 8.0, ionic strength 0.025. Histochemical stain for acid phosphatase (Burstone, 1962): Naphothol-AS-MX-phosphoric acid (Sigma), it is insoluble in water, therefore 20 mg is dissolved in 0.5 ml of N,N-dimethylformamide. Then, 20 ml of 0.2 M acetate or citrate buffer (pH 5.0) is added. To this, 20 mg of Fast Garnet GBC (O-aminoazotoluene, diazonium salt, Sigma) is

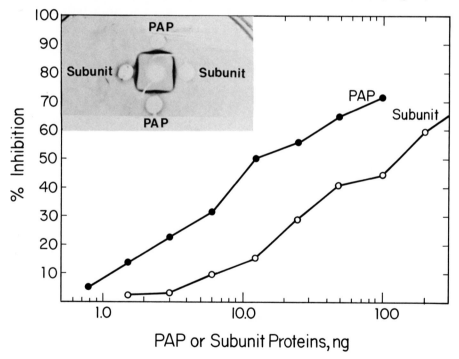

FIG. 2. Antigenic determinants of human prostatic acid phosphatase. PAP and subunit showed line of identity in the Ouchterlony double diffusion plates when reacted against anti-PAP antibody. Competitive inhibitions of binding of ^{125}I-labeled PAP or subunit to anti-PAP antibody in the presence of various concentrations of unlabeled PAP or subunit. Parallel regression lines suggest antigenic identity.

dissolved. If an insoluble dye residue persists, the solution is filtered before use. The stain is prepared fresh every day.

b. Procedure.

1. Molten 2% agarose solution is diluted with an equal volume of prewarmed (55°C) electrophoresis buffer and mixed carefully. Approximately 8 ml of 1% agarose is spread on a 5.5 × 7-cm size slide with a prewarmed pipet and the agar is allowed to solidify for 20 to 30 minutes and stored.

2. Prior to use, wells (2 mm diameter) are punched 5 mm apart in a row. Another parallel row of wells is punched at a distance of 8 to 10 mm opposite the first row of wells.

3. The slide is placed in an electrophoresis apparatus in such a way that one row of wells faced the anode and the other row faced the cathode. Wet filter paper wicks are attached to the edges of the agar slide and electrophoresis buffer is added.

4. Five microliters of standard PAP is added to the wells on the cathode side and 5 μl of serially diluted anti-PAP serum is added to the wells on the anode side.

5. Electrophoresis is carried out at 4°C for 50 minutes or longer at a constant current of 15 mA. At the end of the run, the slide is immersed into the Burston's histochemical staining solution for acid phosphatase activity for 60 minutes at room temperature. A purple or violet precipitin line develops if a PAP–anti-PAP complex is present, and the staining reaction is stopped by immersing the slide in 4% acetic acid solution.

An anti-PAP serum showing precipitin lines at a 100-fold dilution or higher will be useful for radioimmunoassay, immunoenzyme assay, and immunohistological studies. When such antisera are available, it is necessary to examine the specificity. The specificity of the antiserum is evaluated by testing against human serum, crude enzyme preparation, and the purified PAP either by immunoelectrophoresis or by double diffusion precipitation in agar gel.

C. Murine Monoclonal Antibodies to Prostatic Acid Phosphatase

The hybridoma technique pioneered by Köhler and Milstein (1975) provides a tool to generate hybrid lines secreting monoclonal antibodies of different classes and of specificities. Application of this technique to human PAP (Lillehoj *et al.*, 1980) produced several monoclonal antibodies to PAP. These reagents provide us with an opportunity to map the antigenic determinants and identify the functional domains of the PAP molecule. In this technique spleen cells of mice, previously immunized with PAP, are fused by polyethylene glycol with murine myeloma cells. Resulting hybrid clones are examined for their secretion of anti-PAP antibodies.

1. Materials

Washing medium: RPMI 1640 (GIBCO, Grand Island, NY).

Growth medium: Iscove modified Dulbecco–Eagle's minimal essential medium (IMEM) (GIBCO) supplemented with gentamycin (Schering Corp., Kenilworth, NJ), L-glutamine (4 mM), and 15% fetal calf serum, is designated complete IMEM.

Polyethlene glycol (PEG) MW 1000 to 1500 (Baker, Phillipsburg, NJ). A bottle of PEG is warmed in a 60–65°C water bath to melt the PEG. Molten PEG is dispensed into 1-ml portions in glass tubes and autoclaved. For fusion experiments a stock tube of PEG is melted and mixed with 2.33 ml of prewarmed sterile RPMI 1640 to obtain 30% (v/v) and maintained at 42°C in a water bath until use.

Murine myeloma cells: P3-X63/NS-1 (NS/1), a k chain secreting P3-X 63-Ag 8 subline (Köhler et $al.$, 1976) and X-63-Ag8. 653, a nonsecreting subclone of P3-X63-Ag8 (Kearney et $al.$, 1979) is maintained in an Iscove medium containing 20 μg/ml of 8-azaguanine. These myeloma cell lines and their parental line, P3-X63-Ag8, have lost hypoxanthine-phosphoribosyltransferase (HGPRT) activity and therefore die in HAT medium.

Aminopterin (100×): to 1.74 mg of aminopterin add 25 ml of distilled water and 1.2 ml of 2 N NaOH; when dissolved, add distilled water to 100 ml and neutralize the solution slowly with 0.2 ml of 2 N HCl.

Hypoxanthine (100×): 136.1 mg/100 ml distilled water, heat at 45°C for 1 hour to dissolve.

Thymidine (100×): 38.7 mg/100 ml distilled water.

8-Azguanine (8-AG) (100×): Add 152 mg 8-AG to 100 ml of 6 M HCl and boil under the hood until dissolved. Aliquot 5/ml tube and store frozen.

Glutamine (50×): 200 mM glutamine (GIBCO).

Glycine (100×): 112.5 mg/100 ml distilled water.

Iscove–HAT medium: 1 part each of hypoxanthine (H), aminopterin (A), thymidine (T), and glycine are added to 96 parts of a complete Iscove medium and filter sterilized by a 0.22-μm membrane (Littlefield, 1964).

8-Azaguanine medium: 1 ml of 8-azaguanine is added to a complete Iscove medium containing 2 mM glutamine and neutralized slowly with 1 ml of 6 M NaOH. Filter sterilize through a 0.22-μm membrane.

NH$_4$Cl (0.17 M): Medium for lysis of erythrocytes. Washed spleen cells are resuspended in 5 ml of 0.17 M NH$_4$Cl, kept on ice for 5 to 10 minutes, then 10 ml of cold medium with 20% serum is added. Pellet the spleen cells and count the viable cells.

2. Procedures

Fusion and feeding of hybrid cells and the cloning of antibody-secreting hybridomas are performed as described by Kenneth et al. (1980). The hybridoma technique and its applications have been reviewed by several authors recently (Melchers et al., 1978; Kenneth et al., 1980).

The steps involved in the procedure to generate hybrid lines are outlined in Fig. 3. A few steps particularly important to the generation of hybrid cells secreting anti-PAP antibodies will be described.

a. Immunization of Mice.   Five- to seven-week-old female BALB/c mice are injected subcutaneously with 100 μg of PAP emulsified in complete Freund's adjuvant. Booster injections are given 40 to 60 days after the primary injection; 100 μg PAP emulsified in incomplete Freund's adjuvant is given subcutaneously. Three days prior to fusion 100 μg of PAP (dissolved in saline) is given intravenously to each mouse.

b. Fusion.   The fusion does not always work. Often a repetition of the fusion procedure without obvious changes results in successful hybridization. The conditions of treatment are critical for successful hybridization. With a low concentration of PEG (e.g., 0.3 ml of 30% PEG) the treatment period lasts for 5 to 8 minutes. However, if a higher concentration (e.g., 1 ml of 50% PEG) is used the treatment period may be reduced to 1 to 3 minutes, timed from the moment of addition of fusogen to the washing step.

c. Screening for the PAP Antibody-Producing Clones.   Culture supernatants are tested for the presence of PAP antibody by the immunoenzyme assay which will be described in detail in the next section. Briefly, 100 μl of supernatant is incubated for 2 hours at 4°C with 10 ng/100 μl of PAP (a partially purified preparation is adequate for this screening assay). Antibodies bound to PAP are precipitated by anti-mouse Ig rabbit serum. After washing the precipitate the pellets are assayed for enzyme activity. Clones which do not secrete anti-PAP antibodies are eliminated from the feeding schedule at an early stage.

d. Growth of Hybrid Myeloma Cells.   Cloned hybrid cells producing monoclonal anti-PAP antibodies are grown into mass cultures and the secreted antibodies are characterized for their specificity and binding characteristics by a radioimmunoassay which will be described in the next section. Hybrid cells grown in Iscove–HAT medium are transferred to fresh Iscove–HT medium. Davidson and Ephrussi (1970) noted that sudden transfer of cells grown in HAT to HAT-free medium resulted in cell degeneration and that this cell death could be prevented by transfer into an intermediate, HT medium. The HT-adapted cells are then transferred to normal Iscove MEM. When the hybrid cells are grown in a 100-mm petri dish, the cells can be preserved by freezing in small vials (1 ml/vial) or inoculated into peritoneum of a normal BALB/c mouse. When the vials

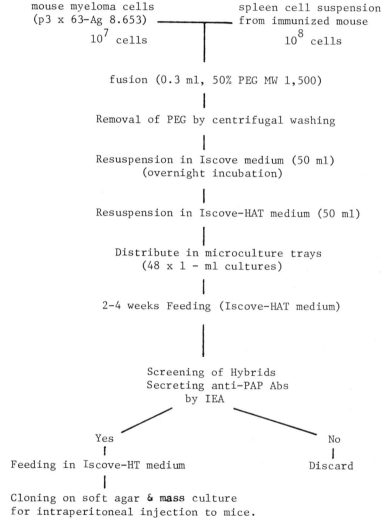

FIG. 3. Flow chart of the procedure for Köhler–Milstein's hybridoma technique.

of frozen cells are thawed the cells are resuspended in 5 ml of Iscove MEM and plated in 60-mm dishes. Successful fusions have been obtained in syngeneic, allogeneic, and xenogeneic combinations. Fusion of NS-1 cells to immunized mouse spleen cells resulted in three hybridoma-secreting PAP antibodies which do not cross-react with lysosomal acid phosphatase (Lillehoj *et al.*, 1980; Choe *et al.*, 1980c).

IV. Immunological Assays

A. METHODOLOGY

Immunochemical assay methods for PAP are based either on competitive binding or on enzymological assays of immune complexes. Radioimmunoassay (RIA) represents a competitive binding assay and a double antibody RIA has been used by many investigators. The RIA has been widely applied to the clinical investigations and it is now possible to evaluate its performance in the light of clinical findings (Choe *et al.*, 1980b). Extensive reviews of theory and practice of RIA for diverse systems have been published (Berson and Yalow, 1973; Ekins *et al.*, 1968; Hunter, 1973; Jaffe and Behrman, 1974).

A solid-phase fluorescent immunoassay (Lee *et al.*, 1978) and immunoenzyme assay (Choe *et al.*, 1980a) measure the concentration of antigen by its catalytic activity after the precipitation of antigen–antibody complexes. There are advantages and disadvantages of both the competitive binding assay (e.g. RIA) and the enzymological immunoassay (e.g., fluorescent immunoassay and immunoenzyme assay). The immunologic enzyme assays are as sensitive as or superior to RIA in their performance. However, the clinical application of these techniques has not been extensive.

B. DOUBLE-ANTIBODY RADIOIMMUNOASSAY (CHOE *et al.*, 1980a,b)

1. Radioiodination of PAP

Prostatic acid phosphatase is iodinated by a modification of the procedure of Hunter and Greenwood (1962). The lactic dehydrogenase method (Thorell and Johansson, 1971) yields a degree of iodination similar to the chloramine-T method. To a small plastic test tube are added in sequence 50 μl of 0.5 *M* phosphate, pH 7.4, 10 μl of a 1.0 mg/ml solution of pure acid phosphatase, 20 μl of Na ^{125}I, 10 mCi/200 μl (in NaOH), and 10 μl phosphate buffer containing chloramine-T, 2.0 mg/ml. To minimize damage to the protein, the iodination is terminated within 30 seconds by the addition of 10 μl sodium metabisulfite, 3.0 mg/ml in phosphate buffer. The reaction mixture is applied to a 0.6 × 20-cm column of Sephadex G-75 (superfine). The column can be conveniently prepared in a 10-ml plastic disposable pipet plugged with siliconized glass-wool. The column is usually equilibrated with 0.1 M phosphate buffer, pH 7.4 and a small quantity (usually 1–2 mg in a 100 to 500 μl volume) of bovine serum albumin is passed through the column, then washed and equilibrated before the separation of ^{125}I-labeled PAP. ^{125}I-labeled PAP is eluted with 0.1 M phosphate buffer, 0.5-ml fractions are collected, and 5-μl aliquots are sampled and counted. The labeled PAP emerges in the first peak of radioactivity in the void volume. The ^{125}I-labeled PAP is diluted in buffer containing bovine serum albumin, 2 mg/ml, and stored in the refrigerator or frozen.

The aliquots were examined for enzyme activity and immunoreactivity after incubating them overnight at 4°C in the presence of excess antibody. Binding by excess antibody has averaged about 85%. The specific activity of the preparation can be estimated by the self-displacement method according to the RIA procedure; evaluation of the mass of radioiodinated PAP, from the specific enzyme activity of the preparation, gives similar specific radioactivity. The calculated specific activity of our preparations has averaged 10 to 22 μCi/μg. The ^{125}I-labeled PAP, stored frozen or at 4°C, is stable for 6 to 8 weeks.

2. Prostatic Acid Phosphatase Standard

PAP standards are provided in commercial RIA kits. However, PAP can be purified in the laboratory and tested for its impurities and specific enzyme activity as described in the previous sections. Concentrations of purified enzyme solutions are determined by absorbance measurement at 280 nm, assuming $E_{1\,cm}^{1\%} = 14.4$ according to Ostrowski (Derechin et al., 1971). A 1 mg/ml stock solution is made in 0.1 M acetate, pH 5.0 containing 30% glycerol, aliquoted, and stored frozen. Further dilutions can be made from the stock using proper diluents; in cases of clinical assays of serum or plasma PAP, normal human female serum is used; in case of PAP measurement in cell culture supernatant or cell extracts, tissue culture medium containing fetal calf serum or bovine serum albumin has been used as the diluent. Conveniently, 10 μl of stock solution is diluted into 3.99 ml of plasma to obtain 250 ng/ml, then serial dilutions are made to generate 250, 125, 62.5, 31.2, 15.6, 7.8, 3.9, 1.9, and 0.98 ng/ml solutions. Aliquots (100 μl) were placed in many 10 × 75-mm tubes and stored at −20°C until used. The control tubes contained 100 μl of the PAP-free plasma from women. The same standards were used for both RIA and IEA.

3. Evaluation of Antisera

The optimal titer of antibody, either rabbit antisera or monoclonal murine hybridoma antibodies, is determined by testing serum dilutions of antisera in a series of tubes containing small amounts (10 to 100 pg) of labeled PAP. Tubes are incubated at 4°C for 1 to 3 days before separation of bound and free PAP. The range to be covered can be determined by making a wide range of dilutions. The dilution of the antibody used in the assay may be taken as the dilution at which 50% of label is bound to antibody (B/F—1.0).

4. Assay Procedure

The radioimmunoassay should be performed in duplicate; in addition to the assay tubes, each sample is measured with a control tube to which normal serum is added in place of antiserum. The primary immune complex is to be separated with precipitating second antibody; to form a precipitate of satisfactory size, 1.0–5.0 μg of carrier normal γ-globulin from the same species of animal from which the primary antibody was derived is added in the diluent. The diluent used is phosphate-buffered saline, pH 7.4, containing 0.01 M EDTA.

Approximately 0.05 to 0.1 ng (100 μl) of ^{125}I-labeled PAP is added to 100 μl of the unknown serum samples or standards and the antigen–antibody interaction was initiated by adding of 100 μl of diluted anti-PAP serum. Anti-PAP rabbit serum (R22-3) is diluted in normal rabbit γ-globulin (1 : 100 in diluent) as carrier. The 20,000-fold dilution of R22-3 used in the standard assays gives approximately 65% of binding of ^{125}I-labeled PAP in the absence of competing unlabeled antigen. To improve the sensitivity of the assay, we have used 40,000-fold diluted R22-3 on some occasions. Optimal incubation times for the PAP radioimmunoassay range from 1 to 3 days (Fig. 4).

After a primary incubation (48 hours at 4°C), 100 μl of a 10-fold diluted goat antiserum to rabbit immunoglobulins is added and the tubes are further incubated for 10 minutes at 4°C. The dilution of antiserum is based on preliminary titration experiments. The 10-fold diluted anti-rabbit Ig goat serum can precipitate essentially all PAP–anti-PAP immune complexes within 5 minutes at 4°C. Cold diluent, 1 ml, is added to each tube which is then centrifuged at 3000 g for 15 minutes at 4°C. After aspirating the supernatants, the radioactivity of the pellets is measured by a gamma counter. Standard curves are prepared by plotting the percentage bound (after the correction with nonspecific binding blank) on the ordinate and the concentration of PAP standard per milliliter on the abscissa (Fig. 4). Unknown values are read from the curve by finding the concentration of

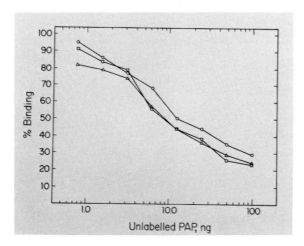

FIG. 4. A typical standard curve for our PAP radioimmunoassay. Various dilutions of rabbit anti-PAP serum (R22-3) are used: (○) 1:10,000; (□) 1:20,000; (△) 1:40,000.

PAP that produces the percentage binding obtained with the sample. If the original samples have been already diluted, this value is multiplied by the dilution of specimen to derive the concentration of PAP in the original specimen. Currently, nanograms per milliliter based on purified PAP as the standard is used by most investigators.

C. DOUBLE-ANTIBODY IMMUNOENZYME ASSAY
   (CHOE et al., 1980a,b)

1. PAP Standards and Antiserum

Materials used for the double antibody RIA are applicable to IEA with little modification. Additional reagents for enzyme assay (see Section II,A) are required.

2. Assay Procedure

To one of triplicate assay tubes containing 100 μl of either standard PAP or clinical serum sample is added 100 μl of 100-fold diluted normal rabbit serum. This series of tubes is the control group. For the assay group, 100 μl of 100-fold diluted anti-PAP serum is placed in the two remaining triplicate assay tubes.

After incubation at 4°C for 60 minutes to precipitate the immune com-

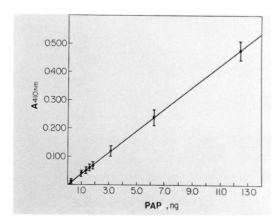

FIG. 5. A standard curve of double-antibody immunoenzyme assay of PAP.

plexes, 100 μl of 100-fold diluted anti-rabbit Ig goat serum is added to each tube. After an additional 10-minute incubation at 4°C, 1 ml of cold phosphate-buffered saline is added to each tube, which is then centrifuged (4°C, 15 minutes, 1500 g) to sediment the antigen–antibody complexes.

After removing the supernates, the pellets are dissolved in 100 μl of 0.1 M citrate buffer, pH 5.0, at room temperature by vortex mixing to yield a clear solution. After warming these dissolved immune complexes for 2 minutes at 37°C water bath, 100 μl of p-nitrophenyl phosphate (10 mM) is added to each tube to initiate the enzyme assay, and the enzyme reaction is allowed to proceed for 10 minutes at 37°C. The reaction is stopped by adding 0.7 ml of 0.2 N NaOH. To determine the resulting p-nitrophenol release, the absorbance is measured at 410 nm. The concentrations of p-nitrophenol are plotted against PAP concentration to establish a standard correlation curve (Fig. 5).

D. Appraisal

Radioimmunoassay and immunoenzyme assay have been used for the characterization of antigenic structure of prostatic acid phosphatase (Choe *et al.*, 1981b) as well as to the clinical investigation of serum prostatic acid phosphatase determination (Choe *et al.*, 1980a). The sensitivity of assays, defined as the least detectable concentration (two standard deviations from the average), was 1.95 ng/ml for both methods. Values obtained by the two methods yielded relatively good correlations (Fig. 6).

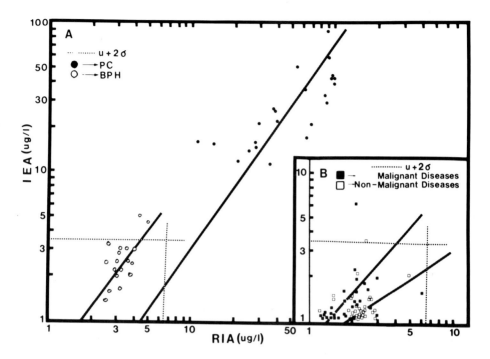

Fig. 6. Correlation between radioimmunoassay (y) and immunoenzyme assay (x) values. (A) For 23 sera from advanced prostatic carcinoma (PC), $y = 0.87 x + 7.2$; for 18 sera from benign prostatic hyperplasis (BPH), $y = x + 0.72$. (B) For 29 sera from malignant diseases of nonprostatic origin, $y = 0.47 x + 0.68$; for 32 sera from miscellaneous nonmalignant disorders, $y = 0.35 x + 0.66$. Correlation coefficients (r) range from 0.912 to 0.981 for each group, and the probability associated with r for each degree of freedom is $p \ll 0.002$. Reproduced from Choe *et al.* (1980a) with permission of the publisher.

The lowest prostatic acid phosphatase concentration detectable by the immunological assays cannot be lowered to a few picograms per milliliter, unless one can produce an extraordinarily high affinity antibody (e.g., 10^{10} to 10^{11} liters per mole). For example, with a concentration of specific antibody (IgG) of 1 mg/ml (most of immune rabbits produce this level of antibodies, most of monoclonal antibodies from hybridomas are 10 μg/ml), the IgG concentration is approximately 7×10^{-6} M. Even if the specific antibodies have high affinity, relatively high concentrations of antibody must be used. This can be seen from the basic relationship (Fazekas de St. Groth, 1979), $K = b/(f \cdot [\text{Ab}])$, where b and f represents molar concentrations of bound and free antigen at equilibrium; [Ab] is the molar concentration of antigen-combining sites (Fab) of specific antibodies remaining unoccupied at equilibrium, and K is the equilibrium constant or relative affinity constant. If the $K = 10^{10} M^{-1}$, and the total concentration of antibody combining sites is $7 \times 10^{-9} M$ (this is a 1000-fold dilution of original antiserum), then the value of b/f will be $10^{10} M^{-1} \times 7 \times 10^{-9}$ or 0.7, in other words, a maximum of 70% antigen binding occurs. This consideration is only a theoretical one, however, it serves to prove the point.

Ekins *et al.* (1968) showed that the antibody concentration should be about $3/K$ and the concentration of the labeled antigen approximately $4/K$ in order to obtain most sensitive yet statistically reliable assay conditions in radioimmunoassay. However, since the prostatic acid phosphatase is a high-molecular-weight protein, the use of concentration level equivalent to the reciprocal of K is impractically high ($10^{-9} M$, i.e., 100 ng/ml). As a rule of thumb, the lowest antibody concentration that will bind a measurable fraction of antigen has been adopted by almost all investigators for maximal sensitivity. The lower limit of prostatic acid phosphatase measured under such assay condition reaches $10^{-11} M$ or 1–2 ng/ml. However, assays run under such conditions suffer from poor precision, a point Berson and Yalow (1973) have already emphasized.

As discussed above, the sensitivity of radioimmunoassay is highly affected by antibody affinity, because it measures free and bound antigen in equilibrium. However, the immunoenzyme assay is less affected by the affinity of antibodies. In this assay, relatively high concentrations of antibody (e.g., 100-fold dilution) are used to establish zero-order kinetics for the antigen binding, and the sensitivity of the assay becomes dependent on the catalytic activity of the bound antigen. In fact, its sensitivity can be further improved by prolonging the incubation period or by use of fluorogenic or radioactive isotope-labeled substrates.

V. Immunohistological Methods

A. CELLS AND TISSUES PRODUCING PROSTATIC ACID PHOSPHATASE

Human red blood cell acid phosphatase is a small molecular weight protein, 15,000–20,000 (Fenton and Richardson, 1967). The structural gene for this enzyme (ACP_1) is located on chromosome 2 (Ferguson-Smith *et al.*, 1973; Mace and Robson, 1974; Povey *et al.*, 1974). Most of the differentiated cells, however, synthesize and store in the lysosomes an acid phosphatase of molecular weights approximately 100,000 (Yam, 1974). Because of its ubiquitous presence in the lysosomes, this enzyme has been regarded as a marker for this organelle (Novikoff, 1976). Recently, the structural gene for this enzyme (ACP_2) has been assigned to chromosome 11 by somatic cell hybridization study (Shaws *et al.*, 1976).

Acid phosphatase activity in the prostate is over 1000 times greater than that of any other human tissues (Gutman and Gutman, 1939; Woodward, 1942). Much of the enzyme activity is in the glandular epithelium and in the lumen of the gland as the secretion (Brandes and Bourne, 1956; Kirkheim *et al.*, 1964; Aso *et al.*, 1972). Furthermore Shulman and co-workers (1965) demonstrated that acid phosphatase of the human prostate gland is antigenically unique. Ultrastructural and cytochemical studies of prostatic epithelial cells revealed two separate forms of acid phosphatase, presumably representing lysosomal and secretory forms (Brandes and Kirkheim, 1977). They suggested that the secretory enzyme is regulated by androgens and estrogens since it is decreased by orchiectomy or hypophysectomy (Rosenkrantz, 1969; Serrano *et al.*, 1977). Recently, Choe and co-workers (1980c) used immunohistological methods to demonstrate that the PAP is expressed exclusively by the prostatic epithelial cells in cultures and tissues. These antigenic and functional differences between the lysosomal and prostatic secretory isoenzymes suggest, but do not prove, the genetic nonidentity of the two enzymes. Probably, both red cell and prostatic enzymes are expressed only by groups of differentiated cells and genetic expression of these genes may be under the control of organ-specific effectors. Immunohistological methods will be particularly suitable for the elucidation of genetic control of acid phosphatase biosynthesis.

The PAP-immunohistology has been applied to (1) the identification of prostatic epithelial cells in culture (Rose *et al.*, 1978; Pontes *et al.*, 1979) and (2) identification of metastatic prostatic carcinoma cells in biopsies (Burns, 1977; Jobsis *et al.*, 1978; Pontes *et al.*, 1978). In the next section the three main techniques of PAP-immunohistology are described in some detail. The methods are based on double-antibody technique or indirect staining method in which the second antibodies are conjugated to fluorescein isothiocyanate (FITC) or peroxidase. Although FITC- or peroxidase-conjugated antibodies are available from commercial sources, a few conjugation procedures we have used are described in the following sections.

B. Immunofluorescence Method

1. Fluorescent Antibody

a. FITC Conjugation by the Method of McKinney et al. (1964). FITC (1 mg/ml) is dissolved in 0.15 M Na$_2$HPO$_4$ (pH 9.0) immediately before use. One milliliter of solution per 100 mg protein is added to the IgG solution (at least 25 mg/ml) while stirring at room temperature. The pH is adjusted to 9.5 by the addition of 0.1 M Na$_3$PO$_4$ while stirring, and the reaction allowed to run for 60 minutes at room temperature. The conjugate is separated on Sephadex G-25 column.

b. *Alternative Method* (*Marshall et al., 1958*).   Protein (10 mg/ml) solution is prepared in carbonate-buffered saline (9 vol 0.15 M NaCl and 1 vol carbonate buffer). Carbonate buffer is prepared by mixing 5.8 ml of 5.3% Na_2CO_3 and 10 ml of 4.2% $NaHCO_3$ and pH is adjusted to 9.5. Dry FITC is added to the concentration range 20–40 μg/ml of protein. The mixture is gently rotated on a mixer for 1 hour at room temperature during which time the dye dissolves. The conjugate is isolated as described above.

2. *Purification of FITC Conjugate on DEAE-Cellulose*

About 1 gm of the cellulose should be used for 2 ml of conjugate containing 20 mg of protein. The conjugated IgG is equilibrated with starting buffer overnight.

Elution is performed with (1) starting buffer, 0.0175 M phosphate, pH 6.3, (2) 0.0175 M phosphate, pH 6.3, containing 0.125 M NaCl, and (3) 0.0175 M phosphate, pH 6.3, containing 0.250 M NaCl. The fractions should be concentrated immediately by vacuum dialysis. The IgG–FITC fractions are examined by Ouchterlony double diffusion precipitation. Some fractions may have been under- or overlabeled and cause inhibition of specific staining or nonspecific staining.

3. *Evaluation of FITC Conjugate*

a. *Conjugate*.   Conjugate (suitably diluted to 1:40) is measured at 495 and 280 nm to obtain *F/P ratio*. Satisfactory conjugates have optical density ratios approaching unity. Values below 0.5 indicate low labeling while a conjugate giving a value over 1.5 is overlabeled and is likely to cause nonspecific staining.

b. *Presence of Free Dye*.   A slide glass is prepared with thin layer of Sephadex G-25 or G-50 in PBS. A filter paper wick is attached to each end of the slide and a few microliters of IgG–FITC is applied about 1 cm from one end of slide. Elute the labeled protein for 15–20 minutes with PBS. When scanned under the UV lamp, the conjugate has migrated several centimeters, whereas the free dye remains at the point of application. If there is free dye release, the conjugate should be purified on Sephadex G-50 column.

4. *Fixation of Tissue and Cultured Cells*

Cells grown as a monolayer on a coverslip or on a microscopic slide are fixed in ice-cold acetone for 5 to 10 minutes. The biopsy materials are fixed in formalin and sectioned like paraffin-embedded tissue. Formalin-fixed paraffin sections have rarely been used in immunohistology, because the antigenicity of many proteins is impaired by the formalin treatment. However, PAP remains stable, catalytically and antigenically, through the formalin fixation (Jobsis *et al.*, 1978); therefore paraffin sections are recommended for PAP-immunohistology rather than frozen sections. Paraffin sections are deparaffinized according to the routine histological procedure before the immunohistological stainings. Briefly, the slides are deparaffinized for 50 seconds to 1 minute in xylene, then slides are dipped in a series of ethanol solutions (absolute ethanol to 50% ethanol) for a minute more or less to remove xylene. The slides are finally placed in PBS and washed for over 30 minutes. Acetone-fixed cell cultures are also washed in PBS before the immunohistological procedures which include immunoperoxidase and Sternberger staining. Phosphate-buffered saline containing 0.2% bovine serum albumin (PBS–BSA) has been used for dilution of antisera and for washing of slides.

5. *Procedure*

1. Slides are incubated for 30 minutes with anti-PAP antiserum in a humid chamber at room temperature. Dilution of antiserum is determined by preliminary experiments, which is usually 100- to 500-fold dilutions. Then, the excess antibodies are removed by washing in PBS for 30 minutes to 1 hour at room temperature.

2. The slides are further incubated with FITC-conjugated second antibody for 30 minutes at room temperature. Then, the slides are washed with PBS–BSA for 30 minutes to 1 hour. The concentration of FITC-conjugated second antibody has to be determined by preliminary experiments.

3. After the addition of a drop of glycerol–phosphate (9:1 mixture of glycerol and phosphate buffer), slides are sealed with cover glass and observed under the fluorescence microscope.

C. IMMUNOPEROXIDASE METHOD

Among the various enzymes, horseradish peroxidase MW 40,000 is best suited for the immunohistology; mainly because of its small size, the penetration of the peroxidase-labeled antibodies into cells is very satisfactory. In addition this enzyme is remarkably resistant to heat, organic solvents, and embedding materials. Peroxidase activity, after the immunohistological reactions, can be visualized with various reagents, such as benzidine, α-naphthol, and p-phenylendiamine, and various leuko dyes.

1. Conjugation of IgG to Peroxidase by Glutaraldehyde
(Avrameas, 1969)

To 1 ml of 0.1 M phosphate buffer, pH 6.8, containing 5 mg of IgG and 12 mg of horseradish peroxidase (type II, Sigma), 0.05 ml of 1% glutaraldehyde is added dropwise while the solution is stirred gently. The mixture is stirred gently at room temperature for 2 hours.

The mixture is dialyzed overnight against two changes of 5 liters of PBS at 4°C. Then the conjugate is centrifuged at 20,000 rpm for 30 minutes to remove any precipitated proteins. The specificity of conjugated IgG is examined by immunodiffusion and immunoelectrophoresis. Enzymatically and immunologically active conjugate can be stored at 4°C for up to 3 months.

2. Conjugation of IgG to Peroxidase by Carbodiimide
(Kurstack et al., 1969)

Fifteen milligrams of horseradish peroxidase ($\sim$ 656 units/mg) is dissolved in 1 ml of 0.05 M Tris acetate buffer, pH 7.2, containing 5 mg of the specific antibody preparation. To this solution are added 40 mg of 1-cyclohexyl-3-(2-morpholino-ethyl)carbodiimide methoparatoluene sulfonate (MCDI) dissolved in 1 ml of 0.05 M Tris acetate buffer, pH 7.2. The solution is mixed and stirred gently from 2 to 12 hours at 4°C. The light precipitate formed during the reaction is eliminated by centrifugation. The peroxidase–antibody conjugate is separated from unconjugated antibody and peroxidase either by precipitation with $(NH_4)_2SO_4$ at 50% saturation or by gel filtration through Sephadex or Sephacryl columns.

3. Immunoperoxidase Procedure

1. The fixed specimens are incubated with a drop of anti-PAP serum (diluted in PBS variously) at 25°C for 30 minutes to 1 hour. Then the slides are washed twice for 1 minute and once for 30 minutes in PBS at room temperature.

2. The reacted slides are further incubated with a drop of PBS containing peroxidase-conjugated anti-IgG (second Ab) globulin (0.5 mg protein/ml) at 25°C for 30 minutes. The slides are washed twice for 1 minute and once for 30 minutes in PBS at room temperature.

3. The slides are stained for peroxidase activity for 5 to 20 minutes. For peroxidase activity, two substrates have been used in our laboratory, benzidine or α-naphthol.

Benzidine solution is prepared as follows: To 10 ml of 0.05 M Tris buffer, pH 7.6, containing 5 mg of 3,3′-diaminobenzidine tetrachloride

(Sigma) H_2O_2 is added to a final concentration of 0.01% immediately before use. Sucrose (0.25 M) improves the cellular morphology.

The alternative staining solution is prepared as follows: Dissolve 15 mg of α-naphol and 22 mg of p-phenylenediamine in 20 ml of 0.07 M phosphate buffer, pH 5.8 or 7.2, added to 1% NaCl. The solution is filtered and two to three drops applied immediately to smears or sections. The reaction occurs immediately, the site of peroxidase activity appearing in the form of purple spots. The reaction can be stopped by placing on the preparation a few drops of 0.05 M acetic acid.

4. The stained cells can be counterstained with 1% methyl green-pyronin with 1% methylene blue or 0.1% toluidine blue. The slide is dehydrated in two changes of alcohol and cleared in two changes of xylene for 1 minute each. After coverslip, examine it with light microscope.

D. Sternberger's Unlabeled Antibody Peroxidase– Antiperoxidase Method (Sternberger et al., 1970; Sternberger, 1979)

1. Preparation of Soluble Peroxidase–Antiperoxidase Complex

1. Highly purified horseradish peroxidase (RZ = 3.0) is available from Miles Laboratories (Kankakee, IL). High titer antiperoxidase sera are easily prepared by immunization of animals with 500 μg to 1 mg of peroxidase in complete Freund's adjuvant according to the schedule described under Section III,B.

2. As a preliminary test to determine qualitatively the equivalence zone of antiperoxidase serum, to a series of tubes (8 to 10) containing varying amounts of peroxidase (0.05 to 0.5 mg in saline) are added equal volumes of undiluted antiperoxidase serum. After overnight incubation at 4°C the tubes are centrifuged and the pellets are resuspended into 1 ml volume with saline. By reading the absorbance at 400 nm and plotting, the zones of antigen excess, equivalence, and antibody excess are determined.

3. For the preparation of soluble peroxidase–antiperoxidase complex, the amounts of peroxidase and antiserum to give rise to maximal precipitation (zone of equivalence estimated from the preliminary test) are scaled up to 10 to 150 ml level depending on the need. With a batch of rabbit antiperoxidase in our laboratory, we have proceeded as follows: in a 40-ml centrifuge tube containing approximately 60 mg horseradish peroxidase (RZ = 2.0) in 10 to 15 ml saline, 20 ml of rabbit serum is added dropwise with gentle stirring. One hour after the incubation at room temperature the tube is centrifuged for 20 minutes at 2000 rpm at 4°C. The

immune precipitate is washed three times with ice-cold saline by re-suspension and centrifugation.

4. The immune precipitates are resuspended in 10 ml of the 0.4% solution of peroxidase by a thorough repeated pipetting. With mild stirring the suspension is brought to pH 2.3 by the addition of 1 N HCl at room temperature, then neutralized immediately to approximately pH 7.4 using 1 N NaOH. These steps of acidification in the presence of excess peroxidase and immediate neutralization are necessary to obtain soluble and stable immune complexes (Sternberger, 1979).

5. The solubilized immune complexes are chilled in the ice bath and an equal volume of a solution of $(NH_4)_2SO_4$ is added to remove peroxidase.

6. The immune complex is dissolved in 5 ml of distilled water and dialyzed against 4 liters of 0.1 M acetate buffer, pH 5.0, under protection from light for 2 days.

7. The soluble peroxidase–antiperoxidase complex thus prepared is stable for several days in solution. For storage, we add glycerol to the final concentration of 30% to the complex; aliquots are placed in 1.0 ml volume in vials and frozen at $-70°C$. Once one of these vials is thawed, it is divided into small aliquots, 25 to 100 μl each, in tightly stoppered vials and stored at $-20°C$. For each experiment a single vial is diluted and used. The diluted solution is not reused in order to avoid complications arising from the degradation of peroxidase–antiperoxidase complex.

2. Sternberger Staining

1. Washing slides: Slides are washed for 30 minutes at room temperature with buffered saline (phosphate or Tris, pH 7.2–7.6) containing 3% normal serum of the species from which the second antibody (or link antibody) is obtained.

2. Primary incubation: The primary antiserum is diluted (proper dilution having been determined by preliminary experiments testing, e.g., 1:100 to 1:1000 dilutions) in buffer containing 1% normal serum of the species from which the second antibodies are obtained. The slides covered with primary antibodies are incubated for 30 minutes to as long as 48 hours at 4°C, depending on the concentration and affinity of the antibodies. At low concentration and affinity, antibodies require a long period of incubation to approach equilibrium in their interaction with antigen. At the end of primary incubation, slides are washed in buffer containing 1% normal serum as indicated above for 15 to 30 minutes at room temperature.

3. Second incubation: Slides are covered with the second antibodies (or link antibodies) diluted in buffered saline (e.g., 1:10 to 1:100) for 5 to 30

minutes at room temperature, then washed with normal serum containing buffer for 15 to 30 minutes.

4. Third incubation: Slides are incubated with properly diluted peroxidase–antiperoxidase complex for 5 to 30 minutes at room temperature, followed by washing and blotting. The soluble peroxidase–antiperoxidase complex is diluted usually 1:50 to 1:100 in the same normal serum containing buffer as mentioned above.

5. The slides are then stained for peroxidase activity for 3 to 8 minutes followed by washing in distilled water. The reaction mixtures for the benzidine and Nadi reactions are described in Section V,C. The stained cells may be counterstained with hematoxylin or any other stain. Then they may be dehydrated in xylene or cedar wood oil, and mounted in Permount, or alternatively they may be mounted in glycerol-buffer without dehydration for microscopy.

E. COMMENT

Immunofluorescence or peroxidase reaction is localized in the cytoplasm of prostatic acid phosphatase-producing cells (Fig. 7). It is easy enough to distinguish prostatic acid phosphatase synthesizing cells from nonproducer or positive slides from the controls. However, it is advantageous to discuss a few misleading observations that may result from nonspecific staining. The first source of the nonspecific staining is electrostatic and hydrophobic bonding of immunoglobulins with tissue as described in detail by Von Mayersbach (1967). A net positive charge of tissue, particularly in the cytoplasm of the cells, relative to that of immunoglobulin increases after various fixative treatment, therefore, causing varying degrees of nonspecific staining. One measure to remedy the condition is the addition of bovine serum albumin or gelatin to the diluents of reagent and washing buffer. In the indirect or second antibody method, pretreatment of tissue sections with normal serum of the species that donated second antibody also minimizes nonspecific adsorption of the primary antibody. A second source of staining nonspecificity is the presence of Fc receptors not only on mononuclear cells but also conceivably in solid tissue. However, Fc receptors of mononuclear cells react mainly, if not exclusively, with IgG molecules when aggregated by physical means or in the form of antigen–antibody complexes (Basten et al., 1972). If the antisera have been centrifuged for 1 hour at 100,000 g and freed from any oligomeric aggregates larger than 40 S, this type of nonspecific staining can be avoided. Furthermore, it has been reported that FITC-labeled

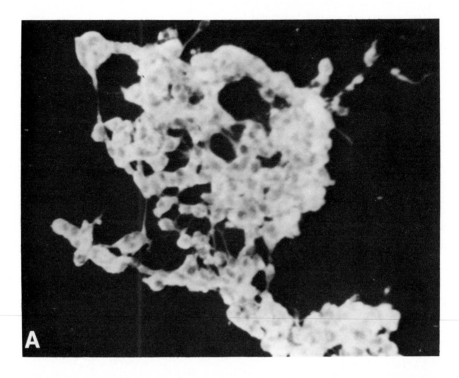

Fɪɢ. 7. Immunofluorescence method for the cells and tissues producing prostatic acid phosphatase. Rabbit anti-PAP antiserum (R32, 1:1000 dilution) and fluorescein isothiocyanate-conjugated goat anti-rabbit IgG antibody (G5, 1:1000 dilution) are used as described in the text. (A) Human prostatic epithelial cell primary culture (×200); (B) metastatic prostatic adenocarcinoma cells in bone marrow biopsies (×400); (C) prostatic adenocarcinoma, transurethral resection specimen (×100); (D) prostatic adenocarcinoma, transurethral resection specimen (×100); (E) prostatic adenocarcinoma metastasized to bladder (×100).

IgGs lose the ability to bind to Fc receptors and protein A and the ability to fix complement (Trasher *et al.*, 1975).

A third source of staining nonspecificity is peculiar to the indirect method. The second antibody preparation is made by immunization with isolated IgG and probably contains contaminants that react directly with tissue, that is, even when the primary antibody has been omitted. Therefore, it is important to use highly purified IgG preparations or subunits as the immunogen when the second antibody is made. For the conjugation of second antibodies with FITC or peroxidase, the use of purified antibody, rather than IgG, could further improve the specificity of the method.

Peroxidase-labeled antibodies are about equally sensitive as immunofluorescence and similar fixatives and staining procedure are used for both

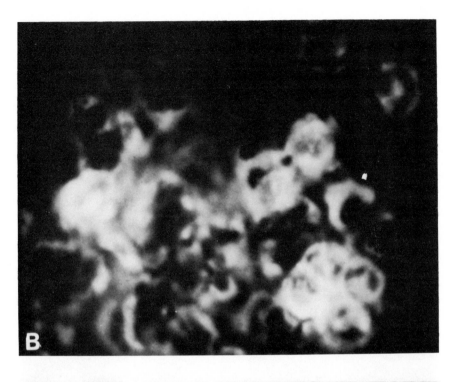

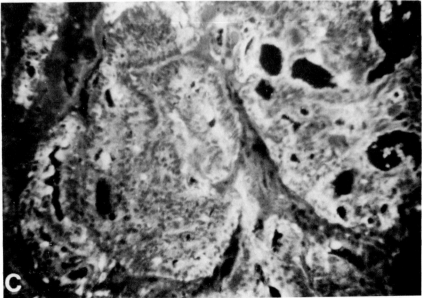

FIG. 7B and C.

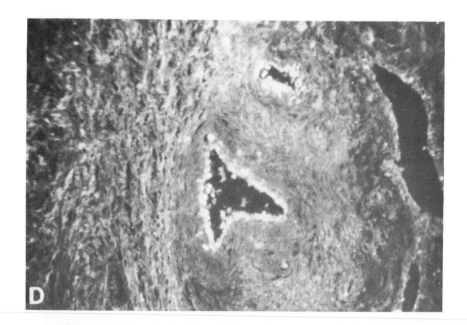

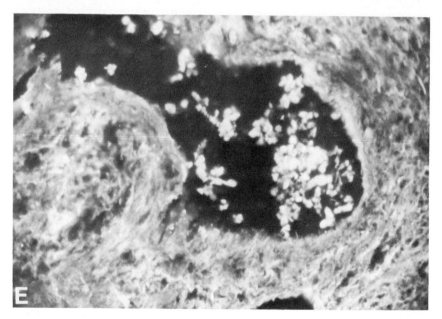

FIG. 7D and E.

methods. Sternberger's peroxidase–antiperoxidase technique (1979) is far more sensitive than the former two methods. From the practical point of view, requirements of UV microscopy and photographic recording are restrictions to immunofluorescence. On the other hand, the immunoperoxidase and Sternberger techniques offer the advantage of storing the stained preparations for the records. Photography is essential for immunofluorescence slides, as fluorescence wanes on storage. Total light intensity is often low in dark-field microscopy, especially when only a small part of the section is immunofluorescent. In order to avoid long exposure times, film with high ASA ratings are recommended. In an attempt to preserve FITC fluorescences it is common practice to photograph tissue sections before observing details. When one returns to the area of the tissue section after photography, fluorescence may have been reduced, and evaluation depends mostly on the photography. Therefore, we save these immunofluorescence slides for further evaluation by the Sternberger technique. It is our routine practice to prepare hematoxylin–eosin stained step section slides to identify the morphological details of the tissues in comparison with the immunohistological slides.

Although the microscopic characteristics of metastatic prostatic cancer have been reported to resemble those of primary tumors (McCullough *et al.*, 1974), frozen section examination of lymph nodes is rather inaccurate (McLaughlin *et al.*, 1976). Therefore, immunohistological evaluation of metastatic prostatic cancer can be a helpful investigative methodology in surgical staging (Jobsis *et al.*, 1978; Pontes *et al.*, 1979). Histochemical as well as ultrastructural studies of prostatic epithelial cells have established the secretory process of acid phosphatase (Brandes and Kirkheim, 1977; Kirkheim *et al.*, 1974). However, immunoelectron microscopy has never been applied to the organelles synthesizing prostatic acid phosphatase. These techniques can be useful for the study of the regulation of prostatic acid phosphatase biosynthesis in several tissues in which only a group of special cells is synthesizing this enzyme.

ACKNOWLEDGMENTS

The authors wish to acknowledge the roles played by Mrs. Mi-Kyung Dong and Drs. Hyun-Sun Lillehoj, Michael Baron, and Steve Bloink in the development of those immunological methods. These studies have involved the generous collaboration of a number of investigators, particularly Dr. Edson J. Pontes, Roswell Park Memorial Institute, Buffalo, New York, and Dr. Robert Riehle, Department of Urology, Wayne State University Medical Center, Detroit, Michigan. This work was supported in part by Public Health Grants CA 16426 and CA 18748 from the National Cancer Institute.

REFERENCES

Aso, Y., Yokoyama, M., Okada, K., Tokue, A., Koise, K., Murahayashi, I., and Takayasu, H. (1972). *Invest. Urol.* **9**, 329–334.

Avrameas, S. (1969). *Immunochemistry* **6**, 43–52.

Basten, A., Miller, J. F. P., Sprent, J., and Pye, J. (1972). *J. Exp. Med.* **135**, 610–626.

Berson, S. A., and Yalow, R., eds. (1973). "Methods in Investigative and Diagnostic Endocrinology," pp. 84–135. North-Holland Publ., Amsterdam.

Bodansky, O. (1972). *Adv. Clin. Chem.* **15**, 43–147.

Brandes, D., and Bourne, G. H. (1956). *J. Pathol. Bacteriol.* **71**, 33–36.

Brandes, D., and Kirkheim, D. (1977). *In* "Urologic Pathology: The Prostate" (M. Taunenbaum, ed.), pp. 99–128. Lea & Febiger, Philadelphia, Pennsylvania.

Burns, J. (1977). *Biomedicine* **27**, 7–12.

Burstone, M. W. (1962). "Enzyme Histochemistry and its Application in the Study of Neoplasms." Academic Press, New York.

Choe, B. K., Pontes, E. J., McDonald, I., and Rose, N. R. (1978a). *Prep. Biochem.* **8**, 73–89.

Choe, B. K., Pontes, E. J., Rose, N. R., and Henderson, M. D. (1978b). *Invest. Urol.* **15**, 312–318.

Choe, B. K., Pontes, E. J., Dong, M. K., and Rose, N. R. (1980a). *Clin. Chem.* **26**, 1854–1859.

Choe, B. K., Pontes, E. J., and Rose, N. R. (1980b). *In* "Manual of Clinical Immunology" (N. R. Rose and H. Friedman, eds.), pp. 951–962. Amer. Soc. for Microbiologist, Washington, D.C.

Choe, B. K., Pontes, E. J., Lillehoj, H. S., and Rose, N. R. (1980c). *Prostate* **1**, 383–398.

Choe, B. K., Rose, N. R., and Pontes, E. J. (1981a). *In* "Prostatic Carcinoma, Biology and Diagnosis" (E. S. E. Hafez and E. Spring-Mills, eds.), pp. 131–140. Nijhoff, The Hague.

Choe, B. K., Dong, M. K., Walz, D., and Rose, N. R. (1981b). *Mol. Immunol.* **18**, 451–454.

Davidson, R., and Ephrussi, B. (1970). *Exp. Cell Res.* **61**, 222–226.

Derechin, M., Ostrowski, W., Galka, M., and Barnard, E. A. (1971). *Biochim. Biophys. Acta* **250**, 143–154.

Ekins, R. P., Newman, G. B., and O'Riordan, J. L. H. (1968). *In* "Radioisotopes in Medicine: *In Vitro* Studies" (R. L. Hayes, F. A. Goswitz, and B. E. P. Murphy, eds.), p. 58. US Atomic Energy Commission, Oak Ridge, Tennessee.

Fazekas de St. Groth, S. (1979). *In* "Immunological Methods" (I. Lefkovits and B. Pernis, eds.), pp. 1–42. Academic Press, New York.

Fenton, M. R., and Richardson, K. E. (1967). *Arch. Biochem. Biophys.* **120**, 332–341.

Ferguson-Smith, M. A., Newman, B. F., Ellis, P. M., Thomson, D. M. G., and Riley, I. D. (1973). *Nature (London) New Biol.* **243**, 271–274.

Foti, A. G., Cooper, J. F., Herschman, H., and Malvaez, R. R. (1977). *New Engl. J. Med.* **297**, 1357–1361.

Franks, L. M. (1980). *In* "Methods in Cell Biology" (C. Harris, B. F. Trump, and G. D. Stoner, eds.), Vol. 21, pp. 153–169. Academic Press, New York.

Goldstein, I. J., Reichert, C. M., and Misaki, A. (1974). *Ann. N.Y. Acad. Sci.* **234**, 283–296.

Gutman, A. B., and Gutman, E. B. (1938). *Proc. Soc. Exp. Biol. Med.* **41**, 277–281.

Heatfield, B. M., Sanefuji, H., and Trump, B. F. (1980). *In* "Methods in Cell Biology" (C. Harris, B. F. Trump, and G. D. Stoner, eds.), Vol. 21, pp. 171–194. Academic Press, New York.

Hunter, W. M. (1973). *In* "Handbook of Experimental Immunology" (D. M. Weir, ed.), 2nd Ed., pp. 17.1–17.36. Davis, Philadelphia, Pennsylvania.

Hunter, W. M., and Greenwood, F. C. (1962). *Nature (London)* **194**, 495.
Jaffe, B. M., and Behrman, H. R., eds. (1974). "Methods of Hormone Radioimmunoassay." Academic Press, New York.
Jobsis, A. C., DeVries, G. P., Anholt, R. R. H., and Sanders, G. T. B. (1978). *Cancer* **41**, 1788–1793.
Kastendieck, H., and Altanähr, E. (1979). *Arch. Androl Suppl.* **2**, 64–70.
Kearney, J. F., Radbruch, A., Liesegang, B., and Rajewsky, K. (1979). *J. Immunol.* **123**, 1548–1550.
Kennett, R. H., McKearn, T. J., and Bechtol, K. B., eds. (1980). "Monoclonal Antibodies, Hybridoma: A New Dimension in Biological Analyses." Plenum, New York.
Kirkheim, D., Gyorkey, F., and Brandes, D. (1964). *Invest. Urol.* **1**, 403–421.
Kirkheim, D., Brandes, D., and Bacon, R. L. (1974). *In* "Male Accessory Sex Organs, Structure and Function in Mammals" (D. Brandes, ed.), pp. 397–423. Academic Press, New York.
Köhler, G. (1979). *In* "Immunological Methods" (I. Lefkovits and B. Pernis, eds.), pp. 391–401. Academic Press, New York.
Köhler, G., and Milstein, C. (1975). *Nature (London)* **256**, 495–497.
Kurstack, E., Coté, J. R., and Bellonick, S. (1969). *C. R. Acad. Sci. (Paris)* **268**, 2309.
Lee, C., Wang, M. C., Murphy, G. P., and Chu, T. M. (1978). *Cancer Res.* **38**, 2871–2878.
Lillehoj, H. S., Choe, B. K., and Rose, N. R. (1980). *J. Cell Biol.* **87**, 301a. (Abstr.)
Littlefield, J. W. (1964). *Science* **145**, 709–710.
Lowry, O. H., Rosebrough, N. R., Farr, A. L., and Randall, R. J. (1951). *J. Biol. Chem.* **193**, 265–275.
Luchter-Wasyl, E., and Ostrowski, W. (1974). *Biochim. Biophys. Acta* **365**, 349–359.
McCullough, D. L., Prout, G. R., and Daly, J. J. (1974). *J. Urol.* **111**, 65–71.
Mace, M., and Robson, E. B. (1974). *In* "Human Gene Mapping." New Haven Conference (1973), Birth Defects Original Article Series, Vol. 11, No. 3, pp. 176–178.
McKinney, R. M., Spillane, J. T., and Pearce, G. W. (1964). *J. Immunol.* **93**, 232–240.
McLaughlin, A. P., Saltzstein, S. L., McCullough, D. L., and Gittes, R. F. (1976). *J. Urol.* **115**, 89–94.
Marshall, J. D., Eveland, W. C., and Smith, C. W. (1958). *Proc. Soc. Exp. Biol. Med.* **98**, 898–901.
Melchers, F., Porter, M., and Warner, N., eds. (1978). "Lymphocyte Hybridomas." Springer-Verlag, Berlin and New York.
Novikoff, A. B. (1976). *Proc. Natl. Acad. Sci. U.S.A.* **73**, 2781–2787.
Ostrowski, W. (1963). *Bull. Acad. Pol. Sci. Cl. 6* **11**, 271.
Ostrowski, W. (1980). *In* "Male Accessory Sex Glands" (E. Spring-Mills and E. S. E. Hafez, eds.), pp. 197–213. Elsevier, Amsterdam.
Ostrowski, W., Wasyl, Z., Weber, M., Guminska, M., and Luchter, E. (1970). *Biochim. Biophys. Acta* **221**, 397–406.
Pontes, E. J., Choe, B. K., Rose, N. R., and Pierce, J. M., Jr. (1977). *J. Urol.* **117**, 459–463.
Pontes, E. J., Choe, B. K., Rose, N. R., and Pierce, J. M., Jr. (1978). *J. Urol.* **119**, 772–776.
Pontes, E. J., Choe, B. K., Rose, N. R., and Pierce, J. M., Jr. (1979). *Invest. Urol.* **16**, 483–485.
Povey, S., Swallow, D. M., Bobrow, M., Craig, I., and van Heyningen, V. (1974). *Ann. Hum. Genet.* **38**, 1–5.
Rose, N. R., Pontes, E. J., and Choe, B. K. (1978). *Natl. Cancer Inst. Monogr.* **49**, 29–30.
Rosenkrantz, H. (1969). *N.Y. Acad. Sci.* **166**, 466–481.
Serrano, J. A., Paul, B. D., Wasserkrug, H. L., and Serrano, A. A., (1977). *Proc. Electron Microsc. Soc. Am.* **35**, 434–435.
Shaws, T. B., Lalley, P. A., and Brown, J. A. (1976). *J. Cell Biol.* **70**, 98a. (Abstr.)

Shulman, S., Mamrod, L., Gonder, M., and Soanes, W. A. (1964). *J. Immunol.* **93**, 474–480.

Smith, J. K., and Whitby, L. G. (1968). *Biochim. Biophys. Acta* **151**, 607–618.

Sternberger, L. A. (1979). "Immunocytochemistry." Wiley, New York.

Sternberger, L. A., Hardy, P. H., Cuculis, J. J., and Meyer, H. G. (1970). *J. Histochem. Cytochem.* **18**, 315–333.

Thorell, J. I., and Johansson, B. G. (1971). *Biochim. Biophys. Acta* **251**, 363–369.

Trasher, S. G., Bigazzi, P. E., Yoshida, T., and Cohen, S. (1975). *J. Immunol.* **114**, 762–764.

Van Etten, R. L., and Saini, M. S. (1978). *Clin. Chem.* **24**, 1525–1530.

Vihko, P., Kontturi, M., and Korhonen, L. K. (1978). *Clin. Chem.* **24**, 466–470.

Von Mayersbach, H., ed. (1967). *Acta Histochem. (Jena) Suppl.* **7**.

Wang, M. C., Valenzuela, L. A., Murphy, G. P., and Chu, T. M. (1980). *Invest. Urol.* **17**, 159–163.

Woodward, H. Q. (1942). *Cancer Res.* **2**, 497–508.

Yam, Y. T. (1974). *Am. J. Med.* **56**, 604–616.

CHAPTER VI

HUMAN COLON TUMOR ANTIGENS

LYNN C. YEOMAN, CHARLES W. TAYLOR, AND SUBHAS CHAKRABARTY

I. Introduction to Antigens of the Colon

A. The Importance of Cancer Markers

The detection, staging, and management of human colon cancer remains one of the major challenging problems facing oncology today. The development of suitable markers for the early detection of neoplasms, their properties, and their application have been discussed by Vaitukaitis (1975), by Ruddon (1978), and more recently by McIntire (1980). In their listing of criteria to be used for the selection and development of useful markers for the detection and staging of cancer it becomes apparent that both the specificity for tumor type as well as the sensitivity for the earliest possible detection are of significant importance.

B. Experimental Animal Models for Colon Cancer

One approach to the development of markers for cancer of the digestive tract has been the induction of experimental adenocarcinomas of the colon in mice by carcinogens. Administration of 1,2-dimethylhydrazine to mice at a dose of 15 mg/kg body weight results in the production of adenocarcinomas of the colon (Boffa *et al.*, 1980). In previous studies using computer-assisted microdensitometry, Allfrey *et al.* (1978) identified two nuclear nonhistone proteins with molecular weights 44,000 (TNP$_1$)* and 62,000 (TNP$_2$) which showed accelerated rates of synthesis at early stages of carcinogenesis. Recently Pumo *et al.* (1980) have identified tumor-specific antigens in both transplantable and in dimethylhydrazine-induced colon tumors in rats. These authors described an antigen which was common to colon tumor chromatin and normal baby rat colon chromatin as assayed by microcomplement fixation.

---

* Abbreviations: CA, colon antigen; CCA, colon carcinoma antigen; CEA, carcinoembryonic antigen; CEA-B, carcinoembryonic antigen breast; CEA-M, carcinoembryonic antigen membrane; CIE, crossed immunoelectrophoresis; Con A, concanavalin A; CRIE, crossed radioimmunoelectrophoresis; CSA, colon-specific antigen; CTA, colon tumor antigen; CTSA, colon tumor-specific antigen; GP, glycoprotein; GP-I, glycoprotein I; HMW, high molecular weight; HNoAG-1, human nucleolar antigen-1; LMW, low molecular weight; NCA, normal colon antigen; NFA, normal fecal antigen; PBS, 0.15 M NaCl/20 mM phosphate, pH 7.2; QIE, quantitative immunoelectrophoresis; RIA, radioimmunoassay; RSB, 10 mM Tris/10 mM NaCl/1.5 mM MgCl$_2$, pH 7.4; SDS, sodium dodecyl sulfate; TEX, a MW 110,000 glycoprotein described by Kessler *et al.* (1972); TKM, 50 mM Tris/25 mM KCl/5 mM MgCl$_2$, pH 7.4; TNP, tumor nuclear protein; VHMW, very high molecular weight.

C. Carcinoembryonic Antigen of the Colon

For the most part, however, the area of human colon tumor antigens has been dominated by studies on carcinoembryonic antigen. Originally discovered by Gold and Freedman (1965) both the chemistry (Egan *et al.*, 1976) and the marker potential of this antigen (Wanebo *et al.*, 1978; Waalkes *et al.*, 1980) have been the source of considerable investigation and difference of opinion (Lane and Savage, 1975). This has been biochemically supported by the comparison of CEA from normal patients with that material isolated from tumors (Shively *et al.*, 1978). It becomes clear from these studies that not only is CEA expressed in normal and in nonneoplastic disease states, but that its molecular features are identical. Nevertheless, immunodiagnosis based upon CEA immunolocalization has evolved from earlier studies utilizing GW-39 tumor-bearing hamsters as described by Goldenberg *et al.* (1974). More recently this approach has been taken in the immunolocalization of CEA-producing tumors in human cancer patients (Goldenberg *et al.*, 1980). Using specific antibodies against CEA and sophisticated computer-assisted imaging technology tumor visualization has been achieved for relatively small tumor masses.

D. Human Colon Tumor Model Systems

1. Cultured Cell Lines and Transplantable Solid Tumors

Due to the need for additional (McIntire, 1980) and more reliable markers for human colon cancer (Lane and Savage, 1975) several approaches have been taken to establish laboratory transplantable human colon cancers that grow either in tissue culture (Drewinko *et al.*, 1976; Tom *et al.*, 1976) or as solid tumors (Goldenberg *et al.*, 1966; Carrel *et al.*, 1976). Of interest is some of the difficulty experienced in the establishment of cultured or transplantable tumor lines from human primary tumors of the colon. One major difficulty is the high level of bacterial contamination that is often present when specimens are collected for the purpose of establishing a culture. Another is the large population of fibroblast-like cells which can rapidly overgrow the colon tumor cells in a matter of months.

2. The GW-39 Adenocarcinoma Cell Line

An unusual adenocarcinoma of the colon is the GW-39 cell line established as a permanent heterograft in Golden Syrian Hamsters by Goldenberg *et al.* (1966). This line was derived from the sigmoid region of the colon of a 58-year-old female patient and represents one of a limited num-

TABLE I

COLON-ASSOCIATED ANTIGENS

Antigen	Chemical properties	Reference
CEA	Cell surface GP (47–57% carbohydrate), MW 175,000 pI 4.5–5.5	Gold and Freedman (1965); Egan et al. (1977); Kosaki and Yamamoto (1975)
Colon carcinoma antigen III	MW 60,000	Franchimont et al. (1973)
CCA-II	CEA related GP, MW 60,000 does not cross Rx with CEA in RIA	Newman et al. (1974)
CSA-LMW	Cell surface GP, MW 46,000	Goldenberg et al. (1976)
CSA-HMW	Cell surface GP, MW 170,000 to 900,000	Goldenberg et al. (1976)
CSA-VHMW	Cell surface GP, MW 5,000,000 to 10,000,000	Goldenberg et al. (1976)
CEA-M	MW 200,000, pI 4.2, GP (carbohydrate/protein = 2:1)	Leung et al. (1977)
CSAp	40,000–150,000 MW, organ specific	Pant et al. (1978)
GPI	CEA related 200,000 MW GP	Tsao and Kim (1978)
TEX	MW 110,000, GP, binds to Con A is 35% carbohydrate, similar amino-terminal amino acid sequence to CEA, cross-reacts with CEA	Kessler et al. (1978)
HNoAG-1	Nucleolar protein, 68/6.3	Davis et al. (1979); Chan et al. (1980)
TNP$_1$	MW 44,000; pI 7.0 & 7.2; nuclear	Boffa et al. (1980)
TNP$_2$	MW 62,000, pI 6.2; nuclear	Boffa et al. (1980)
CTA	Lipoprotein, MW bands at 12,000, 40,000, and 60,000	Thomson et al. (1980)
CEA-B	120,000 MW GP related to CEA	Santen et al. (1980)
CTSA	Nuclear; associated with inactive chromatin	Pumo et al. (1980)
NFA-1	20,000–30,000, CEA-related GP	Kuroki et al. (1981)
NFA-2	160,000–170,000 CEA-related GP	Kuroki et al. (1981)
NCA	80,000–90,000, GP	Kuroki et al. (1981)
CA-3	Cytonuclear protein, pI 4.5–4.9, MW > 150,000	Chakrabarty et al. (1981b)

ber of permanent heterografts that will grow in immunocompetent animals. Another example is the Co-115 line which was grafted and maintained in nude mice by Carrel et al. (1976). In addition, several human colon tumors have been adapted to tissue culture, in particular the LoVo cell line (Drewinko et al., 1976) as well as numerous cells lines and their clones established by Tom *et al.* (1976), Rutzky *et al.* (1979), and Tsao and Kim (1978). These include the LS174 and LS180 colon tumor cell lines and their subclones.

More recently strong efforts have been made to adapt these cultures to serum-free growth medium in order to better evaluate the effects of nutrition on cell growth and marker production as well as to reduce the number of complicating elements which are introduced by components of the serum and the medium (Rutzky, 1979; Van der Bosch *et al.*, 1981).

E. Neoantigens and Other Antigens of the Colon

A wealth of neoantigens has resulted from careful examination of the cell surface preparations and total cellular extracts of these and other colon tumor cell lines (Kahan *et al.*, 1979). A tabulation of a number of antigens, their characteristics, and literature citations are presented in Table I.

II. Production of Subcellular Fractions, Antibodies, and Preabsorptions

A. Methods for Tumor Cell Extraction

The antigens extracted from tumor cells are a result of the solubilizing properties of the extracting medium, the integrity of the biological material being extracted, and the portion of the tumor cell used as a starting material. The 0.9% NaCl and 3 M KCl extraction procedures and subsequent purification steps have been described by Reisfeld *et al.* (1977) in a discussion of rational approaches to the ellucidation of tumor-associated antigens. Other popular approaches to the extraction of tumor antigens include extraction with 1.0 M perchloric acid or 1% sodium deoxycholate (Howell *et al.*, 1979). Another extraction method is the phenol–alcohol procedure (Goldenberg *et al.*, 1976). Tumors are homogenized in water and mixed with an equal volume of 90% phenol. After mixing at 65°C for 30 minutes and overnight at 4°C the top aqueous layer is collected. From 3 to 4 volumes of 95% ethyl alcohol are added and the precipitate is collected by centrifugation. From 0.1 to 2.0% SDS has been used to solubilize the antigens present in cell membrane preparations (Kahan *et al.*, 1976). A summary of these extraction procedures and appropriate references are listed in Table II. The effects that these various approaches can have upon a specific group of related antigens have been assessed for CEA and CEA-related antigens by Kimball and Brattain (1978). They

TABLE II
EXTRACTION MEDIA FOR CELLULAR AND MEMBRANE TUMOR ANTIGENS

Extractant	Reference
0.9% NaCl	Reisfeld *et al.* (1977)
3 *M* KCl	Reisfeld *et al.* (1977)
1.0 *M* perchloric acid	Howell *et al.* (1979)
Sodium deoxycholate	Howell *et al.* (1979)
Phenol-alcohol	Goldenberg *et al.* (1976)
Sodium dodecyl sulfate	Kahan *et al.* (1976)
2% *n*-butanol	Kahan *et al.* (1979)

found that the number of peaks obtained from gel filtration columns and the heterogeneity of the electrophoretic products obtained as analyzed by isoelectric focusing on polyacrylamide gels were a function of the extract employed.

B. PREPARATION OF SUBCELLULAR FRACTIONS

One approach to the detection of previously undetected tumor antigens that we have used has been the production of subcellular fractions prior to the point of extraction and immunization (Yeoman *et al.*, 1976). In previous studies on the nuclear antigens of Novikoff hepatoma ascites cells nuclei were isolated by the 0.5% Nonidet P-40 method as described by Yeoman *et al.* (1976) and chromatin was prepared according to the procedure of Marushige and Bonner (1966). Nuclear antigens A, 1, 2, and 3 were extracted from Novikoff hepatoma nuclear chromatin with 0.6 *M* NaCl in 0.01 *M* Tris at pH 8 (Yeoman and Busch, 1978).

C. IMMUNIZATION WITH NUCLEI, NUCLEOLI, AND NUCLEAR SUBFRACTIONS

Prior to these studies the production of antibodies to nuclear antigens began with the isolation of cell nuclei. Early studies of this type began with whole nuclei or nucleoli from a normal or tumor cell as the immunogen (Busch *et al.*, 1974). Subsequently antibodies with specificity for the "tissue of origin" were obtained by the immunization of rabbits with non-histone–protein–DNA complexes that had been salt extracted in order to remove loosely bound nuclear proteins (Chytil and Spelsberg, 1971; Wakabayashi and Hnilica, 1972). This change represented a substantial reduction in antigenic complexity over and against the use of whole nuclei or nucleoli as an immunogen. Second, the use of chromatin and its tightly associated proteins was reasoned to facilitate the selection of those molecules potentially involved in critical and specific protein–DNA interactions. It was from these studies that it became clear from an immunological standpoint that the cell nucleus did contain tissue-specific nonhistone proteins and that they could be used as a source of tumor markers. The two previous methods present the antigens to the xenogeneic immune system complexed with a substantial amount of nucleic acid. From the studies of Nicolini (1975) it was thought that certain structural elements of the protein–nucleic acid complexes were required in order to maintain immunological cell specificity. It was Zardi *et al.* (1973) who were able to obtain antibodies to nonhistone proteins alone. More recently antibodies have been prepared against single, highly purified nonhistone proteins (Catino *et al.*, 1979) as an aid to the study of their cellular localization and function.

D. SUBCELLULAR FRACTIONATION OF THE GW-39 TUMOR CELL

1. Organoid Growth Characteristics—"Sacs"

Application of much of the preceding methodology to the cellular fractionation of GW-39 adenocarcinoma cells, a permanent heterograft of a human adenocarcinoma of the sigmoid region of the colon (Goldenberg *et al.*, 1966), was initially met with substantial difficulty. The organoid clusters of cells which grow in mucin-filled laceunae ("sacs") were resistant to both the 0.025 *M* citric acid method for nuclear isolation (Taylor *et al.*, 1973) as well as the Nonidet P-40 method as directly applied to Novikoff hepatoma cells (Yeoman *et al.*, 1976). In addition, the Nonidet P-40/deoxycholate method of Muramatsu *et al.* (1974) and the Triton X-100 method of Berkowitz *et al.* (1969) were also unsuccessful as applied directly to the GW-39 tumor tissue.

2. Enzymatic and Detergent Weakening of "Sacs"

In order to generate cytoplasmic and nuclear fractions for subsequent extractions and immunizations the clusters of cells were weakened by enzymatic means (Drewinko *et al.*, 1976) and disrupted from their sacs by homogenization. Tissues from tumor-bearing hamsters was ground in a Hobart meat grinder and dispersed in 10 volumes of modified Eagle's medium containing 0.05% neuraminidase and 0.05% β-glucosidase. The suspension of tissue in medium was incubated at 37°C for 3 hours with gentle agitation prior to washing with PBS. The selection of neuraminidase and β-glucosidase in combination was chosen from a series of experiments in

TABLE III

ENZYMATIC AND CHEMICAL AGENTS EMPLOYED IN COMBINATION AND
ALONE TO AID THE DISRUPTION OF GW-39 TUMOR SACS

Agent	Effectiveness
Collagenase[a]	−
Collagenase and hyaluronidase	+
Hyaluronidase[b]	+
Hyaluronidase and neuraminidase	+
Neuraminidase[c]	+
Neuraminidase and β-glucosidase	+ +
β-Glucosidase	+
"Mucomyst"[d]	−

[a] Both collagenase and collagenase/dispase (a Boehringer–Mannheim trade name) were used.

[b] Useful, but prohibitively expensive.

[c] Judged to be more effective alone and in combination than hyaluronidase.

[d] Mead Johnson's product name for N-acetyl-L-cysteine.

which the agents shown in Table III were evaluated. Although hyaluronidase was effective, its prohibitive cost prevented its consideration for use on a routine preparative basis.

Weakened sacs were washed in RSB for 10 minutes and subsequently homogenized in RSB containing 0.5% Nonidet P-40. The conversion of the organoid clusters of cells to dispersed cells is illustrated in Fig. 1. The dispersed cells were further homogenized in fresh RSB/NP40 until nuclei were obtained. The nuclei were purified through 0.33 and 0.88 M sucrose solutions.

3. Preparation of GW-39 Cell Extracts

Dispersed cells were extracted with 0.05 M Tris, pH 7.4, containing 0.025 M KCl and 0.005 M MgCl$_2$ and spun at 100,000 g for 4 hours to remove mitochondria and polysomes. Nuclei were extracted with 0.075 M NaCl/0.025 M EDTA and subsequently with 0.01 M Tris pH 8. The dilute Tris extracts of cells and of nuclei were studied for their potential as

FIG. 1. Photomicroscopic analysis of GW-39 cells at various stages in the disruption of their organoid clusters and preparation of nuclei. (A) Suspension of the ground GW-39 tumor tissue in PBS to reveal the clustered organization of the cells, "sacs." × 900. (B) Disrupted cells after treatment with glycosidases and Nonidet P-40 detergent. × 400.

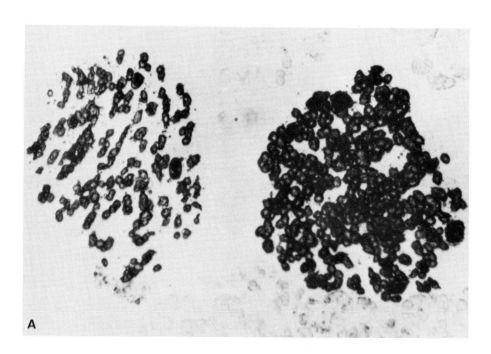

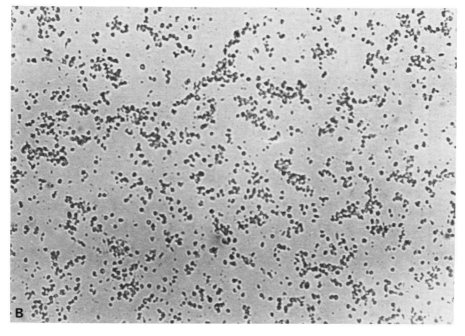

tumor markers in terms of cytoplasmic, nuclear, and common (cytonuclear) antigens (Chakrabarty *et al.*, 1981b).

E. Immunization Protocols for GW-39 Cell Antigens

1. Standard Immunization Schedules

Tris–cytosol (TKM) and Tris–nuclear fractions were concentrated to 10 mg/ml and used for the immunization of rabbits. Two immunization schedules were used. The first utilized weekly injections of 10 mg of extract mixed with an equal volume of complete Freund's adjuvant for 3 weeks and bleeding 10 days later (Yeoman *et al.*, 1976). Booster immunizations using Freund's incomplete adjuvant followed at 30-day intervals with bleedings taken 10 days after each booster.

2. Hyperimmunization

More recently the technique of hyperimmunization has been employed in order to raise the titer of the antiserum for the existing antigens as well as to increase the number of antigens detected (Harboe and Ingild, 1973). This procedure requires immunization on a continuous biweekly basis with the first bleeding taken in 2 months. Between 200 μg and 1 mg of tumor cell extract was suspended in 1 ml of Freund's complete adjuvant for each immunization. Subsequent bleedings were taken at monthly intervals.

F. Preabsorption of Anti-GW-39 Cell Antisera

Due to the presence of infiltrating lymphocytes and serum proteins in the GW-39 tumors an exhaustive series of preabsorptions were employed to greatly reduce or eliminate the recognition of hamster antigens. Acetone powders were prepared from the liver, spleen, lung, and kidney of normal Golden Syrian hamsters (Potter, 1972). These absorptions are similar to those employed by Pant *et al.* (1978). These powders were hydrated with PBS to a final concentration of 50 mg/ml for each tissue employed. Preabsorption was for 2 hours at 25°C and for 16 hours at 4°C. After centrifugation to remove the immunoprecipitate the preabsorption was repeated and immunoglobulin fractions were prepared by ammonium sulfate precipitation.

Attempts to replace the acetone powder preabsorptions with preabsorbant-Sepharose columns (Wofsy and Buff, 1969) or with water-insoluble protein polymers (Avrameas and Ternynck, 1967) were unsuccessful in our hands. While these insoluble absorbant systems can be reused and do not tend to contaminate serum, they were only partially effective in the removal of anti-CEA reactivity from the anti-GW-39 sera.

III. Crossed and Crossed Radioimmunoelectrophoresis

A. QUANTITATIVE IMMUNOELECTROPHORETIC METHODS AND THEIR APPLICATION

Quantitative immunoelectrophoresis (QIE), employing standardized polyclonal reference antisera, offers great potential in the analysis of complex antigenic systems. This technique allows the quantification of individual antigens without previous separation and the elucidation of antigenic complexity, immunological reactivity, and relative antigenic concentrations (Verbruggen, 1975; Axelsen *et al.*, 1973). It is also possible to determine the immunodominant antigenic species within a complex antigenic mixture in terms of the density and staining intensity of their immunoprecipitates. Generally, larger and more immunogenic molecules often give rise to denser precipitates (i.e., more antibodies bound to the antigen) than smaller and less immunogenic molecules (Lowenstein, 1978). This point is illustrated more clearly for one of the GW-39 tumor-associated antigens (antigen 3) identified in a latter section of the article.

QIE techniques have been successfully employed in the study of complex cell surface antigens, biological membranes, microbial antigens, and allergens (Schulman and Karpatkin, 1980; Bjerrum and Bog-Hansen, 1976; Johansson and Hjerten, 1974; Smyth *et al.*, 1976, 1978; Owen and Salton, 1977; Bog-Hansen *et al.*, 1975; Axelsen, 1976). QIE techniques are nondenaturing and are 10–100 times more sensitive than SDS-containing polyacrylamide gels (Nurden and Caen, 1974). QIE can be adopted to study the human immune response to individual antigens within a complex antigenic mixture without their prior isolation. For example, the human IgE antibody response to individual antigens within an antigenic mixture can be studied by QIE technique (Axelsen *et al.*, 1973; Lowenstein, 1978; Chakrabarty *et al.*, 1981a).

It is beyond the scope of this article to give a detailed review of the development of QIE. However, a brief review of its development is given in order to better understand the technique. The technical details of QIE have been described in detail by Axelsen *et al.* (1973).

B. Ouchterlony Immunodiffusion Reactions

One of the more simple and convenient methods for demonstration of immunochemical relationships between soluble antigens and antibodies is the double diffusion method described by Ouchterlony (1948, 1949). Precipitin bands are formed at equivalence points where optimal concentrations of antigen and antibody are present. The number of precipitin bands indicates the minimum number of individual antigen–antibody systems. The precipitates formed are generally identified by the use of a reference antigen. There are three basic precipitin patterns underlying the antigen–antibody interactions: reactions of identity, nonidentity, and partial identity.

C. Analytical Immunoelectrophoresis

Immunoelectrophoresis (Grabar and William, 1953) was developed from the technique of double diffusion. The relatively low resolving power of double diffusion techniques was increased by separating the antigens by electrophoresis prior to diffusion. The analytical immunoelectrophoretic method for the study of antigens and antibodies is based upon their characteristic mobility in an electric field. Each antigen–antibody system will form one precipitin band which can be stabilized in a suitable matrix such as agarose. There are many applications for the immunoelectrophoretic technique. These include (1) identification of the minimum number of antigenic components present in a mixture, and (2) determination of the antigenic purity of a fractionated material by comparing it with the immunoprecipitated bands obtained with the unfractionated material.

D. Crossed Immunoelectrophoresis–"Rocket"
   Immunoelectrophoresis

The immunoelectrophoretic technique described above is a qualitative method. In 1960, Ressler showed that antigens could be forced, by an electric current, into an agar gel bed containing antiserum (Ressler, 1960). The quantitation of the protein in a single antigen–antibody system is given by the rocket-shaped precipitate formed, hence the term "rocket immunoelectrophoresis." However, the precipitates resulting from more than one antigen–antibody system were seen as multiple rocket-shaped curves superimposed upon each other. Thus the precipitin arcs formed were not distinct from one another. However, rocket immunoelectrophoresis performed with a monospecific antiserum is particularly useful in monitoring purification procedures employed in antigen isolation. A few years later high-resolution quantitative crossed immunoelectrophoresis was developed (Laurell, 1965). In the CIE technique, antigens are first separated by electrophoresis in one dimension followed by electrophoresis into antibody-containing gel in a second dimension perpendicular to the first. Immunoprecipitates are formed during the second dimension of electrophoresis. The area given in each immunoprecipitate can be correlated with the concentration of an individual antigen. The high resolving power and the possibility of quantification of individual antigens without previous separation have provided for its acceptance and widespread application (Axelsen *et al.*, 1973). Precipitin reactions of identity, nonidentity, and partial identity can be identified by CIE. For a complete analysis of a complex antigen–antibody system, the first dimension of electrophoresis as performed in CIE can be supplemented by isoelectrofocusing (for determination of p*I*s) or by isotachophoresis (Chakrabarty *et al.*, 1981b).

E. APPLICATION OF CIE TO THE ANALYSIS OF GW-39 CELL ANTIGENS

1. Cytosol–Anticytosol System

The application of CIE to the analysis of GW-39 colon tumor antigens is shown in Figs. 2–5. The antigens detected in the cytosol–anticytosol system are illustrated in Fig. 2. Approximately 20 antigens were detected by the anticytosol antibodies (Fig. 2A). The important antigens, in terms of immunogenicity as detected by the intensity of staining and quantity, appeared to be antigens 1, 2, and 3 (Fig. 2B). Antigen 5 was a well-separated antigen from antigen 1 and 2 and was present in fairly high amount in the antigenic mixtures. Antigens 6, 7, and other antigens which were present in smaller amounts were classified as "group A" antigens and are shown in Fig. 2B. These antigens were not detected when smaller amounts of cytosol antigens were employed in the CIE analysis. Cytosol antigens 1 and 2 were found upon further analysis to be immunologically related.

2. Nuclear–Antinuclear System

The antigens detected in the nuclear and antinuclear system are illustrated in Fig. 3. Essentially 4 antigens were detected (Fig. 3A). Nuclear antigens 3A and 3B appeared to be the important antigens in terms of immunogenicity (intensity of staining) as illustrated in Fig. 3B. Nuclear antigens 3A and 3B appeared to migrate in approximately the same position as cytosol antigen 3 in the cytosol–anticytosol system

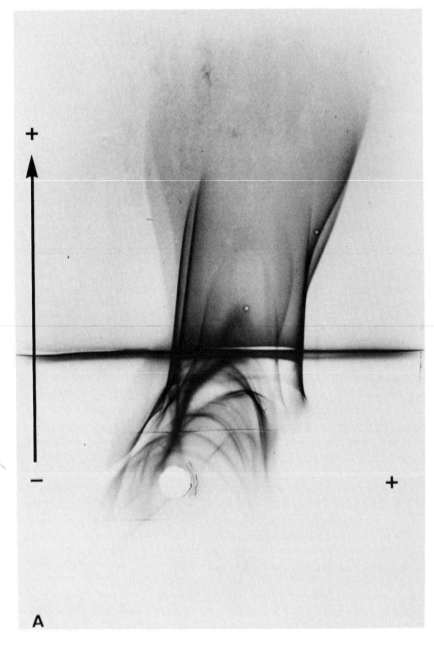

A

Fig. 2. CIE analysis of cytosol antigens employing anticytosol antibodies. (A) Cytosol antigens (20 μl) were employed in the analysis. (B) Schematic drawing of the antigens identified in (A). Broken lines indicate weakly stained immunoprecipitin peaks.

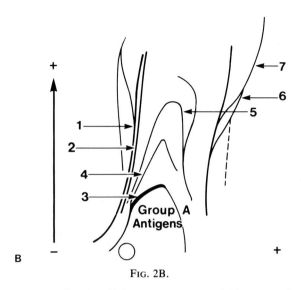

FIG. 2B.

3. Cross-Reactivity of Subcellular Fractions and Their Antibodies

The cross-reactivity between the cytosol and nuclear antigens was also studied by the CIE technique. The anticytosol antibodies recognized at least five nuclear antigens while antigens 3A and 3B appeared to be the same in both extracts.

F. Crossed Immunoelectrophoresis Employing Preabsorbed Antisera

Attempts were made to detect and identify GW-39 tumor-associated antigens by the CIE technique employing the preabsorbed anticytosol and antinuclear antibodies. Figure 4 illustrates the results of these experiments. The number of cytosol antigens that were recognized by the preabsorbed anticytosol antibodies was greatly reduced in comparison to the nonabsorbed anticytosol antibodies (Fig. 2A). The prominent cytosol antigens recognized by the preabsorbed anticytosol antibodies included cytosol antigens 1, 3, and 5. Antigens 1 and 5 were identified by superimposing the immunoplate (Fig. 4A) (cytosol preabsorbed anticytosol) onto the other immunoplate (Fig. 2A) (cytosol–anticytosol). A few other minor antigens were also detected by the preabsorbed antibodies. The preabsorbed anticytosol antibodies recognized essentially two nuclear antigens—3A and 3B (Fig. 4B). The possibility that nuclear antigen 3A consisted of more than one antigen was quite probably because of the diffuse staining pattern observed. Figure 3A and B actually revealed that nuclear antigen 3

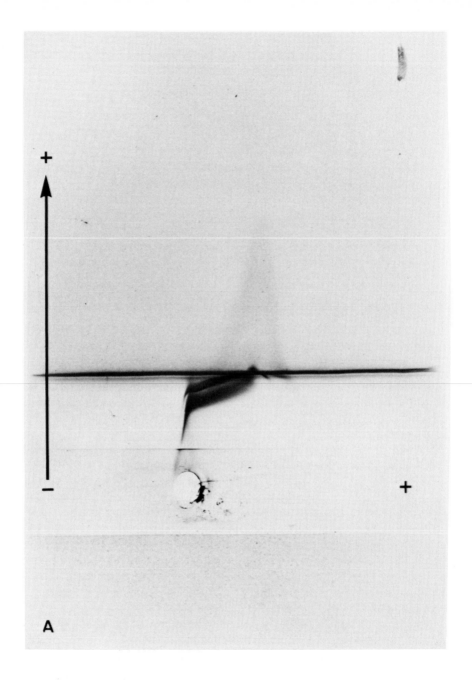

FIG. 3. CIE analysis of nuclear antigens employing antinuclear antibodies. (A) Nuclear antigens (20 μl) were employed in the analysis. (B) Schematic drawing of the antigens identified in (A). Broken lines indicate weakly stained immunoprecipitin peaks.

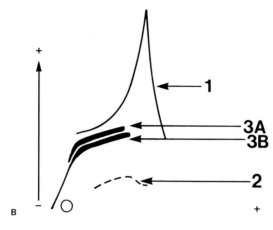

FIG. 3B.

contained at least two antigens. It now appeared that only one of these antigens was recognized by the preabsorbed anticytosol antibodies. The results of the analysis of cytosol and nuclear antigens employing preabsorbed antinuclear Tris antibodies are illustrated by Fig. 5A and B. The preabsorbed antinuclear antibodies recognized essentially three cytosol antigens, the prominent antigen being cytosol antigen 3 (Fig. 5A). The nuclear antigens 3A and 3B were also recognized by the preabsorbed antinuclear antibodies (Fig. 5B). The crossed immunoelectrophoretic results are summarized for preabsorbed and nonpreabsorbed antibodies in Table IV.

G. Identification of CEA in GW-39 Cell Extracts—Elimination of CEA Recognition by Preabsorption of Antisera

Due to the large number of colonic antigens (both normal and neoplastic colon) that display complete or partial immunological identity with CEA (see Table I) it was important to determine whether any of these colon antigens selected for further characterization showed any cross-reactivity with CEA. This possibility was ruled out by performing crossed radioimmunoelectrophoresis (Norgaard-Pedersen, 1973) and demonstrating that the preabsorbed antibodies had no capacity for the recognition of ^{125}I-labeled CEA (obtained commercially from Hoffmann-LaRoche). The Tris extract of GW-39 cytoplasm was mixed with 10^6 cpm of ^{125}I-labeled CEA. Crossed radioimmunoelectrophoresis was performed and autoradiography was run.

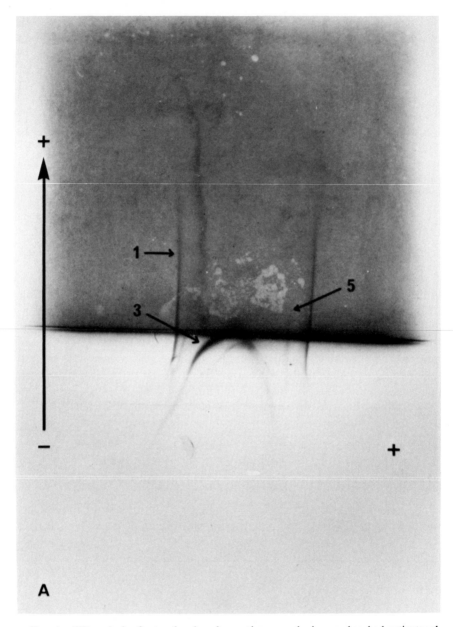

Fig. 4. CIE analysis of cytosol and nuclear antigens employing preabsorbed anticytosol antibodies. Amounts of cytosol and nuclear antigens employed in the analysis were the same as in Figs. 2A and 3A. (A) CIE analysis of cytosol antigens employing preabsorbed anticytosol antibodies. (B) CIE analysis of nuclear antigens employing preabsorbed anticytosol antibodies.

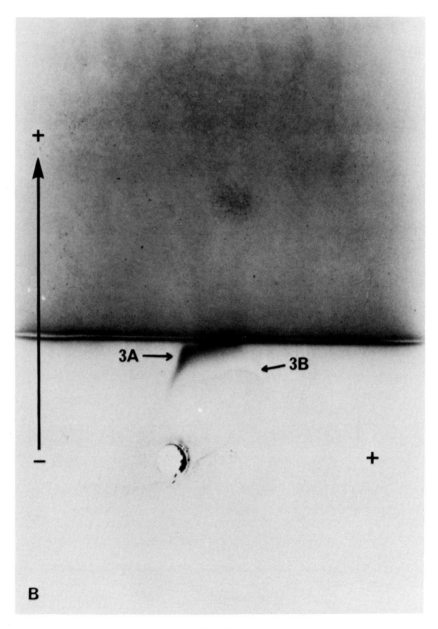

Fig. 4B.

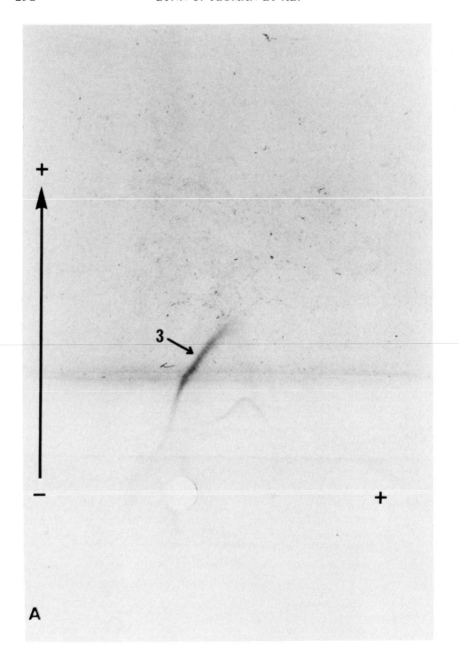

FIG. 5. CIE analysis of cytosol and nuclear antigens employing preabsorbed antinuclear antibodies. (A) CIE analysis of cytosol antigens employing preabsorbed antinuclear antibodies. (B) CIE analysis of nuclear antigens employing preabsorbed antinuclear antibodies.

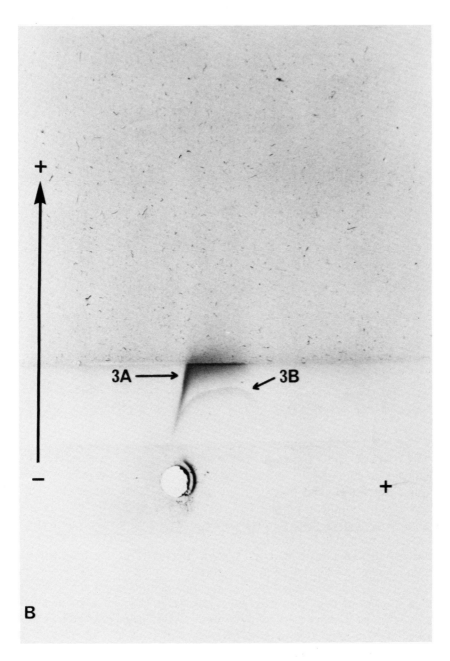

Fɪɢ. 5B.

TABLE IV
CYTOSOL AND NUCLEAR ANTIGENS OF GW-39

Antigen–antibody system[a]	Number of antigens detected	Comments
Cytosol Ags/anti-cytosol Abs	Approximately 20	Ags 1, 2, and 3 are immunogenic Ags in terms of intensity of staining. Ags 1 and 2 are present in the highest amount and are partially identical to each other
Nuclear Ags/anti-nuclear Abs	4	Nuclear Ags 3A and 3B are immunogenic Ags in terms of intensity of staining
Cytosol Ags/pre-absorbed anticytosol Abs	Approximately 5	Cytosol Ags 1, 3, and 5 are precipitated, suggesting that these Ags may be tumor associated
Nuclear Ags/pre-absorbed anticytosol Abs	2	Nuclear 3A and 3B are precipitated, suggesting that these cross-reactive Ags may be tumor associated
Cytosol Ags/pre-absorbed anti-nuclear Abs	3	Cytosol Ag 3 is precipitated; suggesting that this cross-reactive Ag may be tumor associated
Nuclear Ags/pre-absorbed anti-nuclear Abs	2	Nuclear Ags 3A and 3B are precipitated, suggesting that these cross-reactive Ags may be tumor associated

[a] Ags, antigens; Abs, antibodies.

The results of these experiments are shown in Fig. 6. At least two radiostained immunoprecipitins were detected in the cytosol–anticytosol and nuclear–antinuclear systems after 13 hours of autoradiography. The anti–cytosol antibodies recognized CEA that was present in both the cytosol and nuclear extracts. No radiostained immunoprecipitins were observed for both the Tris–cytosol and Tris–nuclear antigens when the preabsorbed anticytosol antibodies were employed in the crossed radioimmunoelectrophoretic analysis. No radiostaining was observed with the preabsorbed antibodies even after 30 hours of autoradiography. Overlaying the autoradiographs onto the Coomassie Blue-stained immunoplates revealed that none of the important cytosol or nuclear antigens described above contained CEA. CEA was observed to migrate in the position of immunoprecipitins belonging to the minor group A antigens (Fig. 2B).

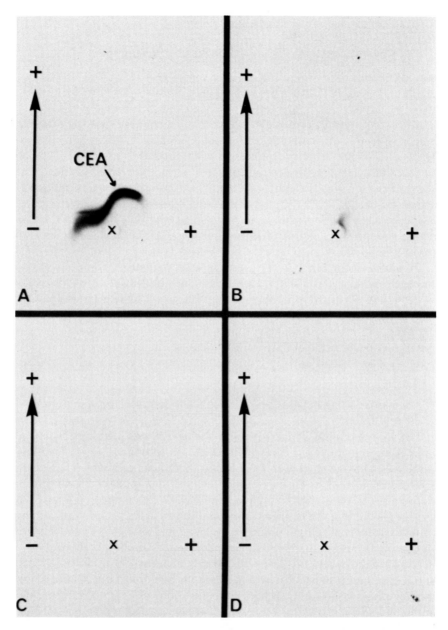

FIG. 6. Crossed radioimmunoelectrophoretic analysis of cytosol and nuclear antigens—identification of CEA following 13 hours of autoradiography. (A) Radiostaining observed in the cytosol and anticytosol system. (B) Radiostaining observed in the nuclear and antinuclear system. (C and D) Absence of radiostaining in the cytosol and nuclear antigens, respectively, when preabsorbed anticytosol antibodies were employed in the crossed radioimmunoelectrophoretic analysis.

IV. Immunolocalization of GW-39 Colon Tumor Antigens

A. THE INDIRECT IMMUNOFLUORESCENT STAINING TECHNIQUE

Since the antisera obtained against cytoplasmic and nuclear Tris extracts showed both common and unique immunoreactivities in the extracts of GW-39 cells it was of interest to examine the immunolocalization of these antigens in a limited number of other colon tumor cell lines. The method chosen was the indirect immunofluorescent staining technique of Hilgers *et al.* (1972). In the case of cultured human colon tumor cells (provided by Drs. B. Tom and L. Rutsky) the cells were dried onto microscope slides at 4°C and fixed for 5 minutes with acetone. In the case of cryosections the specimens were put onto gelatin-coated slides and fixed with 0.05% formaldehyde to preserve ultrastructure according to the method of Lazarides (1976). This particular concentration of formaldehyde (made fresh from paraformaldehyde) was found to be optimal for preservation of ultrastructure while retaining the immunoreactivity of the antigens. At 0.1% formaldehyde and higher the immunoreactivity was greatly reduced, while at 0.01% formaldehyde and lower the cellular morphology was obscured.

B. IMMUNOLOCALIZATION OF CYTOSOL COLON ANTIGENS

The immunofluorescence obtained for six human colon cell culture lines using the anti-Tris–cytosol antibodies is shown in Fig. 7. The fluorescence is localized in each case to the cytoplasm although it differs in fluorescent intensity. This difference in intensity probably results from differences in antigen production on the part of individual cell lines or in the accessibility of the antigens to the antibodies in each case. The coating of fluorescence at cell membranes observed in Fig. 7a–c, e, and f is not thought to be artifactual but to in fact represent a very bright fluorescence in the cytoplasm and up to the membrane of these cells. However, cell surface concentrations of these antigens cannot be ruled out. Controls imploying preimmune serum at high concentrations of FITC-labeled second antibody did not show any fluorescence intensely above that general subliminal image which results from autofluorescence or filter leakage of excitation light. A few cell lines displayed some low intensity nucleolar fluorescence (Fig. 7f). It will be shown later using anti-3 antibody that this nuclear fluorescence probably results from the expression of antigen 3. A summary of the fluorescent intensities observed for anti-Tris–cytosol antibodies is presented in Table V.

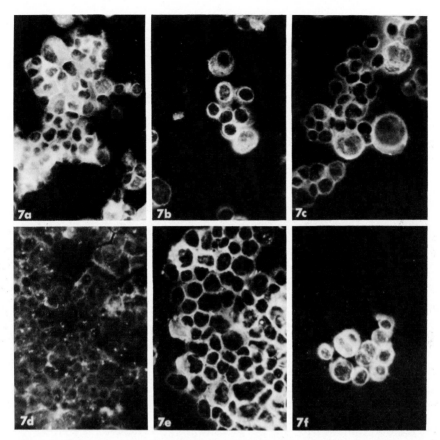

Fig. 7. Indirect immunofluorescence observed in cultured human colon tumor cells with preabsorbed anti-Tris–cytosol antibodies. Cells were fixed on the slides with acetone at 4°C and stained for immunofluorescence as described in the text. The cells are (a) LS174T TC26, (b) clone 10-1, (c) clone 10-3, (d) clone 10-4, (e) SW480, and (f) clone 3-5. Specimens were photographed with a Zeiss fluorescence microscope equipped with an epi-illuminator. All photographs represent a 900-fold magnification.

TABLE V

INDIRECT IMMUNOFLUORESCENCE OBSERVED WITH 7× PREABSORBED ANTI-GW-39
TRIS–CYTOSOL SERUM IgG

Colon tumor specimen	Brightness
1. LS174T TC26	4
2. Clone 10-1	3
3. Clone 10-3	2
4. Clone 10-4	1
5. SW 480	3
6. Clone 3-5	4

C. Immunolocalization of Nuclear Colon Antigens

A similar approach was taken with anti-Tris–nuclear antibodies which were shown to recognize predominantly antigen 3 by CIE analysis. The same series of cultured human colon tumor cell lines was examined as shown in Fig. 8. Although less intense, one can still see a marked cytoplasmic fluorescence in the cells shown in Fig. 8a–c, e, and f and to a lesser extent in Fig. 8d. The detection of nuclear structure in the form of a

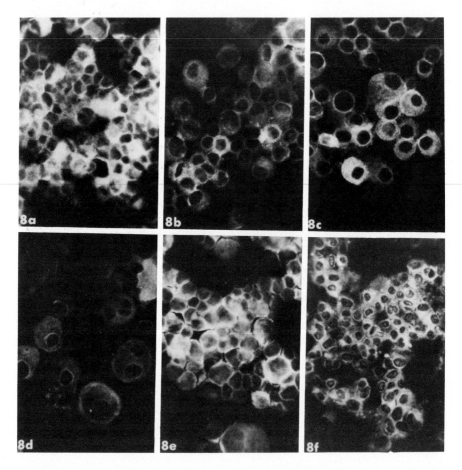

FIG. 8. Indirect immunofluorescence observed in cultured human colon tumor cells with preabsorbed anti-Tris–nuclear antibodies. See Fig. 7 for the description of cells and methods.

TABLE VI

INDIRECT IMMUNOFLUORESCENCE OBSERVED WITH 7× PREABSORBED
ANTI-GW-39 NUCLEAR TRIS SERUM IgG

Colon tumor specimen	Brightness
1. LS174T TC26	4
2. Clone 10-1	2
3. Clone 10-3	3
4. Clone 10-4	1
5. SW 480	4
6. Clone 3-5	3

matrix in Fig. 8a, b, e, and f as well as nucleoli in Fig. 8f is thought to represent nuclear concentrations of antigen 3. A summary of the fluorescent intensities observed is presented in Table VI.

D. IMMUNOFLUORESCENT ANALYSIS OF PRIMARY HUMAN COLON TUMORS

In order to establish that the same kinds of cellular fluorescence were seen in primary human colon tumors, cryosections of tumors were treated according to the procedure of Lazarides (1976). The results are shown in Fig. 9.

All of the colon tumor cells and tissues examined displayed some immunofluorescence. As already mentioned, the intensity and localization are probably a function of antigen production, accessibility and permeability of the specimen. The bright cytoplasmic fluorescence observed for the anti-Tris–cytosol antibodies in Figs. 7 and 9 is quite reasonable. The nuclear localization is probably the result of nuclear concentrations of antigen 3.

Since, fluorescence obtained for anti-Tris–nuclear antibodies is quite similar to that obtained from anti-Tris–cytosol antibodies an explanation is in order. This is thought to result from the immunodominant quality of antigen 3 as well as its presence in both nuclear and cytosol fractions. This phenomenon is not unique to antigen 3. Nuclear antigen 2 from Novikoff hepatoma cells was isolated from nuclear extracts by affinity chromatography (Yeoman and Busch, 1978) as well as from the cytoplasm by more conventional protein isolation methodology (Taylor *et al.*, 1979). GW-39 colon cell antigen 3 may represent one of a class of cellular proteins designated as "cytonuclear" proteins (DiBerardino and Hoffner, 1975; Bonner, 1978).

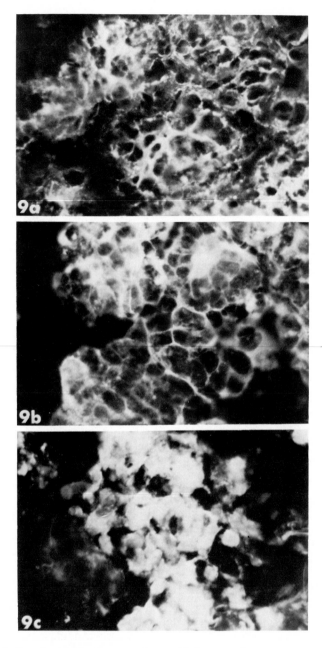

FIG. 9. Indirect immunofluorescence observed in human colon tumor cryosections with anti-GW-39 TKM cytosol antiserum. Sample (a) is specimen 10-66/10-9-79, (b) specimen 10-85/10-24-79, and (c) is specimen 10-61/10-18-79. Specimens were fixed for immunofluorescence as described by Lazarides (1976). See Fig. 7 for a description of the photomicroscopy.

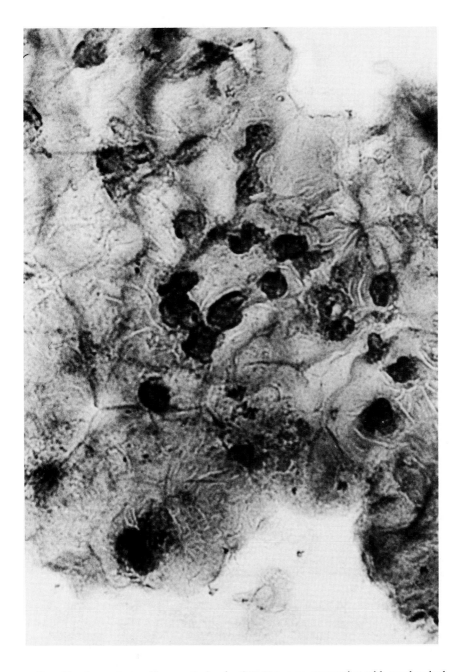

FIG. 10. Immunoperoxidase analysis of a GW-39 tumor cryosection with preabsorbed anti-CA-3 antibodies. The specimen was photographed under bright field illumination with a Zeiss photomicroscope.

E. Immunoperoxidase Analysis for Colon Antigen 3 Localization

That antigen 3 does occur in the cell nucleus is more clearly shown in an immunoperoxidase analysis of a GW-39 tumor cryosection (Weir *et al.*, 1974) in Fig. 10. The immunoperoxidase reactivity in the nucleus and surrounding the nucleolus is more clearly demonstrated in this figure. It is important to point out, however, that substantial immunoreactivity is still apparent within the cytoplasm.

V. Purification and Properties of Colon Antigens

A. Enzymatic Analysis for Protein, Carbohydrate, and Nucleic Acid

In order to proceed with the isolation and characterization studies on these antigens it was important to determine the classes of macromolecules involved. By establishing whether these molecules contained protein, carbohydrate, or nucleic acid, the selection of potential separation methods could be made. Too often the assumption is made that the major products in saline extracts are proteins or glycoproteins. While this may frequently be the case, there are reports of other types of antigenic species. One recent example of this is the report by Breimer (1980) on neutral glycolipids isolated from gastric adenocarcinoma cells. These were mixtures of glycosphingolipids which contained five to nine sugar moieties. The results of a digestion experiment are shown in Fig. 11. It is clear that the rocket pattern is altered drastically by treatment with proteinase K and to a lesser extent by neuraminidase. Digestion with RNase A and DNase I had no effect on the pattern obtained. It was clear from this study that the antigens of the Tris extract of GW-39 cell cytoplasm were proteins and that some of them were glycoproteins.

B. Preparative Isoelectric Focusing in Granulated Gels

Initial attempts at purification of GW-39 antigens 1, 3, and 5 from Tris–cytosol utilized isoelectric focusing in Ultrodex as described by Radola (1973). This method has proven useful in the purification of nuclear antigen 2 from Novikoff hepatoma cells (Taylor *et al.*, 1979). Figure 12 shows the fractionation of protein and immunoreactivity achieved in pH 3.5 to 10 focusing of the Tris–cytosol extract. A pH gradient running from pH 4.2 to 8.4 was obtained. Although the distribution of protein was fairly uni-

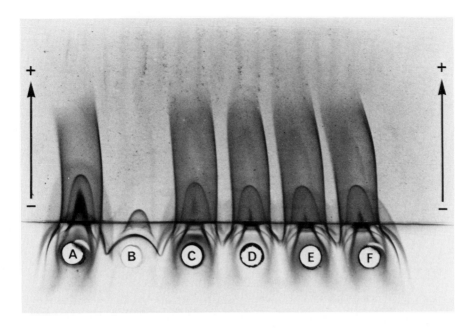

FIG. 11. Rocket immunoelectrophoretic analysis of enzymatic digests of GW-39 cell Tris extracts. A 500-μg quantity of GW-39 cell Tris–cytosol extract was digested for 16 hours at 25°C with (A) neuraminidase, (B) proteinase K, (C) insoluble protease, (D) RNase A, (E) DNase I, and (F) an incubated control. Rocket plates were stained with Coomassie Blue.

form throughout the gradient, the immunoreactivity, as measured by rocket height, was concentrated in fractions 1–17 with the strongest immunoreactivity shown in fractions 7–11. More information was obtained when individual fractions were analyzed by immunoelectrophoresis. The results are shown in Fig. 13. Analysis of these same fractions with preabsorbed antisera showed antigen 1 to focus from pH 4.3 to 5.3, antigen 5 to focus at pH 4.8, and antigen 3 to focus in a broad range. Although it was possible to isolate substantial amounts of antigenically pure antigen 3 from fractions 22 through 25 of the Ultrodex "flat-bed" it was this broad range of focusing that prompted the exploration of more efficient approaches to the isolation of antigen 3.

C. G-100 SEPHADEX GEL FILTRATION OF CYTOSOL ANTIGENS

The separation of Tris–cytosol by gel filtration on G-100 Sephadex is shown in Fig. 14. Analysis of the individual peaks from this column for their antigen content by CIE showed antigen 3 to be exclusively present in

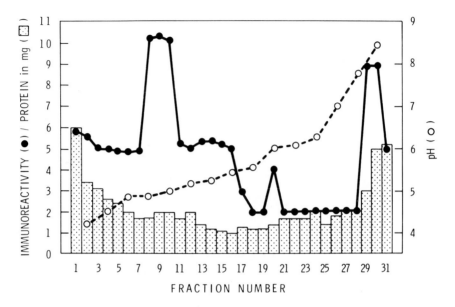

FIG. 12. Preparative isoelectric focusing of GW-39 tumor cell cytosol extract in Ultrodex. Approximately 80 mg of Tris–cytosol extract was mixed with Ultrodex and pH 3.5 to 10 range Ampholine. Focusing was completed in 42,600 volt hours. The pH (O‑‑‑‑O) was measured with a microsurface pH electrode. The immunoreactivity (●——●) was determined by net rocket height and the protein content was measured by the absorbance at 280 nm.

fractions 20–23. The bulk of antigen 1 and antigen 5 reactivity was contained in the region eluting between fractions 25 and 37. Not only did this provide a simple and direct approach to the isolation of antigen 3, but it provided the first indication of its size. Antigen 3 was shown from its migration relative to molecular weight standards to be greater then or equal to 150,000. The antigens coming off between fractions 25 and 29 were bracketed between molecular weights 60,000 and 75,000. This measurement was fortunate since detection of antigenic reactivity after western transfer (Towbin *et al.*, 1979) from SDS-containing Laemmli gels (Laemmli, 1970) was not possible for these antigens. This finding indicated their sensitivity to denaturation by sodium dodecyl sulfate. A CRIE analysis of antigenic purity for antigen 3 is shown in Fig. 15. Fractions 20–23 from the G-100 Sephadex column shown in Fig. 14 were pooled and labeled with ^{125}I by the iodogen procedure (Fraker and Speck, 1978). This product was mixed with cold GW-39 Tris–cytoplasmic extract in order to generate a rocket of substantial size. The predominant antigen product in this fraction at both short and long exposures to X-ray film is antigen 3. A

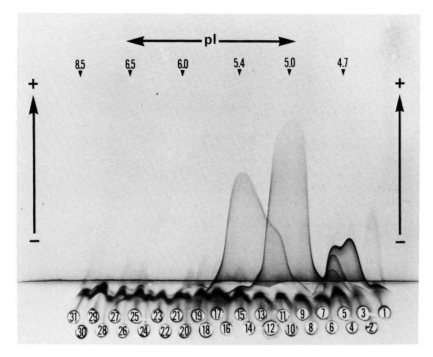

FIG. 13. Rocket immunoelectrophoretic analysis of preparative IF flat-bed fractions. The individual fractions numbered in Fig. 12 were collected, eluted with PBS, and concentrated. Samples were subjected to one-dimensional rocket immunoelectrophoretic analysis. Rocket plates were stained with Coomassie blue.

summary of those properties which have been attributed to antigen 3 is presented in Table VII.

D. ANTIBODY–SEPHAROSE AFFINITY CHROMATOGRAPHY

The purification of antigens by affinity methods frequently represents a substantial fold purification in a single purification step. Options in this catagory include the use of lectins (Lis and Sharon, 1977) as well as the use of antibodies coupled to CNBr activated agarose (March *et al.*, 1974). This approach was very useful in the isolation of the nuclear antigens from Novikoff hepatoma cells (Yeoman, 1978). Recent attempts at the purification of GW-39 antigen 3 have yielded antigen 3 products which are similar in antigenic purity to that shown for G-100 Sephadex purified antigen 3 in Fig 15.

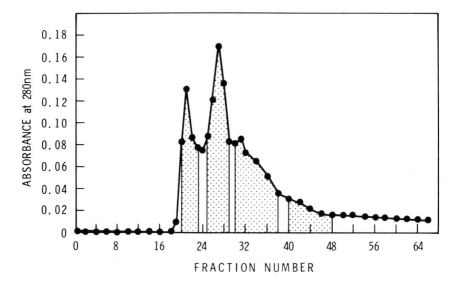

F_{IG}. 14. G-100 Sephadex chromatography of the GW-39 cell Tris–cytosol extract. A 10-mg load (1.0 ml) of Tris–cytosol extract was brought to 0.15 *M* NaCl and loaded on a 1.5 × 95-cm column. The flow rate was 6 ml/hour and 3.0-ml fractions were collected. The absorbance was measured at 280 nm and the indicated regions were pooled for further analysis.

VI. Summary

A. A S_{LIGHTLY} D_{IFFERENT} A_{PPROACH}

It has been our goal to take a slightly different approach in the selection of cellular extracts for the extraction of potential tumor markers. By the subcellular fractionation of GW-39 colon adenocarcinoma cells into cytoplasmic and nuclear fractions, antigens have been extracted which may have been dominated by other molecules when presented to a xenogeneic host as a group. It is of interest that by this approach three potential antigen markers have been detected which share no immunological cross-reactivity with CEA. Of these three antigens, antigen 3 is the most highly purified and characterized at this writing. It is not known whether antigen 3 will prove to be more useful then antigens 1 or 5 (G-100 fraction 2) when more normal and tumor specimens have been examined. Whether this antigen corresponds to any of the antigens described by other workers is not clear. By size and tumor of origin, one would clearly have to consider the HMW-CSA antigen (MW 170,000–900,000) or the VHMW-CSA (MW 5 million to 10 million) of Goldenberg *et al.* (1976) as a possibility. The demonstration of cytoplasmic and nuclear concentrations of colon antigen 3

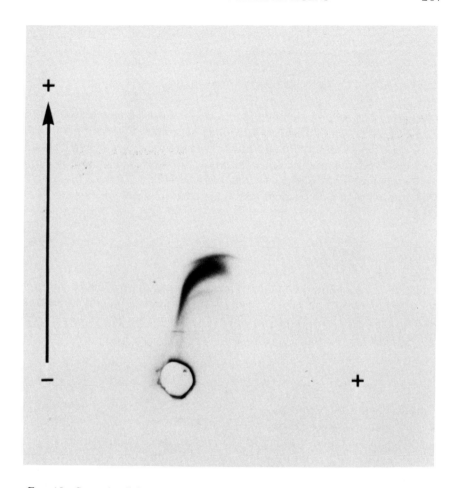

Fig. 15. Crossed radioimmunoelectrophoretic analysis for G-100 Sephadex purified antigen 3. Electrophoresis in agarose at pH 8.6 in Svendsen's buffer was performed in the horizontal direction. Electrophoresis at pH 8.6 into anti-Tris–cytosol antibodies was run in the vertical dimension. Rockets were visualized by exposure to RP-Royal X-omat X-ray film for 3 hours.

TABLE VII
PROPERTIES OF GW-39 ANTIGEN 3

Protein
GP
pI 4.5–4.9
MW ≥ 150,000
Immunodominant in both nuclear
   and cytoplasmic Tris extracts
No cross-reactivity with CEA

would tend to contrast it with HMW-CSA, hence we think that it has not been observed previously.

B. Progress in the Purification of Colon Antigen 3

Progress has been made in the purification of this antigen by both standard protein isolation methods as well as by affinity chromatography. In each case the product is highly purified by immunological criterion and well on its way to purity by other criterion. It has already been shown that it is a glycoprotein of MW > 150,000, has a pI from 4.5 to 4.9, is present in both cytoplasmic and nuclear extracts, and does not cross-react with CEA.

C. Colon Antigens as Markers

The marker potential of antigen 3 is currently under evaluation through the development of an RIA as well as by crossed radioimmunoelectrophoretic examination of specimens obtained from patients with colon and ovarian cancer.

D. The Biological Significance of Tumor Antigen Studies

Of particular interest to us is the biological significance of this product to the cancer cell and its aberrant gene control. Further purification and biochemical characterization will be required to determine unusual molecular features or similarities of this antigen to other known cancer markers (see Table I). It is our goal to ascertain the chemical and functional impact that these molecules have upon cancer cells so that a more basic understanding of their importance can be perceived at the molecular level. It is through a careful search for valid and useful cancer markers that molecules of critical importance to the biological mechanism involved in either tumor promotion, carcinogenesis, or maintenance of the cancer phenotype can be singled out for further studies. The development of model systems where the presence, synthesis, or transport of specific tumor markers is affected by the administration of antineoplastic agents will be especially useful for the development of new approaches to the rational therapy of cancer. Although no deliberate effort has been made to select for cell surface antigens in these studies, those which fall into such a catagory would be useful for the development of immunologically targeted modes of cancer therapy.

ACKNOWLEDGEMENT

The original research included in this report was supported by United States Public Health Service Grant CA-10893, P-6 awarded to L.C.Y. by the National Cancer Institute.

REFERENCES

Allfrey, V. G., Boffa, L. C., and Vidali, G. (1978). *In* "Biological Markers of Neoplasia: Basic and Applied Aspects" (R. W. Ruddon, ed.), pp. 351–366. Amer. Elsevier, New York.

Avrameas, S., and Ternynck, T. (1967). *J. Biol. Chem.* **242**, 1651–1659.

Axelsen, N. H. (1976). *Scand. J. Immunol.* **5**, 177–190.

Axelsen, N. H., Krøll, J., and Weeke, B. (1973). *Scand. J. Immunol.* **2**, Suppl. 1.

Berkowitz, D. M., Kakefuda, T., and Sporn, M. B., (1969). *J. Cell Biol.* **42**, 851—854.

Bjerrum, O. J., and Bog-Hansen, T. C. (1976). *Biochim. Biophys. Acta* **455**, 66—89.

Boffa, L. C., Diwan, B. A., Gruss, R., and Allfrey, V. G. (1980). *Cancer Res.* **40**, 1774–1780.

Bog-Hansen, T. C., Bjerrum, O. J., and Ramlau, J. (1975). *Scand. J. Immunol.* **4** (Suppl. 2), 141–147.

Bonner, W. M. (1978). *In* "The Cell Nucleus" (H. Busch, ed.), Vol. VI, pp. 97–148. Academic Press, New York.

Breimer, M. E. (1980). *Cancer Res.* **40**, 897–908.

Busch, R. K., Daskal, I., Spohn, W. H., Kellermayer, M., and Busch, H. (1974). *Cancer Res.* **34**, 2362–2367.

Carrel, S., Sordat, B., and Merenda, C. (1976). *Cancer Res.* **36**, 3978–3984.

Catino, J. J., Busch, H., Daskal, Y., and Yeoman, L. C. (1979). *J. Cell Biol.* **83**, 462–467.

Chakrabarty, S., Lowenstein, H., Ekramoddoullah, A. K. M., Kisil, F. T., and Sehon, A. H. (1981a). *Int. Arch. Allergy Appl. Immunol.* **65**, 377–389.

Chakrabarty, S., Taylor, C. W., and Yeoman, L. C. (1981b). *J. Immunol. Methods* **43**, 301–311.

Chan, P. K., Feyerbend, A., Busch, R. K., and Busch, H. (1980). *Cancer Res.* **40**, 3194–3201.

Chytil, F., and Spelsberg, T. C. (1971). *Nature (London) New Biol.* **233**, 215–218.

Davis, F. M., Gyorkey, F., Busch, R. K., and Busch, H. (1979). *Proc. Natl. Acad. Sci. U.S.A.* **76**, 892–896.

DiBerardino, M. A., and Hoffner, J. J. (1975). *Exp. Cell Res.* **94**, 235–252.

Drewinko, B., Romsdahl, M. M., Yang, L. Y., Anhearn, M. J., and Trujillo, J. M. (1976). *Cancer Res.* **36**, 467–475.

Egan, M. L., Coligan, J. E., Pritchard, D. G., Schnute, Jr., W. C., and Todd, C. W. (1976). *Cancer Res.* **36**, 3482–3485.

Egan, M. L., Pritchard, D. G., Todd, C. W., and Go, V. L. W. (1977). *Cancer Res.* **37**, 2638–2643.

Fraker, P. J., and Speck, J. C. (1978). *Biochem. Biophys. Res. Commun.* **80**, 849–857.

Franchimont, P., Debruche, M. L., Zangerle, P. F., and Pryard, I. (1973). *Ann. Immunol.* **124c**, 619–630.

Gold, P., and Freedman, S. O. (1965). *J. Exp. Med.* **122**, 467–481.

Goldenberg, D. M., Witte, S., and Elster, K. (1966). *Transplantation* **4**, 760–763.

Goldenberg, D. M., Preston, D. R., Primus, J., and Hansen, H. J. (1974). *Cancer Res.* **34**, 1–9.

Goldenberg, D. M., Pant, K. D., and Dahlman, H. L. (1976). *Cancer Res.* **36**, 3455–3463.

Goldenberg, D. M., Kim, E. E., Deland, F. H., Bennett, S., and Primus, F. I. (1980). *Cancer Res.* **40,** 2984–2992.

Grabar, P., and William, C. A. (1953). *Biochim. Biophys. Acta* **10,** 193–194.

Harboe, N., and Ingild, A. (1973). *Scand J. Immunol.* **2** (Suppl. 1), 161–164.

Hilgers, J., Nowinski, R. C., Geering, G., and Hardy, W. (1972). *Cancer Res.* **32,** 98–105.

Howell, J. H., Russo, A. J., and Goldrosen, M. H. (1979). *Cancer Res.* **39,** 612–618.

Johansson, K.-E., and Hjerten, S. (1974). *J. Mol. Biol.* **86,** 341–348.

Kahan, B. D., Rutzky, L. P., Berlin, B. S., Tomita, J. T., Wiseman, F., LeGrue, S., Noll, H., and Tom, B. H. (1976). *Cancer Res.* **36,** 3526–3534.

Kahan, B. D., Rutzky, L. P., Legrue, S. J., and Tom, B. H. (1979). *In* "Methods in Cancer Research" (H. Busch, ed.), Vol. XVII, pp. 197–275. Academic Press, New York.

Kessler, M. J., Shively, J. E., Pritchard, D. G., and Todd, C. W. (1978). *Cancer Res.* **38,** 1041–1048.

Kimball, P. M., and Brattain, M. G. (1978). *Cancer Res.* **38,** 619–623.

Kosaki, G., and Yamamoto, T. (1975). *Ann. N.Y. Acad. Sci.* **259,** 366–376.

Koura, M., and Isaka, H. (1980). *Cancer* **71,** 313–318.

Kuroki, M., Koga, Y., and Matsuoka, Y. (1981). *Cancer Res.* **41,** 713–720.

Laemmli, U. K. (1970). *Nature (London)* **227,** 680–685.

Lane, M., and Savage, H. (1975). "Methods in Cancer Research" (H. Busch, ed.), Vol. XI, pp. 367–375. Academic Press, New York.

Laurell, C. B. (1965). *Anal. Biochem.* **10,** 358–361.

Lazarides, E. (1976). *J. Cell Biol.* **68,** 202–219.

Leung, J. P., Eshdat, Y., and Marchesi, V. T. (1977). *J. Immunol.* **119,** 664–669.

Lis, H., and Sharon, N. (1977). *In* "The Antigens" (M. Sela, ed.), Vol. IV, pp. 429–529. Academic Press, New York.

Løwenstein, H. (1978). *In* "Progress in Allergy" (P. Kallos, B. H. Waksman, and A. L. DeWeck, eds.), Vol. 25, pp. 1–62. Karger AG, Basel.

McIntire, K. R. (1980). *Cancer Res.* **40,** 3083–3085.

March, S. C., Parikh, I., and Cuatrecasas, P. (1974). *Anal. Biochem.* **60,** 149–152.

Marushige, K., and Bonner, J. (1966). *J. Mol. Biol.* **15,** 160–174.

Muramatsu, M., Hayashi, Y., Onishi, T., Sakai, M., Takai, K., and Kashiyama, T. (1974). *Exp. Cell Res.* **88,** 345–351.

Newman, E. S., Petras, S. E., Georgiadis, A., and Hansen, H. J., (1974). *Cancer Res.* **34,** 2125–2130.

Nicolini, C. (1975). *Physiol. Chem. Phys.* **7,** 571–576.

Norgaard-Pedersen, B. (1973). *Clin. Chim. Acta* **48,** 345–346.

Nurden, A. T., and Caen, J. P. (1974). *Br. J. Haematol.* **28,** 253–260.

Ouchterlony, O. (1948). *Acta Pathol. Microbiol. Scand.* **25,** 186–191.

Ouchterlony, O. (1949). *Acta Pathol. Microbiol. Scand.* **26,** 507–515.

Owen, P., and Salton, M. R. J. (1977). *J. Bacteriol.* **132,** 974–985.

Pant, K. D., Dahlman, H. L., and Goldenberg, D. M. (1978). *Cancer* **42** (Suppl. 1), 1626–2634.

Potter, V. R. (1972). *In* "Manometric and Biochemical Techniques" (W. W. Umbreit, R. H. Burris, and J. F. Stauffer, eds.), pp. 147–148. Burgess, Minneapolis, Minnesota.

Pumo, D. E., Gottnick, D., Little, B. W., and Chiu, J. F. (1980). *Cancer Lett.* **9,** 285–291.

Radola, B. J. (1973). *Biochim. Biophys. Acta* **295,** 412–428.

Reisfeld, R. A., David, G. S., Ferrone, S., Pellegrino, M. A., and Holmes, E. C. (1977). *Cancer Res.* **37,** 2860–2865.

Ressler, N. (1960). *Clin. Chim. Acta* **5,** 359–365.

Ruddon, R. W. (1978). *In* "Biological Markers of Neoplasia: Basic and Applied Aspects" R. W. Ruddon, ed.), pp. 1–7. Amer. Elsevier, New York.

Rutzky, L. P. (1979). *In* "Nutritional Requirements of Vertebrate Cells in Culture" (R. Ham and C. Waymonth, eds.), Cambridge Univ. Press, London and New York.

Rutzky, L. P., Tomita, J. T., Calenoff, M. A., and Kahan, B. D. (1979). *J. Natl. Cancer Inst.* **63**, 893–902.

Santen, R. J., Collette, J., and Franchimont, P. (1980). *Cancer Res.* **40**, 1181–1188.

Schulman, S., and Karpatkin, S. (1980). *J. Biol. Chem.* **225**, 4320–4327.

Shively, J. E., Todd, C. W., Go, V. L. W., and Egan, M. L. (1978). *Cancer Res.* **38**, 503–505.

Smyth, C. J., Friedman-Kien, A. E., and Salton, M. R. J. (1976). *Infect. Immun.* **13**, 1273–1288.

Smyth, C. J., Siegel, J., Salton, M. R. J., and Owen, P. (1978). *J. Bacteriol.* **133**, 306–319.

Taylor, C. W., Yeoman, L. C., Daskal, I., and Busch, H. (1973). *Exp. Cell Res.* **82**, 215–226.

Taylor, C. W., Yeoman, L. C., Woolf, L. M., and Busch, H. (1979). *Biochemistry* **18**, 4049–4054.

Thomson, D. M. P., Tataryn, D. N., Weatherhead, J. C., Friedlander, P., Rauch, I., Schwartz, R., Gold, P., and Shuster, J. (1980). *Eur. J. Cancer* **16**, 539–551.

Tom, B. H., Rutzky, L. P., Jakstys, R., Oyasu, C., Kay, C., and Kahan, B. D. (1976). *In Vitro* **12**, 180–191.

Towbin, H., Staehelin, T., and Gordon, J. (1979). *Proc. Natl. Acad. Sci. U.S.A.* **76**, 4350–4354.

Tsao, D., and Kim, Y. S. (1978). *J. Biol. Chem.* **253**, 2271–2278.

Vaitukaitis, J. L. (1975). *New Engl. J. Med.* **26**, 1370–1371.

Van der Bosch, J., Masui, H., and Sato, G. (1981). *Cancer Res.* **41**, 611–618.

Verbruggen, R. (1975). *Clin. Chem.* **21** (1), 5–43.

Waalkes, T. P., Abeloff, M. D., Woo, K. B., Ettinger, D. S., Ruddon, R. W., and Aldendertu, P. (1980). *Cancer Res.* **40**, 4420–4427.

Wakabayashi, K., and Hnilica, L. S.(1972). *J. Cell Biol.* **55**, 271.

Wanebo, H. I., Rao, B., Pinsky, C. M., Hoffman, R. G., Stearns, M., Schwartz, M. K., and Oettgen, H. F. (1978). *New Engl. J. Med.* **299**, 448–451.

Weir, E. E., Pretlow, T. G., Pitts, A., and Williams, E. E. (1974). *J. Histochem. Cytochem.* **22**, 51–54.

Wofsy, L., and Burr, B. (1969). *J. Immunol.* **103**, 380–382.

Yeoman, L. C. (1978). *In* "The Cell Nucleus" (H. Busch, ed.), Vol. V, pp. 263–306. Academic Press, New York.

Yeoman, L. C., and Busch, H. (1978). *Scand. J. Immunol. Suppl.* Nos. 6, 7, pp. 47–61.

Yeoman, L. C., Jordan, J. J., Busch, R. K., Taylor, C. W., Savage, H. E., and Busch, H. (1976). *Proc. Natl. Acad. Sci. U.S.A.* **73**, 3258–3262.

Zardi, L., Lin, J., and Baserga, R. (1973). *Nature (London) New Biol.* **245**, 211–213.

CHAPTER VII

5'-NUCLEOTIDE PHOSPHODIESTERASE AND LIVER CANCER

K. C. TSOU AND K. W. LO

I. Introduction

The interest in our laboratory related to 5'-nucleotide phosphodiesterase stems from our overall interest in the role of nucleases in cancer. The regulatory role of the phosphodiesterase has only recently become important. Much of our work is still in a very early stage of development and therefore a discussion of the background of this area may be of interest to other cancer researchers.

Phosphodiesters occur extensively in nature. They include the nucleic acids (DNA, RNA) where the phosphodiester bonds form the backbone of the nucleic acids, cyclic nucleotides (cAMP, cGMP, and cCMP), phospholipids (phosphatidylcholine, phosphatidylethanolamine, phosphatidylserine), cobamide coenzyme (vitamin B_{12}), CMP-sialic acid, and teichoic acid.

Enzymes which hydrolyze these phosphodiesters are also very abundant. Thus, for nucleic acids, there exist the endonucleases which catalyze the hydrolysis of internal phosphodiester bonds and exonucleases with specificity for terminal phosphodiester bonds. For the cyclic nucleotides, there are specific phosphohydrolases for cAMP (Appleman et al., 1973), cGMP (Appleman et al., 1973), and cCMP (Kuo et al., 1979), respectively. In phospholipids, phospholipase C and D catalyze the hydrolysis of the phosphodiester bonds (Hanahan, 1971).

Among the exonucleases, 5'-nucleotide phosphodiesterase hydrolyzes DNA or RNA from 3' → 5' to give 5'-nucleotides. This enzyme was referred to as phosphodiesterase I by Razzell and Khorana (1959), but since it has specificity toward phosphodiesters containing 5'-nucleosides (Khorana, 1961) and that 5'-nucleotides are formed by the enzymatic hydrolysis of these phosphodiesters, 5'-nucleotide phosphodiesterase (5'-NPD) should be more appropriate. However, it should not be confused

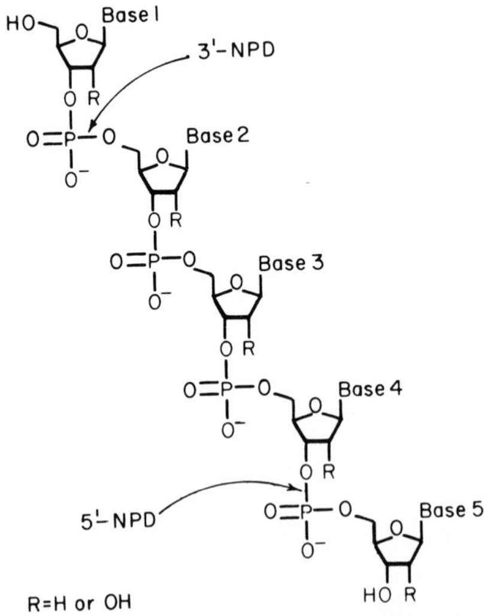

FIG. 1. The modes of cleavage of nucleic acid chains by 5'-nucleotide phosphodiesterase (5'-NPD) and 3'-nucleotide phosphodiesterase (3'-NPD).

with 5'-nucleotidase (5'-ND), an enzyme which catalyzes the hydrolysis of 5'-nucleotides to nucleosides and inorganic phosphate (Drummond and Yamamoto, 1971). Similarly, exonuclease which acts on DNA or RNA from 5' → 3' end to give 3'-nucleotides, commonly referred to as phosphodiesterase II (Razzell and Khorana, 1961), should preferably be called 3'-nucleotide phosphodiesterase (3'-NPD). This enzyme has been found predominantly in the spleen. The modes of cleavage of 5'-NPD and 3'-NPD on nucleic acids are shown in Fig. 1. Even though both 5'-NPD and 3'-NPD have been used extensively in the determination of base sequences in nucleic acids and synthetic oligonucleotides (Ho and Gilham, 1973), their physiological role has remained obscure. As will be seen in this chapter, only recently have we and others begun to inquire about the role of these enzymes in nature.

II. Assay Methods for 5'-Nucleotide Phosphodiesterase

A. BIOCHEMICAL METHODS

Bis-(p-nitrophenyl)phosphate (BNP) was the first chromogenic substrate used for the assay of this enzyme (Sinsheimer and Koerner, 1952). However, BNP is not a specific substrate for 5'-NPD because 3'-NPD also catalyzes its hydrolysis (Koerner and Sinsheimer, 1957). In addition, the product of the enzyme reaction, p-nitrophenylphosphate, is also a substrate for phosphomonoesterases (alkaline and acid phosphatases). Thus, when crude 5'-NPD preparations are assayed, these phosphomonoesterases are invariably present and would give inaccurate results. p-Nitrophenyl phenylphosphonate developed by Butler et al. (Kelly and Butler, 1975, 1977; Kelly et al., 1975) may obviate this difficulty but is still less specific as judged by its high K_m value. The use of oligonucleotides for the assay of 5'-NPD (Lehman and Nussbaum, 1964) is expensive and is not suitable for continuous kinetic measurements.

The chromogenic substrate, p-nitrophenyl 5'-thymidylate, is a specific substrate for 5'-NPD (Razzell and Khorana, 1959; Khorana, 1961). However, it is not sensitive enough to detect low levels of enzyme activity. A number of more sensitive substrates are available. These include 4-methylumbelliferyl 5'-uridylate and 4-methylumbelliferyl 5'-adenylate (March and Tsou, 1970), 4-methylumbelliferyl 5'-thymidylate (Lo et al., 1972), bis-(4-methylumbelliferyl)phosphate and bis-(umbelliferyl)phosphate (Boguslaski, 1974), poly(2-aza-ε-adenosine) (Yip and Tsou, 1979), and guanylyl (3' → 5')-ε-adenosine 2-sulfonate (Tsou and Yip, 1980). The most sensitive of these fluorogenic substrates is 4-methylumbelliferyl 5'-

thymidylate (4MUpT). The biochemical assay based on this substrate is given below.

The assay is performed on a Turner Model 111 fluorometer equipped with a cuvette holder thermostated as $37.0 \pm 0.1°C$ and a Beckman 10-in. recorder. The excitation filters are 7–54 (transmission 254 nm, also passes 313, 365, and 405 nm lines) plus a 40% transmission filter. The emission filters are Wratten No. 2A (transmission > 415 nm) plus transmission filters of 10 and 20%. The slit is set at 3. The assay medium consists of a substrate concentration of 2.55 μM 4MUpT in 0.05 M Tris–HCl buffer, pH 9.0 containing 1 mM MgCl$_2$ in a total volume of 2.2 ml. A 10×75-mm Pyrex test tube (Corning No. 9800-10) is used. After temperature equilibration (5 to 10 minutes), the reaction was initiated by the addition of suitable volumes (50 or 100 μl) of serum or tissue extracts (5 to 100 μl). The increase in fluorescence is continuously monitored on a recorder to give an estimate of the initial rate of enzyme hydrolysis. Enzyme activities are calculated from slopes of these initial rates and from a calibration curve of known concentration of 4-methylumbelliferone. Errors in duplicate assays are usually within 5%.

B. HISTOCHEMICAL METHODS

A more detailed review of the histochemical methods for this enzyme has been reported recently (Tsou, 1974). Therefore, only brief discussions of these methods are given. α-Naphthyl 5'-thymidylate was first used by Sierakowska and Shugar (1963) for the demonstration of this enzyme. More recently, naphtho-ASBI 5'-thymidylate (Sierakowska et al., 1978) has been proposed as a better substrate. These substrates utilized a post-coupling procedure with diazonium salts to yield colored insoluble dye. The diazo-coupling methods are generally satisfactory but they often have high background especially when staining for weak enzyme activities. Thus we sought to improve the histochemical method by introducing an indigogenic method. The importance of this development will be obvious in our isozyme demonstration (see Section VI,A).

The indigogenic methods for enzyme localization was first introduced by Barnett and Seligman (1951) and Holt (1952). The advantages of indigogenic substrates are (1) no coupling agents are required, (2) indigo is very insoluble in aqueous solution, and (3) the bluish-purple color is especially suited for histochemistry. The indigogenic principle for 5'-NPD is illustrated in Fig. 2.

The indoxyl formed by the initial enzyme reaction rapidly dimerizes to indigo. By introducing an iodine atom at the 5-position of the indoxyl moiety (Tsou, 1974; Aoyagi et al., 1974), an electron dense 5,5'-diiodoindigo

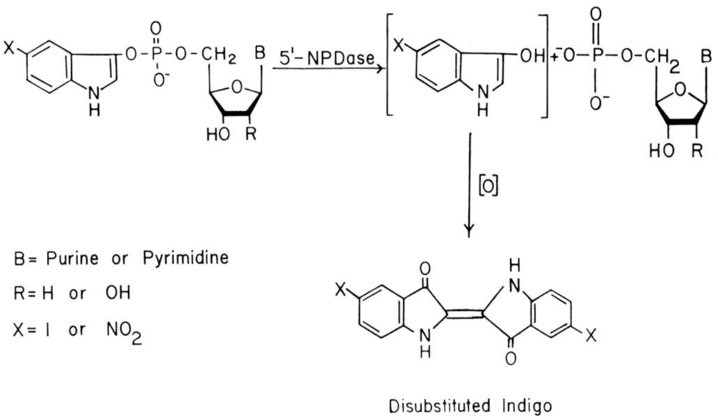

B = Purine or Pyrimidine
R = H or OH
X = I or NO$_2$

Disubstituted Indigo

FIG. 2. The indigogenic principle for 5'-nucleotide phosphodiesterase.

is formed, which can be used not only for the light microscopic localization of 5'-NPD but also at the electron microscopic level (Tsou, 1974; Tsou *et al.*, 1974a). Horwitz *et al.* (1969) also reported the use of 5-bromo-4-chloro-5'-thymidylate for biochemical study, but we found that it is not a good substrate and that it is not suitable for electron microscopy (Tsou, 1974).

III. 5'-Nucleotide Phosphodiesterase and Enzyme Activation for Cancer Chemotherapy

Our interest in this enzyme is in part related to our research on the development of enzyme-activated anticancer agents. A brief discussion here might be appropriate. It is known that the fluorinated pyrimidines, 5-fluorouracil (5FU) or its nucleoside 5-fluoro-2'-deoxyuridine (FUdR) are among the most useful palliative cancer chemotherapeutic agents. The "active" antimetabolite has been shown to be 5-fluoro-2'-deoxy 5'-uridylate (pFUdR) (Cohen *et al.*, 1958; Heidelberger *et al.*, 1960a,b) which is a potent inhibitor for thymidylate synthetase (Hartmann and Heidelberger, 1961). Conversion of FUdR to pFUdR is mediated by thymidine kinase (TK) (Hakala, 1973). Prolonged treatment of 5FU or FUdR, however, leads to resistance of these agents and it was soon recognized that once resistance develops, the TK levels are lowered in some cancer cells (Umeda and Heidelberger, 1968; Miller *et al.*, 1976; Wilkinson *et al.*, 1977). The use of synthetic pFUdR, however, will not overcome this problem because of facile hydrolysis by 5'-nucleotidase or other nonspecific phosphomonoesterases. Concomitant with the decrease in TK in cancer cells resistant to fluorinated pyrimidines there is an increase in 5'-NPD activity (Miller *et al.*, 1976). Therefore, it appears to us that phosphodiesters containing FUdR should be useful in situations where resistance to these antimetabolites is a result of deficiency in TK (Tsou *et al.*, 1970, 1972). The general usefulness of this principle has been extended to other nucleosides.

IV. 5'-Nucleotide Phosphodiesterase and Liver Growth

A. REGENERATING LIVER

The liver has an amazing capacity to regenerate itself. Depletion of hepatocytes by partial hepatectomy (Bucher and Malt, 1971) immediately initiates this process. The regenerating liver has been used as a model for growth by a number of investigators (Bucher and Malt, 1971). It has been commonly assumed that the major difference between the regenerating growth and neoplastic growth is that the former is a controlled process while the latter is a noncontrolled process. Solt and Farber (1976), however, have recently shown that partial hepatectomy is involved in promoting carcinogenesis. Thus these two processes may be related in some yet undefined manner.

We investigated the activities of 5'-NPD in regenerating rat liver and found that they were higher than sham-operated livers (Tsou *et al.*, 1974b) and paralleled to the change of DNA synthesis as measured by the incorporation of [³H]thymidine (Fig. 3). Thus we were led to suggest that the level of 5'-NPD may be intimately related to DNA replication.

B. 5'-NUCLEOTIDE PHOSPHODIESTERASE LEVEL IN RAT HEPATOMA

As a result of the careful work of Dr. H. P. Morris, a series of chemically induced transplantable rat hepatomas are available (Morris, 1965). The growth rates of these tumors are highly predictable, and they are, therefore, ideal models for either biochemical study (Weber, 1963) or chemotherapy of hepatomas (Lo *et al.*, 1973).

Sometime ago, we undertook an investigation of the 5'-NPD level in six Morris hepatomas with divergent growth rates and found that the tumors all had higher 5'-NPD activities than the corresponding host livers (Tsou *et al.*, 1974b). Thus we were convinced of the merit for the successful use of the phosphodiesterase in the enzyme-activation approach to cancer

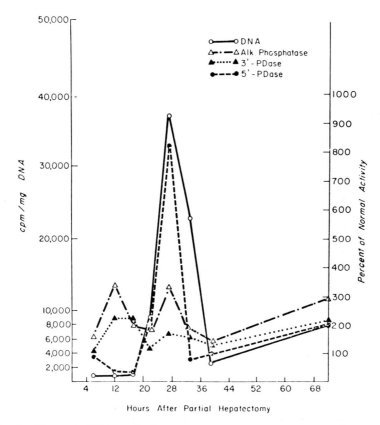

FIG. 3. Changes in DNA synthesis (O——O) as measured by [³H]thymidine incorporation; 5'-nucleotide phosphodiesterase (●----●); 3'-nucleotide phosphodiesterase (▲······▲); and alkaline phosphatase (△—·—·—△) in regenerating rat liver.

chemotherapy (see Section III). In addition, the tumor/host liver enzyme activities ratio provided useful information in distinguishing between fast-, medium-, and slow-growing hepatomas. These data (Table I) again demonstrate that 5'-NPD may be related to growth.

V. Tissue Distribution of 5'-Nucleotide Phosphodiesterase

5'-NPD is widely distributed in nature (Razzell, 1966; Harvey *et al.*, 1970). The enzyme from snake venom is most widely studied (Laskowski, 1966, 1967, 1971, 1980). Highly purified snake venom enzymes for nucleo-

TABLE I

5'-NUCLEOTIDE PHOSPHODIESTERASE ACTIVITIES IN MORRIS HEPATOMAS[a]

Hepatoma	Growth rate	N	5'-Nucleotide phosphodiesterase activity[b]		
			Tumor	Host liver	Tumor/host
7777	Fast	9	281 ± 11[c]	22.3 ± 8.9	15.2 ± 5.4
7800	Medium	1	66.4	14.0	4.7
7794A	Medium	15	126 ± 62	59.1 ± 24.3	2.3 ± 0.9
H16	Slow	1	59.3	14.4	4.1
9618A	Slow	3	204 ± 55	69.7 ± 3.5	3.6 ± 1.7
9633	Slow	9	120 ± 75	24.9 ± 22.8	5.9 ± 3.5

[a] Adapted from Tsou et al. (1974b) with permission.
[b] In pmoles/minute/milligram protein.
[c] Mean ± SE.

tide sequencing are available commercially. The distribution of 5'-NPD in ACI rat tissues is shown in Table II. Among organs with high specific activities are the intestines, prostate, and liver while the lowest specific activity is found in the spleen. The variation in the enzyme in human sera was first reported by us (Lo et al., 1972) by a fluorescent method. A spectrophotometric method was also reported by Hynie et al. (1975). The enzyme that degrades nucleoside diphosphate sugars (Spik et al., 1979) in

TABLE II

DISTRIBUTION OF 5'-NUCLEOTIDE PHOSPHODIESTERASE IN MALE ACI TISSUES[a]

Tissue	Enzyme activity[b] (pmole/minute/milligram protein)
Brain	2.4
Kidney	4.2
Heart	11.8
Pancreas	5.2
Lung	10.3
Small intestine	38.3
Large intestine	123.8
Spleen	0.038
Prostate	69.7
Testis	3.6
Liver	32.8
Serum	46.3

[a] Adapted from Tsou et al. (1974a) with permission.
[b] Except serum, all activities were measured with the 27,000 g supernatant of tissue homogenates at 37.0 ± 0.2°C using ammonium 4-methylumbelliferyl 5'-thymidylate as substrate.

rat serum may also be related to 5'-NPD as pyrophosphatase activity of 5'-NPD has been reported by us (Tsou *et al.*, 1972).

VI. Methods for the Demonstration of Isozymes of 5'-Nucleotide Phosphodiesterase

Polymorphic forms of enzymes and their importance to cancer have been reviewed (Criss, 1971; Schapira, 1973). Thus it was natural for us to inquire further whether there are multiple forms of this enzyme. In addition, based on histochemical studies, we noted the presence of higher levels of enzymes in hepatoma tumor tissue, but less so in normal liver (Tsou *et al.*, 1974a). For this purpose, we use the polyacrylamide gel electrophoresis method. Isozymes of 5'-NPD are thus demonstrated in tissue extracts and sera. The details of this method follow. Gels are casted in 5 (i.d.) × 70-mm tubes. The gel is composed of 1.4 gm Cyanogum 41 (95% monoacrylamide + 5% methylene bis-acrylamide, obtainable from E-C Apparatus Corp., St. Petersburg, FL), 19 ml 0.09 M Tris–boric acid, pH 9.4 (running buffer), and 5 μl N,N,N',N'-tetramethylethylenediamine (TMED). The above mixture is filtered through Whatman No. 1 paper to remove any insoluble materials. Polymerization is started by the addition of 1.0 ml of 20 mg/ml ammonium persulfate (Eastman) in running buffer. The gel tubes are filled to about 1–2 mm from the top and carefully layered with a few drops of running buffer through a bent needle with its tip pressed against the wall of the gel tube. Polymerization will take about 20 minutes. The buffer and unpolymerized gel solutions are carefully removed with a Pasteur pipet and the buffer is replenished. The gels are stored at 10°C until used.

For running the gels, a Shandon two-chamber system (or other similar systems) with circulating ice-cold water is suitable. The samples (20 μl) are loaded, followed by 5 μl of 1.5 gm/ml sucrose and 0.8 mg/ml bromophenol blue tracking dye in running buffer. The samples and dyed sucrose solution are thoroughly mixed with a melting capillary tube and overlaid with buffer. Finally the upper chamber is filled with buffer. The gels are run at a constant current of 2 mA/tube. During the run, cold water (ca. 4°C) is circulated through both chambers. The running time is about 60 minutes. The gels are then removed from the tubes by a fine needle and placed in 10 × 75-mm test tubes (Corning 9800-10). The test tubes are filled with 0.25 mg/ml ammonium 5-iodoindoxyl 5'-thymidylate (IIpT)* in

---

* A by-product in the chemical synthesis of IIpT is 5-iodoindoxyl phosphate (IIp) which is a substrate for alkaline phosphatase. Therefore, it is imperative that the IIpT samples are free of IIp. Pure IIpT has $R_f = 0.85$ (TLC cellulose, 2-propanol:NH$_4$OH:H$_2$O = 7:1:2 v/v) and $A_{232}/A_{270} = 3.00$.

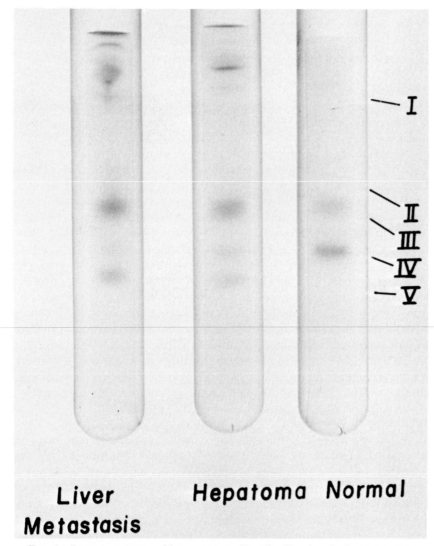

FIG. 4. Isozyme patterns of human serum 5′-nucleotide phosphodiesterase. Note the presence of 5′-NPD-V in hepatoma and liver metastasis. 5′-NPD-II is very weak and is not discernible in this photograph. However, the position of 5′-NPD-II is also indicated in this photograph.

0.05 M Tris–HCl, pH 9.0, containing 1 mM MgCl$_2$ and incubated at 37°C for 18 hours. After removing the substrate solution, the gels are rinsed 2 × 1 hours with H$_2$O and then stored in 8% (v/v) HOAc. The indigo dye is stable for years under this condition. Gels can be read on a light box or scanned by a densitometer at 540 nm.

A. ISOZYME OF HUMAN SERUM

Normal human serum shows four isozymes (Fig. 4) which are identified as 5′-NPD-I, 5′-NPD-II, 5′-NPD-III, and 5′-NPD-IV in the reverse order of their electrophoretic mobility. 5′-NPD-III and 5′-NPD-IV usually account for over 80% of the total serum 5′-NPD activity. 5′-NPD-I is found in the γ-globulin region and is usually weak although still stronger than 5′-NPD-II.* In patients with primary hepatocellular carcinoma (PHC) and liver metastases a faster moving isozyme (5′-NPD-V) is seen (Fig. 4) (Tsou et al., 1937b). The usefulness of 5′-NPD-V for detection of PHC and liver metastases and liver metastasis will be the subject of this chapter.

Gel scanning of the isozyme intensity can be performed with a Gilford Model 2410-S linear transport at 540 nm. One milliunit (mU) of 5′-NPD-V activity is defined as the amount of 5,5′-diiodoindigo formed per millimeter of gel to give an O.D. of 0.05.

The reproducibility of the 5′-NPD-V test is excellent. Coded samples received in duplicates from many laboratories in a span of 1 year were tested. There were perfect agreements in results obtained from serum samples if they had been stored at $-20°C$.

Normal sera from other mammalian species also display isozymes for 5′-NPD. These zymograms are compared with normal human isozymes (Fig. 5). Note that rabbit, goat, rat, horse, calf, sheep, and dog all showed higher total enzyme activities than human.

B. FLUOROGENIC METHODS

A disadvantage of the indigogenic method for enzyme localization is that two molecules of indoxyl are required to produce one molecule of indigo dye and that the extinction coefficients of indigo and substituted indigos in the visible region of the spectrum are rather low (Tsou et al., 1974a). Consequently, there is still a need for an even more sensitive and rapid method for the detection of 5′-NPD isozymes. The inherent sensitivity of fluorescent methods over absorption methods suggests that fluorometric methods would extend the sensitivity of the 5′-NPD-V test or, at least, shorten the time required for the development of the zymograms.

We have adapted the fluorogenic substrate 4MUpT for this purpose. The product of enzymatic reaction, 4-methylumbelliferone (4MU), is

---

* Occasionally, multiple bands are seen in the 5′-NPD-I region. This is especially true in later stages of malignancy but the significance of these extra bands is not known.

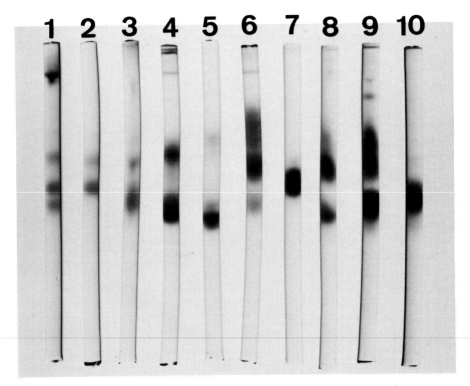

Fig. 5. Comparison of serum 5'-nucleotide phosphodiesterase isozymes from some mammalian species. (1) Liver metastasis (human); (2) normal human; (3) Rhesus monkey; (4) rabbit; (5) horse; (6) calf; (7) dog; (8) goat; (9) sheep; (10) rat. Gels 1–3 were run with 20 μl, gels 4–9 with 15 μl, and gel 10 with 5 μl of serum. Gels 4, 5, 6, 9, and 10 were purposely overloaded to bring out the weaker bands. Note the similarity in isozyme patterns between calf (gel 6) and sheep (gel 9), and the isozyme patterns between normal human (gel 2) and Rhesus monkey (gel 3).

highly fluorescent especially around the pH optimum (i.e., pH 9.0) of 5'-NPD and, therefore, provides an extremely sensitive method. However, 4MU is relatively more soluble than indigo and special precautions have to be taken to prevent product diffusion. These are accomplished by slicing the gel longitudinally into two halves and placing the cut surface on Agarose gel or Whatman 3MM paper impregnated with 1 mg/ml of the substrate in a moist chamber. The gels are incubated at 37°C for 5–10 minutes (depending on the enzyme activity) when fluorescent bands can be seen under long UV (366 nm) light (Camac.) The gels should be photographed within 1 hour for record because a longer delay in time would result in diffuse bands. Figure 6 shows gels of human serum samples stained by 4MUpT. The zymogram patterns are identical with those ob-

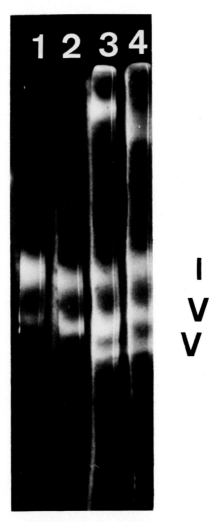

FIG. 6. Zymogram of human serum 5′-nucleotide phosphodiesterase isozymes stained with 4MUpT in filter paper strip. Gels 1 and 2, breast cancer; gels 3 and 4, malignant melanoma. Note the presence of 5′-NPD-V in gels 3 and 4, and the absence of 5′-NPD-II in all four gels.

tained by the indigogenic method. This fluorogenic method is fast and the results of zymograms are usually obtained in 30 minutes after the gel run. Because of the limitation of product solubility, this method cannot be used for long incubation. However, in situations where the results have to be obtained fast, the fluorogenic method is definitely better than the indigogenic method.

C. ISOELECTRIC FOCUSING

Isoelectric focusing is a powerful technique which can separate proteins according to their isoelectric points (pI). At the present state of the art, proteins with pI differing by 0.02 can easily be separated (Sargent and George, 1975). The principle of isoelectric focusing depends on the establishment of a pH gradient by the carrier ampholytes under the influence of an electric field (Righetti and Drysdale, 1976). Proteins will migrate to their respective pIs where they have no net charge and will form sharp bands.

Most commercially available carrier ampholytes contain poly-amino and poly-carboxylate groups. Hence, they are powerful chelators for divalent metal ions (Righetti and Drysdale, 1976). Since we have found that 5'-NPD is a metalloenzyme, the enzyme activity is lost or diminished in the presence of low concentrations of ampholyte. This problem is especially serious in the isozyme study because most 5'-NPD isozymes are focused at pI less than 5, a region where the enzyme is not active. Therefore, the time for electrofocusing should be short. After numerous trials, we have succeeded in partially restoring the enzyme activity after focusing by first washing the gels to remove ampholyte and supplementing the wash buffer with Zn^{2+} and Mg^{2+} (divalent Co^{2+} ion is also effective in restoring the enzyme activity, but it is inferior to Zn^{2+}). However, the majority of enzyme activity is not restored. Consequently, a larger volume of serum has to be used for the development of zymogram.

The method of Bauman and Chrambach (1976) for isoelectric focusing in gel rods can be used with slight modification. A 7% gel is used in this work, and they are made in 100×5-mm (i.d.) glass tubes according to the following procedures:

Gel stock solution: 8.4 ml of 42% (w/v) Cyanogum 41
2.4 ml ampholyte (pH 3.5–10)
6.4 ml 0.5% (v/v) TMED
Polymerization: 11.2 ml gel stock solution
22.4 ml H_2O
60 μl 20% (w/v) ammonium persulfate

After filling the gel tubes, the gel solutins are careful overlaid with water by means of a syringe with a bent needle. (This water is to be removed prior to running.) The gels are stored in a refrigerator overnight and prefocused with a constant power of 10 W and a maximum voltage of 400 V for 30 minutes. The anolyte (lower chamber) consists of 800 ml of 0.06 N H_2SO_4 and the catholyte (upper chamber) 400 ml of 0.06 N NaOH.

After prefocusing, the tops of the gels must be rinsed with distilled water to remove NaOH before sample application. The samples (50 μl) are dyed with bromophenol blue (BPB) and overlaid with a solution containing 5% (v/v) glycerol and 1% (v/v) ampholyte to insulate the samples from denaturation by the catholyte. Focusing can be run exactly under the same condition as for prefocusing and the chambers must be cooled by circulating ice-cold water through to prevent the enzyme from denaturation by the intense heat generated during focusing. The focusing usually reaches equilibrium in 4 hours when the ammeter reading becomes stable

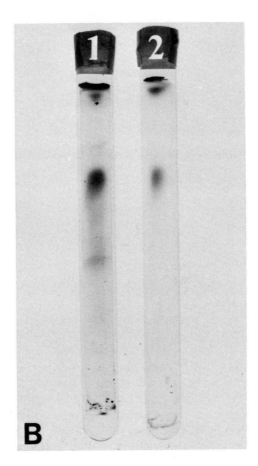

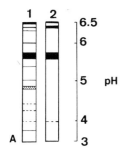

FIG. 7. (A) Schematic drawing of 5'-nucleotide phosphodiesterase from patient J.J. Gel 1 when diagnosis was hepatoma. Gel 2 when diagnosis was cirrhosis. Both samples are positive for 5'-NPD-V. (B) Photograph of zymograms shown schematically in (A).

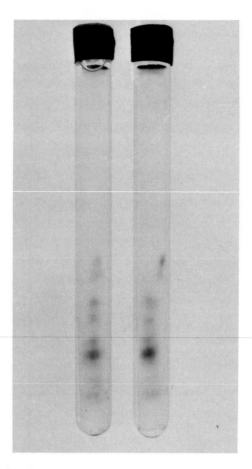

FIG. 8. Results of duplicate 5′-nucleotide phosphodiesterase zymograms after electrofocusing from a patient with breast cancer positive for 5′-NPD-V.

and the BPB-dyed albumin bands become sharp lines. After the run, the gels are extruded from the tubes and washed 4 × 20 minutes with 1 M Tris–HCl pH 9.0 containing 0.23 mM ZnCl$_2$ and 3 mM MgCl$_2$ and then incubated with 2 mg/ml each IIpT and 5-nitroindoxyl 5′-thymidylate (NO$_2$IpT) in the same buffer.* One gel was cut up into 0.25-cm slices and each slice was equilibrated with 1 ml distilled water overnight before measuring for pH.

* The low activities of 5′-NPD after electrofocusing necessitate the use of higher substrate and mixed substrate for incubation. Mixed iodo- and nitroindigo showed higher extinction coefficient in the visible spectrum (Tsou *et al.*, 1974a).

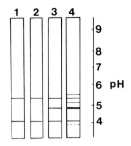

FIG. 9.   Schematic drawing of 5'-nucleotide phosphodiesterase zymograms after electrofocusing of a breast cancer patient as the disease progresses. Gel 1, initial sampling; gel 2,
at 7 months; gel 3, at 8 months; gel 4, at 11 months. The patient expired 2 months after
collecting the sample in gel 4. Note normal serum only contains one band with p*I* about 4.1

Figure 7 depicts the enzyme activity of two serum samples from the
same patient who was first diagnosed as cirrhosis (gel 2) but 6 months
later the diagnosis was changed to hepatoma (gel 1). Both gels show substantial activity on top. The strongest band occurs at a pH of 5.6 and is
present in both gels. There are a number of extra bands not present in gel
2. These include bands at pH of 3.5, 4.3 (very weak), 4.5 (very weak), 4.8
(very weak), 5.0, and 6.0.

The reproducibility of this method is shown in Fig. 8 when the same
sample from a breast cancer patient with liver metastasis was run in duplicate. In addition to the activity on top of the gel (pH 9.0), seven other
activity bands locating at pH 3.9, 5.2, 6.2, 6.8, and 7.2 are seen in both
gels.

The progress of a breast cancer patient was followed in the zymogram
shown in Fig. 9. Gel 1 is from a serum sample of the patient when 5'-
NPD-V was negative. Two weak bands at pH 4.1 and 5.5 are seen. Gel 2 is
from a sample 7 months later when 5'-NPD-V first became positive but
the focusing pattern is the same as in gel 1. Gel 3 is a sample 8 months
after the one in gel 1. Here a new band at pH 4.9 appears. This sample is
also positive for 5'-NPD-V but the band corresponding to 5'-NPD-V is not
yet visible. The last gel (No. 4) is from a sample collected 11 months after
the one in gel 1. The band at pH 4.9 has increased in intensity. In addition,
the band at pH 3.9 is discernible, and there are also two more bands at pH
5.0–5.5. The patient expired 2 months after this sample was collected. It
is clear that the increase in the number of bands is related to the poor
prognosis of the disease. Further, larger panel study will be necessary to
assign each individual band to the tissue of origin even though it was
tempting for us to assign pH 5.5 for breast cancer in this sample.

VII. 5′-Nucleotide Phosphodiesterase Isozyme-V in Primary Hepatocellular Carcinoma (PHC)

A. ETIOLOGY AND DISTRIBUTION OF PRIMARY HEPATOCELLULAR CARCINOMA

Although the incidence of PHC in the United States is relatively low, it is one of the most, if not the most, common cancers in males in Southeast Asia and sub-Sahara Africa. Patients with PHC usually die within 1 year after diagnosis (Okuda and Peters, 1976) because surgery, radiation, and chemotherapy are rarely effective. The extremely poor prognosis and the uneven geographic distribution of PHC have prompted many epidemiological studies as well as studies for the early detection of this form of cancer.

Certain natural products present in food (Schoenthl, 1959; Mugera and Nderito, 1968; Laqueur et al., 1973), mycotoxin contaminants (Wogan, 1973; Kalengayi and Desmet, 1975a,b), and many chemicals such as azo dyes, nitrosamines, and polycyclic hydrocarbons (Fishbein, 1979) are known to induce PHC in experimental animals. Among these compounds, the mycotoxin, aflatoxin B, which has been found to contaminate peanuts, grains, and other foodstuffs, has received the widest attention as a possible environmental agent in PHC in humans.

PHC is usually found in liver that has been damaged by chronic inflammation (chronic active hepatitis) and/or postnecrotic cirrhosis. In addition, etiological relationships between viral hepatitis, cirrhosis, and PHC have been suggested from epidemiological and retrospective studies (Payet et al., 1956; Steiner and Davies 1957; Mikaye, 1961). With the availability of testing methods for hepatitis B infection by means of hepatitis B surface antigen HB_sAg, it became possible to test this hypothesis. High prevalence of HB_sAg in serum from PHC patients over controls was found by many authors (Vogel et al., 1972; Simons et al., 1972; Nishioka et al., 1973; Woodfield et al., 1974; Sakurai and Miyaji, 1975, Prince et al., 1975; Blumberg et al., 1975; Larouzé et al., 1976; MacNab et al., 1976b; Kew et al., 1979). The association of hepatitis B virus (HBV) with HPC is supported by the following findings (see Blumberg and London, 1980 for review): (1) familial clustering of HB_sAg and PHC (Denison et al., 1971; Ohbayashi et al., 1972), (2) production of HB_sAg by a human PHC cell line in culture (MacNab et al., 1976a), and (3) prevalence of HB_sAg and hepatitis B core antigen in livers of PHC patients over those of controls (Nayak et al., 1977). Despite these results, the oncogenic potential of HBV has not been demonstrated. Also, the role of carcinogens in relation to HBV infection in the pathogenesis of PHC in human is not certain, although in animal studies aflatoxins were found to be more potent carcinogens of preexisting liver damage or inflammation (Sun *et al.*, 1971; Lin *et al.*, 1974).

B. α-FETOPROTEIN AND PRIMARY HEPATOCELLULAR CARCINOMA

A protein which migrated under the electrophoretic condition in the α-globulin region was found in the serum of mice with experimentally induced liver cancers by Abelev (1963, 1971, 1974). This protein is also produced by the fetal liver and the yolk sac during embryonic life and is therefore designated as α-fetoprotein (AFP). A homologous protein was also found in human serum with PHC (Tatarinov, 1964.) In humans, AFP synthesis by the liver peaks at about 16 weeks of gestation and gradually decreases. It still can be detected by the relatively insensitive method of double diffusion in cord serum at birth but in normal adults AFP is synthesized by the liver only in minute quantities. Consequently, the detection of AFP is useful for the diagnosis of PHC (Hirai *et al.*, 1973; Hirai and Nishi, 1976). Mass screening on nearly two million people for PHC by AFP has already been instituted in the People's Republic of China (Shanghai Co-ordinating Group for Research on Liver Cancer, 1979). For some unknown reason, the prevalence of AFP among PHC patients in the United States and Western Europe is only about 50%; it is about 80% in Asia and Africa (Masseyeff, 1973).

C. 5'-NUCLEOTIDE PHOSPHODIESTERASE ISOZYME-V AND PRIMARY HEPATOCELLULAR CARCINOMA

Our initial results indicated that 5'-NPD-V was present in the serum samples of all six biopsy proven PHC cases, while none of these patients had elevated AFP (Tsou *et al.*, 1973a). We have subsequently examined the serum samples from 122 PHC patients from the United States and other countries (Uganda, Japan, Philippines) and found that 5'-NPD-V was present in 47 of 54 (88%) patients from the United States and 48 of 68 (71%) from patients outside the United States. The corresponding figures for AFP in excess of 20 ng/ml are 22 of 54 (40%) and 45 of 68 (66%), respectively (Tsou and Lo, 1980). There were also two cases each of cholangiocarcinoma and angiosarcoma in our latter study. 5'-NPD-V was present in all four cases, but AFP was greater than 20 ng/ml in only 1 cholangiocarcinoma patients. Although the samplings are small, 5'-NPD-V may also be of value in the diagnosis of these forms of liver malignancy.

Using the same indigogenic method developed by us, researchers in Shanghai, China also found that 5'-NPD-V to be a highly specific indicator for diagnosis of PHC (Shi *et al.*, 1980). In a more detailed study, they reported (Lu *et al.*, 1980) 5'-NPD-V was present in 83% of 95 PHC patients but only 2 of 15 (13%) of PHC patients after liver resection.

These studies indicated that 5'-NPD-V is a useful diagnostic alternative to AFP for PHC. It is especially valuable in countries where the incidence of elevated AFP is low among PHC patients.

VIII. 5'-Nucleotide Phosphodiesterase Isozyme-V in Liver Metastasis

A. PREVALENCE OF LIVER METASTASES AMONG CANCER PATIENTS

Liver metastases are fairly common among cancer patients, especially those with cancer of the gastrointestinal tract. For example, Swinton *et al.* (1967) described 41 of 334 (12%) patients with sigmoid or rectum cancer having liver metastases at bowel surgery. Similar findings were made by Bengmark and Hafstrom (1969). Our recent study (Pollock *et al.*, 1979) on patients with gastrointestinal cancer found 48 of 122 (39%) liver metastases at surgery. These data confirmed the extensive results of Abrams *et al.* (1950) who found liver metastasis in 49% of 1000 consecutive autopsy cases of cancer deaths, and the more recent studies of over 4000 autopsy cases by Viadana and Au (1975). Viadana *et al.* (1978) also suggested that liver is one of the key disseminating organs in the spread of cancer.

It is well known that cancer patients with liver metastases have a poor prognosis. Thus, a median survival of 75 days was reported by Jaffe *et al.* (1968) for 390 cancer patients with liver metastases and only 7% of these patients survived more than 1 year. Pestana *et al.* (1964) found a mean survival of 9.8 months after diagnosis of liver metastases in 583 patients with carcinomas of the colon or rectum. Consequently, if asymptomatic liver metastases could be diagnosed, hepatic metastectomy (Flanigan and Foster, 1967), or hepatic dearterialization followed by infusion of chemotherapeutic agents (Murray-Lyon *et al.*, 1970; Fortner *et al.*, 1973; Mulcare *et al.*, 1973; Sparks *et al.*, 1975) could be considered.

B. DIAGNOSIS OF LIVER METASTASIS

Liver metastasis is usually diagnosed with radiological liver scans (Hatfield, 1975). False-positive liver scans which are related to space-filling lesions are relatively uncommon. The use of B-mode ultrasonography (Sanders and Sanders, 1977) or computerized tomography with whole body scanner (Alfidi *et al.*, 1976; Stanley *et al.*, 1976) may allow further discrimination between benign and malignant lesions in a positive liver scan. However, liver scans have been found to have a relatively high false-negative rate of 10–30% (Shingleton, 1971; McCready, 1972; Drum and Beard, 1976; McCartney and Hoffer, 1978). The liver scan is probably not sensitive to small (less than 2 cm) metastatic foci or diffusively infiltrating lesions that do not displace functioning Kupffer cells (Castagna *et al.*, 1972). Consequently, a number of serum markers have been proposed to complement liver scans for the detection of liver metastases. These include glutamic oxalacetic transaminase (SGOT; Wroblewski, 1959), alkaline phosphatase (Mendelsohn and Bodansky, 1952), lactic dehydrogenase (LDH; West and Zimmerman, 1958; Munjal *et al.*, 1976), 5'-nucleotidase (Smith *et al.*, 1966), γ-glutamyltranspeptidase (Aronsen *et al.*, 1970; Ohira *et al.*, 1975), glutathione reductase (West *et al.*, 1961), and carcinoembryonic antigen (CEA, Chu and Nemoto, 1973; Lo Gerfo *et al.*, 1973; Neville and Lawrence, 1974; Terry *et al.*, 1974; Martin *et al.*, 1976). The limitations of these tests lie in the high false-positive and false-negative results. For example, elevated alkaline phosphatase is often associated with bone metastasis and CEA is often found elevated in some nonmalignant conditions especially with inflammation (Rule *et al.*, 1972).

C. 5'-NUCLEOTIDE PHOSPHODIESTERASE ISOZYME-V AND LIVER METASTASIS

Not long after the discovery of the association of 5'-NPD-V with PHC, it was found that 5'-NPD-V is also present in cancer patients with liver metastases (Tsou *et al.*, 1973b). The 5'-NPD-V test for liver metastases has since been assessed in a number of coded serum samples provided by the Mayo Clinic through the auspices of the National Cancer Institute. As shown in Table III, the test showed a high degree of agreement (86%) with radiological scan for liver metastasis in patients with breast, lung, and gastrointestinal malignancies. The most significant results came from a panel of breast cancer patients. Here, 5'-NPD-V correctly predicted liver metastases in 26 of 27 (96%) patients but none of the 14 patients with benign breast diseases was positive for 5'-NPD-V. In the same panel, CEA was found elevated in 11 of 12 (92%) breast cancer patients with liver metastases, but it was also elevated in 5 of 12 (42%) patients with benign breast diseases. Therefore, CEA is significantly inferior in specificity than 5'-NPD-V in predicting liver metastases among breast cancer patients.

Large scale studies from samples collected from the Hospital of the University of Pennsylvania (Tsou and Lo, 1980; Tsou *et al.*, 1980a) and Malaysia (Lie-Injo *et al.*, 1980) essentially substantiated the same results obtained from the serum samples provided by NCI/Mayo Clinic. These results are also confirmed by studies in China (Lu *et al.*, 1980).

TABLE III
5'-NPD-V in Cancer Patients with Liver Metastases in Serum Samples
from NCI/Mayo Clinic[a]

Primary Site	Number	Positive 5'-NPD-V	% +
Breast	27	26	96
Stomach	4	2	50
Pancreas	9	7	78
Bile duct	1	1	100
Gall bladder	1	1	100
Colon	14	11	79
Rectum	6	5	83
Carcinoid	2	2	100
Lung	15	13	87
Total	79	68	86

[a] The criterion for liver metastasis is radiological scan. Adapted with permission from Tsou et al. (1973b, 1979, 1980b, c).

D. Prospective Study with 5'-Nucleotide Phosphodiesterase Isozyme-V

It is generally recognized that at the late stages of malignancy, i.e., a more disseminated disease, most biochemical markers are elevated. Therefore, the usefulness of a test can be judged only by a prospective study. This is especially true for liver metastasis, in view of the low sensitivity in detecting liver metastasis by radiological scan (Castagna et al., 1972).

While large scale prospective studies from breast cancer and malignant melanoma are still underway, preliminary results suggest that 5'-NPD-V is useful in predicting liver metastases. This is illustrated by a melanoma patient depicted in Fig. 10. An initial sampling of this patient showed a weak 5'-NPD-V and normal liver function test. The liver scan was also normal.

IX. 5'-Nucleotide Phosphodiesterase Isozyme-V in Benign Diseases

A systematic study of 5'-NPD-V in a variety of nonmalignant liver disorders had been carried out (Tsou and Lo, 1980). Because of the etiological relation between hepatitis B infection, cirrhosis, and PHC (see Section

VII,A) attention was focused between these two forms of nonmalignant liver diseases and 5'-NPD-V. During the acute phase of viral hepatitis, there is a good correlation between HB_sAg in the circulation and 5'-NPD-V (Tsou et al., 1975). However, it should be emphasized that 5'-NPD-V is also present in some hepatitis patients who were negative for HB_sAg (Tsou et al., 1975; Tsou and Lo, 1980). The most interesting result is that only 3 out of 21 (14%) HB_sAg "carriers" are positive for 5'-NPD-V. The results among Down's syndrome patients are equally striking. Patients with Down's syndrome are known to have high incidences of HB_sAg in their circulation (Blumberg et al., 1967; Sutnick et al., 1968;

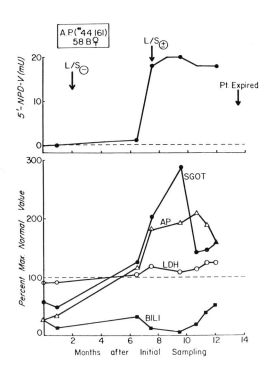

Fig. 10.   Changes in 5'-nucleotide phosphodiesterase isozyme-V and liver function tests of a malignant melanoma patient on follow-up. SGOT, Glutamic oxalacetic transaminase (maximum normal value = 27 IU/liter); AP, alkaline phosphatase (maximum normal value = 108 IU/liter); LDH, lactic dehydrogenase (maximum normal value = 157 IU/liter); Bili, total bilirubin (maximum normal value = 1.5 mg/dl). The initial sampling at 1 month for 5'-NPD-V was weakly positive (< 1 mU). The liver function tests were within normal limits and the liver scan at 2 months was normal. A second sampling at 6.5 months showed slight increase in 5'-NPD-V and mild elevations of SGOT, LDH, and AP. A second liver scan at 7.5 months was questionable but the levels of 5'-NPD-V, AP, and SGOT increased dramatically. The patient also had clinical evidence of liver metastasis.

Szmuness *et al.*, 1970). Among the 20 Down's syndrome patients studied, there were 10 patients positive for HB_sAg but only 1 of these was positive for 5'-NPD-V. All 10 Down's syndrome patients negative for HB_sAg were also negative for 5'-NPD-V (Tsou *et al.*, 1975). Convalescing patients from hepatitis B infection are all negative for 5'-NPD-V.

Among the 29 biopsy-proven late stage cirrhosis studied at the University of Pennsylvania, 17 (59%) were positive for 5'-NPD-V. This result is not surprising because of the postulated etiological reaction between cirrhosis and PHC. We have also studied the presence of 5'-NPD-V from patients in an alcoholic rehabilitation center and found only 34 of 318 patients (11%) positive (Tsou and Lo, unpublished observations). These results are in agreement with those obtained by Lu *et al.* (1980) in China, who found 2 of 24 (8%) cirrhosis patients with 5'-NPD-V. Therefore, unlike γ-glutamyl transpeptidase, the incidence of 5'-NPD-V is low in mild alcoholic cirrhosis.

X. Conclusion

The 5'-NPD-V test is a useful diagnostic aid for PHC and liver metastasis. It has a very low false-negative rate. Because of its noninvasive nature and low cost, it should be recommended in routine follow-up of cancer patients for liver metastasis. When the possibility of cirrhosis can be excluded, a consistent positive 5'-NPD-V in a protracted period is highly indicative of liver metastases.

ACKNOWLEDGMENTS

Original research reported in this chapter was supported by NCI Grants CA-07339, CA-19552, and contract NO1-CB-64029. The successful synthesis of the indigogenic substrate by Drs. S. Aoyagi, S. Matsukawa, M. Chang, and Y. Q. Chen is invaluable. We thank Dr. K. F. Yip, Mr. C. Kilgarriff, Mr. J. Rose, Ms. A. Buchanan-Kadri, Ms. S. Pearson, and Mr. M. Varello for their expert technical assistance. Serum samples were provided by Mayo Clinic, NCI, Hospital of the University of Pennsylvania, Phillipine General Hospital, Albert Einstein Medical Center, and others through the generous collaboration of many physicians. In particular, we wish to thank Drs. J. E. Rhoads, C. Schwegman, E. Rosato, J. Mullen, R. Herberman, K. R. McIntyre, A. Schutt, W. Inouye, R. Creech, M. Mastroangelo, B. Blumberg, T. London, and S. Levick whose collaboration has helped develop this serum test.

REFERENCES

Abelev, G. I. (1963). *Acta Unio Int. Cancrum* **19**, 80–82.
Abelev, G. I. (1971). *Adv. Cancer Res.* **14**, 295–358.
Abelev, G. I. (1974). *Transplant. Rev.* **20**, 3–37.
Abrams, H. L., Spiro, R., and Goldstein, N. (1950). *Cancer* **3**, 74–85.

Alfidi, R. J., Haaga, J. R., and Havrilla, T. R. (1976). *Am. J. Roentgenol.* **127**, 69–74.

Aoyagi, S., March, L., and Tsou, K. C. (1974). *J. Fac. Eng. Chiba Univ.* **26**, 185–191.

Appleman, M. M., Thompson, W. J., and Russell, T. R. (1973). *Adv. Cyclic Nucleotide Res.* **3**, 65–95.

Aronsen, K. F., Noslin, B., and Pihl, V. (1970). *Acta Chir. Scand.* **136**, 17–22.

Barnett, R. J., and Seligman, A. M. (1951). *Science* **114**, 579–582.

Bauman, G., and Chrambach, A. (1976). *Anal. Biochem.* **70**, 32–38.

Bengmark, S., and Hafström, L. (1969). *Cancer* **23**, 198–202.

Blumberg, B. S., and London, W. T. (1980). *In* "Virus in Naturally Occurring Cancers" (M. Essex, G. Todaro, and H. zur Hausen, eds.), Book A, pp. 401–421. Cold Spring Harbor Lab., Cold Spring Harbor, New York.

Blumberg, B. S., Gerstley, B. J. S., Hungerford, D. A., London, W. T., and Sutnick, A. I. (1967). *Ann. Intern. Med.* **66**, 924–931.

Blumberg, B. S., Larouzé, B., London, W. T., Werner, B., Hesser, J. E., Millman, I., Saimot, G., and Payet, M. (1975). *Am. J. Pathol.* **81**, 669–682.

Boguslaski, R. C. (1974). *J. Chem. Eng. Data* **19**, 103.

Bucher, N. L. R., and Malt, R. A. (1971). "Regeneration of Liver and Kidney." Little, Brown, Boston, Massachusetts.

Castagna, J., Benfield, J. R., Yamada, H., and Johnson, D. E. (1972). *Surg. Gynecol. Obstet.* **134**, 463–466.

Chu, T. M., and Nemoto, T. (1973). *J. Natl. Cancer Inst.* **51**, 1119–1122.

Cohen, S. S., Flaks, J. G., Barner, H. D., Loeb, M. R., and Lichtenstein, J. (1958). *Proc. Natl. Acad. Sci. U.S.A.* **44**, 1004–1012.

Criss, W. E. (1971). *Cancer Res.* **31**, 1523–1542.

Denison, E. K., Peters, R. L., and Reynolds, T. B. (1971). *Ann. Intern. Med.* **74**, 391–394.

Drum, D. E., and Beard, J. M. (1976). *J. Nucl. Med.* **17**, 677–680.

Drummond, G. I., and Yamamoto, M. (1971). *In* "The Enzymes" (P. D. Boyer, ed.), 3rd. Ed., Vol. IV, pp. 337–354. Academic Press, New York.

Fiers, W., and Khorana, H. G. (1963). *J. Biol. Chem.* **238**, 2789–2796.

Fishbein, L. (1979). "Potential Industrial Carcinogens and Mutagens." Elsevier, Amsterdam.

Flanigan, Jr., L., and Foster, J. H. (1967). *Am. J. Surg.* **113**, 551–557.

Fortner, J. G., Mulcare, R. J., Solis, A., Watson, R. C., and Golbey, R. B. (1973). *Ann. Surg.* **178**, 162–172.

Hakala, M. T. (1973). *In* "Drug Resistance and Selectivity: Biochemical and Cellular Basis" (E. Mihich, ed.), pp. 263–298. Academic Press, New York.

Hanahan, D. J. (1971). *In* "The Enzymes" (P. D. Boyer, ed.), 3rd Ed., Vol. V, pp. 71–85. Academic Press, New York.

Hartmann, K.-U., and Heidelberger, C. (1961). *J. Biol. Chem.* **236**, 3006–3013.

Harvey, C. L., Olson, K. C., and Wright, R. (1970). *Biochemistry* **9**, 921–925.

Hatfield, P. M. (1975). *Med. Clin. N. Amer.* **59**, 247–276.

Heidelberger, C., Ghober, A., Baker, R. K., and Mukherjee, K. L. (1960a). *Cancer Res.* **20**, 897–902.

Heidelberger, C., Kalder, G., Mukherjee, K. L., and Danneberg, D. B. (1960b). *Cancer Res.* **20**, 903–909.

Hirai, H., and Nishi, S. (1976). *Protides Biol. Fluids* **24**, 621–625.

Hirai, H., Nishi, S., and Watabe, H. (1973). *Gann Monogr.* **14**, 19–34.

Ho, N. W. Y., and Gilham, P. T. (1973). *Biochim. Biophys. Acta* **308**, 53–58.

Holt, S. J. (1952). *Nature (London)* **169**, 271–273.

Horwitz, J. P., Easwaran, C. V., Wolf, P. L., and Kowalczyk, L. S. (1969). *Biochim. Biophys. Acta* **185**, 143–152.

Hynie, I., Meuffels, M., and Poznanski, W. J. (1975). *Clin. Chem.* **21**, 1383–1387.
Jaffe, B. M., Donegan, W. L., Watson, F., and Spratt, J. S. (1968). *Surg. Gynecol. Obstet.* **127**, 1–11.
Kalengayi, M. M., and Desmet, V. J. (1975a). *Cancer Res.* **35**, 2836–2844.
Kalengayi, M. M., and Desmet, V. J. (1975b). *Cancer Res.* **35**, 2845–2852.
Kelly, S. J., and Butler, L. G. (1975). *Biochem. Biophys. Res. Commun.* **66**, 316–321.
Kelly, S. J., and Butler, L. G. (1977). *Biochemistry* **16**, 1102–1104.
Kelly, S. J., Dardinger, D. E., and Butler, L. G. (1975). *Biochemistry* **14**, 4983–4988.
Kew, M. C., Desmyter, K., Bradburne, A. F., and McNab, G. M. (1979). *J. Natl. Cancer Inst.* **62**, 517–520.
Khorana, H. G. (1961). *In* "The Enzymes" (P. D. Boyer, H. Lardy, and K. Myrback, eds.), 2nd. Ed., Vol. V, pp. 79–94. Academic Press, New York.
Koerner, J. F., and Sinsheimer, R. L. (1957). *J. Biol. Chem.* **228**, 1039–1048.
Kuo, J. F., Shoji, M., Helfman, D. M., and Brackett, N. L. (1979). *ICN UCLA Symp. Mol. Cell. Biol.* **123**, 335–355.
Laqueur, G. L., Mickelson, O., Whiting, M. G., and Kurland, L. T. (1973). *J. Natl. Cancer Inst.* **31**, 919–951.
Larouzé, B., London, W. T., Saimot, G., Werner, B. G., Lustbader, E. D., Payet, M., and Blumberg, B. S. (1976). *Lancet* **2**, 534–538.
Laskowski, M., Sr. (1966). *Proc. Nucleic Acid Res.* **1**, 154–187.
Laskowski, M., Sr. (1967). *Adv. Enzymol.* **29**, 165–220.
Laskowski, M., Sr. (1971). *In* "The Enzymes" (P. D. Boyer, ed.), 3rd Ed., Vol. 4, pp. 313–336. Academic Press, New York.
Laskowski, M., Sr. (1980). *Methods Enzymol.* **65**, 276–284.
Lehman, I. R., and Nussbaum, A. L. (1964). *J. Biol. Chem.* **239**, 2628–2636.
Lie-Injo, L. E., Tsou, K. C., Lo, K. W., Lopez, C. G., Balasegaram, M., and Ganesan, S. (1980). *Cancer* **45**, 795–798.
Lin, J. J., Lin, C., and Svoboda, D. J. (1974). *Lab. Invest.* **30**, 267–278.
Lo, K. W., Ferrar, W., Fineman, W., and Tsou, K. C. (1972). *Anal. Biochem.* **47**, 609–613.
Lo, K. W., Miller, E. E., Morris, H. P., and Tsou, K. C. (1973). *Cancer Chemother. Rep.* (Pt 1) **57**, 245–249.
LoGerfo, P., Krupey, J., and Hansen, H. J. (1973). *New Engl. J. Med.* **285**, 138–141.
Lu, H. M. Chen, C., Ming, T. H., Chiang, K. L., Ting, T. S., Pan, L. S., and Yui, C. (1980). *Int. J. Cancer* **26**, 31–35.
McCartney, W. H., and Hoffer, P. B. (1978). *Cancer* **42**, 1457–1462.
McCready, V. R. (1972). *Semin. Nucl. Med.* **2**, 108–127.
MacNab, G. M., Alexander, J. J., Lecatsas, G., Bey, E. M., and Urbanowicz, J. M. (1976a). *Br. J. Cancer* **34**, 509–514.
MacNab, G. M., Urbanowicz, J. M., Geddes, E. W., and Kew, M. C. (1976b). *Br. J. Cancer* **33**, 544–548.
March, L. C., and Tsou, K. C. (1970). *J. Heterocycl. Chem.* **7**, 885–889.
Martin, Jr., E. W., Kirbey, W. E., DiVecchia, L., Anderson, G., Catalano, P., and Minton, J. P. (1976). *Cancer* **37**, 62–81.
Masseyeff, R. F. (1973). *Gann Monogr.* **14**, 3–18.
Mendelsohn, M. L., and Bodansky, O. (1952). *Cancer* **5**, 1–8.
Mikaye, M. (1961). *Acta Unio Int. Canctum* **17**, 892–897.
Miller, E. E., Ledis, S. L., Lo, K. W., and Tsou, K. C. (1976). *J. Pharma. Sci.* **65**, 384–387.
Morris, H. P. (1965). *Adv. Cancer Res.* **9**, 227–302.
Mugera, G. J., and Nderito, P. C. (1968). *In* "Cancer in Africa" (B. Clifford, A. Linsell, and G. L. Timms, eds.), pp. 323–326. East African Publ. House, Nairobi, Kenya.
Mulcare, R. J., Sollis, A., and Fortner, J. G. (1973). *J. Surg. Res.* **15**, 87–95.

Munjal, D., Chawla, P. L., Lokich, J. J., and Zamcheck, N. (1976). *Cancer* **37**, 1800-1807.
Murray-Lyon, I. M., Dawson, J. L., Parsons, V. A., Rake, M. O., Blendis, L. M., Laws, J. W., and Williams, R. (1970). *Lancet* **2**, 172-175.
Nayak, N. C., Dhar, A., Sachdeva, R., Mittal, A., Seth, H. N., Sudarsanam, D., Reddy, B., Wagholikar, U. L., and Reddy, C. R. R. M. (1977). *Int. J. Cancer* **20**, 634-654.
Neville, A. M., and Lawrence, D. J. R. (1974). *Int. J. Cancer* **14**, 1-18.
Nishioka, K., Hirayama, T., Sekine, T., Okochi, K., Mayumi, M., Sung, J. L., Lui, C. H., and Lin, T. M. (1973). *Gann Monogr.* **14**, 167-183.
Ohbayashi, A., Okochi, K., and Mayumi, M. (1972). *Gastroenterology* **62**, 618-625.
Ohira, S., Mazawa, S., and Saito, T. (1975). *Sci. Rep. Res. Int. Tohoku Univ.* **22**, 38-45.
Okuda, K., and Peters, R. (1976). "Hapatocellular Carcinoma," p. 361. Wiley, New York.
Payet, M., Camain, P., and Pene, P. (1956). *Rev. Intern. Hepatol.* **4**, 1-20.
Pestana, A., and Cortina, P. (1966). *Rev. Esp. Fisiol.* **22**, 47-48.
Pollock, T. W., Mullen, J. L., Tsou, K. C., Lo, K. W., and Rosato, E. F. (1979). *Am. J. Surg.* **137**, 22-25.
Prince, A. M., Szmuness, W., Michon, J., Demaille, J., Diebolt, G., Linhard, J., Quenum, C., and Sankale, M. (1975). *Int. J. Cancer* **16**, 376-383.
Razzell, W. E. (1963). *Methods Enzymol.* **6**, 236-258.
Razzell, W. E. (1966). *Biochem. Biophys. Res. Commun.* **22**, 243-247.
Razzell, W. E. and Khorana, H. G. (1959). *J. Biol. Chem.* **234**, 2105-2113.
Razzell, W. E., and Khorana, H. G. (1961). *J. Biol. Chem.* **236**, 1144-1149.
Righetti, P. G., and Drysdale, J. W. (1976). "Isoelectric Focusing." North-Holland Publ., Amsterdam.
Rule, A. H., Straus, E., Vandevoorde, J., and Janowitz, H. D. (1972). *New Engl. J. Med.* **287**, 24-26.
Sakurai, M., and Miyaji, T. (1975). *Ann. N.Y. Acad. Sci.* **259**, 156-167.
Sanders, A. D., and Sanders, R. C. (1977). *J. Nucl. Med.* **18**, 205-220.
Sargent, J. R., and George, S. G. (1975). "Methods in Zone Electrophoresis," 3rd Ed., p. 15. BDH Chemicals, Poole, England.
Schapira, F. (1973). *Adv. Cancer Res.* **18**, 77-153.
Schoenthl, R. (1959). *J. Pathol. Bacteriol.* **77**, 485-580.
Shanghai Co-ordinating Group for Research on Liver Cancer (1979). *Chin. Med. J.* **92**, 801-806.
Shi, B-Z., Ming, T. H., Chang, K.-L., Lu, H.-M., Chen, C., Ting, C.-Y., and Pan, L.-H. (1980). *Chung-hua I Hsueh Chien Yen Tsa Chih* **3**, 75-77.
Shingleton, W. R. (1971). *In* "Nuclear Medicine" (W. B. Blahd, ed.), p. 373. McGraw-Hill, New York.
Sierakowska, H., and Shugar, D. (1963). *Biochem. Biophys. Res. Commun.* **11**, 70-74.
Sierakowska, H., Gahan, P. B., and Dawson, A. L. (1978). *Histochem. J.* **10**, 679-693.
Simons, M. J., Yap, E. H., Yu, M., and Shanmugaratnam, K. (1972). *Int. J. Cancer* **10**, 320-325.
Sinsheimer, R. L., and Koerner, J. F. (1952). *J. Biol. Chem.* **198**, 293-296.
Smith, K., Varon, K. K., Race, G. J., Paulson, D. I., Urschel, H. C., and Mallams, J. T. (1966). *Cancer* **19**, 1281-1285.
Solt, D., and Farber, E. (1976). *Nature (London)* **263**, 701-703.
Sparks, F. C., Mosher, M. B., Hallaner, W. C., Silverstein, M. J., Rangel, D., Passaro, Jr., E., and Morton, D. L. (1975). *Cancer* **35**, 1074-1082.
Spik, G., Six, P., Bouquelet, S., Sawicka, T., and Montreuil, J. (1979). *In* "Glyco-conjugates" (J. D. Gregory and R. W. Jeanloz, eds.), Vol. 2, pp. 933-936. Academic Press, New York.
Stanley, R. J., Sagel, S. S., and Levitt, R. G. (1976). *Am. J. Roentgenol.* **127**, 53-67.

Steiner, P., and Davies, J. N. (1957). *Br. J. Cancer* **11**, 523–524.

Sun, S. C. Wei, R. D., and Schaeffer, B. T. (1971). *Lab. Invest.* **24**, 368–372.

Sutnick, A. I., London, W. T., Gerstley, B. J. S., Cronlund, M. M., and Blumberg, B. S. (1968). *J. Am. Med. Assoc.* **205**, 670–674.

Swinton, N. W., Samaan, S., and Rosenthal, D. (1967). *Surg. Clin. N. Am.* **47**, 657–662.

Szmuness, W., Pick, R., and Prince, A. M. (1970). *Am. J. Epidemiol.* **92**, 51–61.

Tatarinov, Ju. S. (1964). *Vopr. Med. Khim* **10**, 90–91.

Terry, W. D., Henkart, P. A., Coligan, J. E., and Todd, C. W. (1974). *Transplant. Rev.* **20**, 100–129.

Tsou, K. C. (1974). *In* "Electron Microscopy of Enzymes" (M. A. Hayat, ed.), Vol IV, pp. 154–178. Van Nostrand-Reinhold, Princeton, New Jersey.

Tsou, K. C., and Lo, K. W. (1980). *Cancer* **45**, 209–213.

Tsou, K. C., and Yip, K. F. (1980). *Nucleic Acid Res.* **8**, 567–572.

Tsou, K. C., Aoyagi, S., and Miller, E. E. (1970). *J. Med. Chem.* **13**, 765–768.

Tsou, K. C., Lo, K. W., Ledis, S. L., and Miller, E. E. (1972). *J. Med. Chem.* **15**, 1221–1225.

Tsou, K. C., Ledis, S., and McCoy, M. G. (1973a). *Cancer Res.* **33**, 2215–2217.

Tsou, K. C., McCoy, M. G., Enterline, H. T., Herberman, R., and Wahner, H. (1973b). *J. Natl. Cancer Inst.* **51**, 2005–2006.

Tsou, K. C., Hendricks, J., Gupta, P. D., and Lo, K. W. (1974a). *Histochem. J.* **6**, 327–337.

Tsou, K. C., Morris, H. P., Lo, K. W., and Muscato, J. J. (1974b). *Cancer Res.* **34**, 1295–1298.

Tsou, K. C., McCoy, M. G., Lo, K. W., and London, W. T. (1975). *Cancer* **35**, 2361–2364.

Tsou, K. C., Lo, K. W., Tsou, W. H., Herberman, R. B., and Schutt, A. (1979). *In* "Carcino-Embryonic Proteins" (F.-G. Lehmann, ed.), Vol. 1, pp. 429–434. Elsevier, Amsterdam.

Tsou, K. C., Lo, K. W., Mullen, J., Rosato, E., Guintoli, R., Mikuta, J., Mangan, C., and Murphy, J. (1980a). *In* "Prevention and Detection of Cancer" (H. E. Nieburgs, ed.), Pt. II, Vol. 2, pp. 2199–2206. Dekker, New York.

Tsou, K. C., Lo, K. W., Herberman, R. B., and Schutt, A. J. (1980b). *Oncology* **37**, 381–385.

Tsou, K. C., Lo, K. W., Herberman, R. B., Schutt, A. J., and Go, V. L. W. (1980c). *J. Clin. Hematol. Oncol.* **10**, 1–8.

Umeda, M., and Heidelberger, C. (1968). *Cancer Res.* **28**, 2529–2538.

Viadana, A., and Au, K. L. (1975). *J. Med.* **6**, 1–14.

Viadana, E., Bross, I. D. J., and Pickren, J. W. (1978). *Oncology* **35**, 114–126.

Vogel, C. L., Anthony, P. P., Mody, N., and Barker, L. F. (1972). *J. Natl. Cancer Inst.* **48**, 1583–1588.

Weber, G. (1963). *Adv. Enzyme Reg.* **1**, 321–340.

West, M., and Zimmerman, H. J. (1958). *Arch. Intern. Med.* **102**, 103–114.

West, M., Berger, C., Rony, H., and Zimmerman, H. J. (1961). *J. Lab. Clin. Med.* **57**, 946–954.

Wilkinson, D. S., Solomonson, L. P., and Cory, J. G. (1977). *Proc. Soc. Exp. Biol. Med.* **154**, 268–271.

Wogan, G. N. (1973). *In* "The Liver" (E. A. Gall and F. K. Mostofi, eds.), pp. 161–181. Williams & Wilkins, Baltimore, Maryland.

Woodfield, D. G., Endo, Y., and Matsuhashi, T. (1974). *Aust. N.Z. J. Med.* **4**, 3–7.

Wroblewski, F. (1959). *Am. J. Med.* **27**, 911–923.

Yip, K. F., and Tsou, K. C. (1979). *Biopolymers* **18**, 1389–1405.

MODELS AND METHODS FOR DIAGNOSIS AND THERAPY

CHAPTER VIII

SOLID TUMORS AS A MODEL FOR THE DEVELOPMENT OF ANTINEOPLASTIC THERAPY

WILLIAM B. LOONEY AND HAROLD A. HOPKINS

I. Introduction

Solid tumors which comprise the majority of human cancer continue to challenge the best efforts of both the clinician and the experimentalist. We have used two solid tumor models with different growth, morphological, cell kinetic, and metastasizing characteristics to obtain quantitative information on clinical problems. Two treatment modalities alone or in different combinations are being studied for their effects at three organizational levels: cellular, organ, and animal, permitting maximum clinical utilization of data obtained from one solid tumor line which is therapeutically responsive to chemotherapy and radiotherapy, and another which is resistant to both treatment modalities. Changes in multiple parameters have been used as is done in clinical evaluations of therapeutic response. Radiotherapy, chemotherapy, immunotherapy, and surgery must be better coordinated to control growth of both the primary tumor and its metastases if therapeutic efficiency is to significantly improve in therapeutically resistant solid tumors in man.

Clinical protocols employing combined modality therapy are usually designed so that courses of chemotherapy are given followed by radiotherapy, or courses of radiotherapy followed by chemotherapy. In many instances, an experimental basis for the design of these clinical protocols is inadequate or nonexistent. Most chemotherapy is given as multidrug therapy. Often, this makes it difficult or impossible to determine the optimum interaction of radiation with many drugs having various modes of action. The following excerpt from Isselbacher in *Harrison's Principles of Internal Medicine* (1980, p. 1616) applies:

> The sequencing of chemotherapy and radiation therapy has varied from site to site with the use of radiotherapy before, during, and after chemotherapy. It is apparent that there has been little or no consistency in the approach, and the limit of tolerance to radiotherapy of normal tissue, not the ability to control tumor, has been used as a guide to therapy. Further research is needed to determine whether combinations of radiation and drugs are additive, synergistic, or inhibitory.

Two solid tumor lines with different growth, cell kinetic, histological, and metastatic characteristics were selected for our single and combined modality treatment studies. Selection was based on therapeutic response as well as characteristics which would permit studies directed to key clinical questions, e.g., the effect of single and combined modality treatment on the primary tumor, and the relationship of such treatment to control of metastatic dissemination. Hepatoma 3924A has limited effect on the host; metastases are seen only after treatment of the primary. Hepatoma H-4-II-E metastasizes to the lungs and axiliary nodes. It is carried both *in vivo* and *in vitro*, and can be used to evaluate the effects of tumor on host, or of radiation to the tumor and its metastases. *In vitro* plating of tumor cells treated *in vivo* permits determination of tumor cell viability after therapy.

Our experimental studies have shown that effective interaction of single drugs (e.g., 5-FU and cyclophosphamide) with radiation can be realized to produce cure rates $\geq 50\%$. These cure rates were realized by administration of three and four series of combined therapy in which radiation and chemotherapy were separated by 1, 7, or 11 days. The finding that long periods of time (7 to 11 days) between administration of chemotherapy and radiotherapy result in effective utilization of the two modalities is important since diminished host toxicity is also realized.

The results of the successful utilization of sequential combined modality therapy in our experimental solid tumors are providing information for clinical protocols in the treatment of primary and metastatic pulmonary cancer and colorectal cancer. It is evident from these initial efforts that it will require a long-term effort to eventually arrive at successful protocols for sequential combined modality therapy of therapeutically resistant solid tumors in man. It will be necessary to set up on a long-range basis the continuous interchange of information based on results of both clinical and experimental studies. Results of experimental studies will provide the clinician with information which can be utilized in the design of new clinical protocols for sequential combined modality treatments. Results of the clinical protocols will, in turn, provide information which will suggest new experimental protocols to amplify and better understand the clinical results. This continuous interchange of the results of experimental and clinical programs offers one of the more promising approaches to effective management of the major therapeutically resistant solid tumors in man.

II. Radiotherapy

For a tumor in the exponential phase of growth when it is treated, any one of a number of responses can be seen in the growth curves after treatment (Fig. 1). The actual response curves are a continuum, ranging from those tumors which treatment affects only slightly to those which are completely eliminated. The division of this continuum into classes is done primarily for reasons of convenience, and because the classes have some relevance in the design of treatment schedules. Individual growth curves are fitted with polynomials of degree 3–6 through the use of the χ^2 technique (Trefil et al., 1978) and an overall treatment efficiency (OTE) calculated for each tumor from the various parameters taken from the fitted curve. OTE is determined as follows:

$$OTE = 3 - n + \eta$$

where $n = 1, 2, 3$ according to the growth class of the tumor (i.e., I, II, or III)

$$\eta = \text{class efficiency} = 1 - \frac{V_{min}}{V_0} \qquad \text{for Class I}$$

$$= 1 - \frac{V_{min} - V_0}{V_{max} - V_0} \qquad \text{for Class II}$$

$$= 1 - \frac{B_{min}}{\langle bc \rangle} \qquad \text{for Class III}$$

where V_0 = volume at day of treatment, V_{min} = volume at posttreatment minimum, V_{max} = posttreatment volume maximum (occurring prior to V_{min}), B_{min} = minimum posttreatment growth rate, and $\langle bc \rangle$ = average growth rate of controls at day of growth rate minimum. The major advantage of using OTE is that it gives the means for evaluating a continuous spectrum of responses from slowdown (Class III) to regression (Class I). Another method used for comparing treatments is simply to determine the changes in mean tumor volume at specified times after treatment.

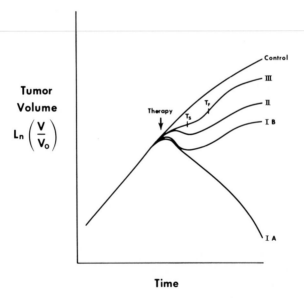

FIG. 1. The classification used to evaluate tumor growth following single and combined modality therapy: Class I, regression—tumor volume becomes smaller than tumor volume (V_0) at time of initial treatment. Class II, pseudoregression—tumor volume is always greater than V_0, but at some point shows a definite diminution from a previously attained maximum. Class III, slowdown—tumor volume never decreases but growth rate slows down.

An extensively used method for assessing therapeutic response is tumor growth delay, defined as the increased number of days required for a treated group of tumors to reach a specific tumor volume, compared to the time for the control group to reach the same size (Thomlinson and Craddock, 1967). The major advantage of converting tumor volume change to "time" is that it offers a simple and easily definable way of expressing the relative effectiveness of different treatment schedules.

The results of local irradiation of the H-4-II-E tumor over a dose range of 750 to 3500 rads are used below to illustrate the different methods for evaluation of tumor growth response. H-4-II-E is a poorly differentiated tumor which has been developed as an *in vito–in vitro* tumor cell system from the H-35 rat hepatoma (Evans and Kovacs, 1977; Kovacs *et al.*, 1977). *In vivo*, H-4-II-E has an actual doubling time of 49.2 hours, a potential doubling time of 34.8 hours, and a cell cycle time of 39.1 hours. T_{G_1} is 30.5 hours, T_S is 6.0 hours, T_{G_2} is 2.1 hours, and T_M is 0.5 hour. The 1-hour [^{3}H]thymidine labeling index is 13.8%, growth fraction is 100%, and cell loss factor is 0.32. It is carried in our laboratory both *in vivo* and *in vitro* and has retained its growth characteristics during passage for the past 4 years (Looney *et al.*, 1978).

Subsequent to radiation, H-4-II-E tumor volumes continue to increase for 2 to 3 days, then become depressed for a period of 5 to 10 days (Fig. 2). Ten to 14 days after treatment, tumor growth is reestablished at rates comparable to those for nonirradiated control tumors. The mean tumor volumes at the time of maximum depression (day 7) and at the time of return to control values (day 14) are shown in Fig. 3. The semilog plot of the tumor volume on day 7 demonstrates smaller incremental tumor volume reduction with increasing radiation doses. The greatest increment of change was between 0 and 750 rads. Mean tumor volume in the 750 rad group was 39% of control values on day 7 and 41% of controls on day 14.

The times after treatment at which minimum tumor volume (T_{min}) and maximum tumor growth rates (T_{max}) occur are shown in Fig. 4. T_{min} increases from 4.87 ± 0.67 days after 750 rads to 8.74 ± 0.87 days after 3500 rads. T_{max} increases from 10.67 ± 0.33 for 750 rads to 15.70 ± 0.62 for 3500 rads. Information on the time of maximum tumor volume change should be helpful in the design of sequential experimental and clinical therapeutic protocols. A second course of treatment at the time of maximum tumor volume change would likely be more effective than if randomly given at other times. A second course of treatment at the time of minimum tumor change would be less likely to be effective. The therapeutic ramifications of T_{max} and T_{min} have not been fully evaluated at present. However, the information may provide the basis for a more rational design of protocols for sequential therapy based on tumor response to the

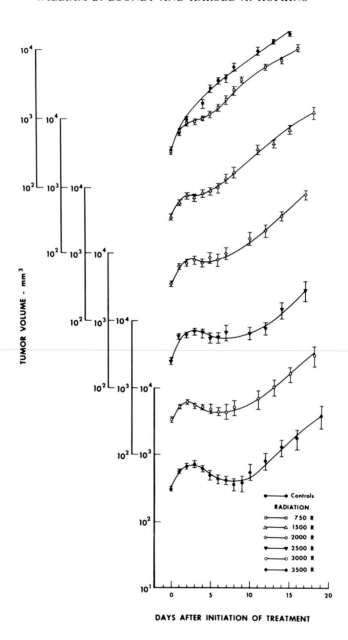

Fig. 2.   Mean tumor volume ± SE for control and radiation-treated H-4-II-E tumors. The curves have been offset for clarity and each has its corresponding logarithmic scale on the ordinate.

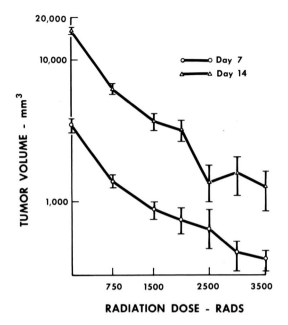

FIG. 3.   Mean tumor volume ± SE 7 and 14 days after radiation treatment of H-4-II-E.

prior treatment series (Looney et al., 1980). Tumor growth delay was calculated using 8 V_0 as the final volume. Increasing the radiation dose from 750 to 3500 rads resulted in an increased tumor growth delay ranging from 3 days for 750 rads to 10 days for 3500 rads (Table I).

All of the tumor responses following 750 rads are Class III or slowdown responses (Table I). The type of response changes from Class III to Class I (regression) and Class II (pseudo-regression) as the radiation dose is increased to 3500 rads. At 3500 rads, 5 of the 10 tumors exhibited a Class I response, 4 a Class II response, and only 1 a Class III response.

The overall treatment efficiency (OTE) increased from 0.35 ± 0.09 after 750 rads to 1.92 ± 0.23 after 3500 rads (Table I). The major increase in OTE occurred as the radiation dose increased from 750 to 2500 rads. Increasing the dose from 2500 to 3500 rads resulted in smaller incremental increases of the OTE.

The mean day of death for the control group was 22 ± 1.9 days. Life span in the group in which the tumors received 2500 rads was 32 ± 7.3 days or 145% of control. Life span in the 3000 rad group was 54 ± 3.8 days (245% of controls). The life span of the 3500 rad group increased to 62 ± 7.0 days (282% of controls). Increasing the tumor radiation dose from 3500 to 4500 rads resulted only in a 3-day increase in mean survival. Life span for the 4500 rad group was 65 ± 10 days (295% of controls). The

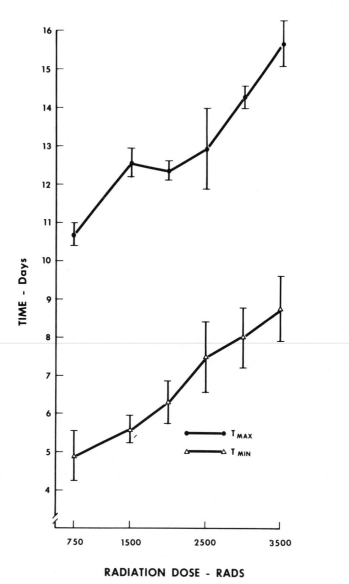

Fig. 4. The times (days) at which minimal volume (T_{min}) and maximal tumor growth rates (T_{max}) occur in H-4-II-E following increasing radiation doses.

increase in mean life span as a function of increasing radiation dose is shown in Fig. 5. Increasing the dose beyond 3000 rads results in relatively small incremental increases in life expectancy. This probably is the result of metastatic dissemination prior to radiation, although local control was also not achieved at these radiation doses.

TABLE I

THE EFFECT OF INCREASING DOSES OF RADIATION ON H-4-II-E TUMOR
RESPONSE AND OVERALL TREATMENT EFFICIENCY

Treatment (rads)	Growth delay (days)[a]	Overall treatment efficiency (OTE) $\pm$ SE[b]	Classification of tumor response to treatment		
			Class I	Class II	Class III
3500	9.54 $\pm$ 0.9	1.92 $\pm$ 0.23	5	4	1
3000	6.06 $\pm$ 2.5	1.87 $\pm$ 0.26	6	1	3
2500	7.76 $\pm$ 0	1.69 $\pm$ 0.20	4	4	2
2000	6.34 $\pm$ 2.3	1.21 $\pm$ 0.23	1	3	5
1500	5.96 $\pm$ 2.5	0.55 $\pm$ 0.17	0	1	5
750	3.28 $\pm$ 1.2	0.35 $\pm$ 0.09	0	0	7

[a] Growth delay shown is the increased time for treated tumors to reach 8 times initial volume (V_0) at time of treatment in excess of the time for control tumors to reach 8 times V_0 of 5.2 $\pm$ 1.2 days.
[b] Standard error of the mean.

Survival of the clonogenic population of cells from this tumor has been determined previously both *in vivo* and *in vitro* (Evans and Kovacs, 1977; Kovacs *et al.*, 1977). The D_0 for cells irradiated *in vitro* under conditions of normal aeration was 190 rads with an extrapolation number of 1.6. The

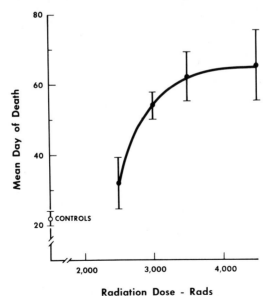

FIG. 5. Mean day of death $\pm$ SE for rats with H-4-II-E and given various doses of radiation.

D_0 for cells irradiated in air-breathing animals was 240 rads with an extrapolation number of 4.

Clonogenic assays made at intervals after 1500 rads (Fig. 6) showed that the clonogenic fraction increased exponentially from 0.03 on day 0 to 1.0 on day 9 or 10 (plating efficiency of control = 0.32). This assay requires the enzymic dissociation of the tumor to a single cell suspension. The mean number of cells per gram of untreated tumor dissociated, the cell yield, was 2.5×10^7 (excluding lymphocytes but not other host cells) and did not show a dependent variation with tumor weight over the range used in these experiments. Yields were reduced from day 1 to day 7 following 1500 rads. Total clonogenic cells per tumor (the product of tumor weight at resection, cell yield and clonogenic fraction for individual tumors) increased in three phases after irradiation (Fig. 7): days 0–7 cell numbers increased 10-fold (doubling time $= T_d = 2.3$ days), days 7–9 cell numbers increased 20-fold ($T_d = 0.46$ days or 11.2 hours), and day 9 onward $T_d = 4.5$ days. Evans and Kovacs (1977) reported for untreated tumors, volume T_d of 49.2 hours and an *in vivo* cell cycle time of 39 hours. Incorporation of [³H]thymidine into tumor DNA during the 1-hour period prior to killing the animal was below control values until day 7 after 1500 rads, then recovered with the recovery phase peaking at twice the control activity (Fig. 8).

Labeling and mitotic indices (Figs. 9 and 10, respectively), initially depressed by irradiation (1500 rads), also recovered at day 7. Mitotic nuclei were always more numerous in the perivascular tissue and decreased in concentration with increasing distance from the vein.

The degree of necrosis in both treated and untreated tumors progressed

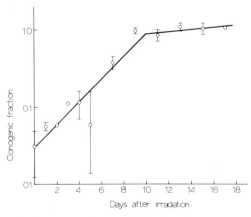

FIG. 6. Changes in the *in vitro* clonogenic fraction of H-4-II-E tumors at intervals after 1500 rads.

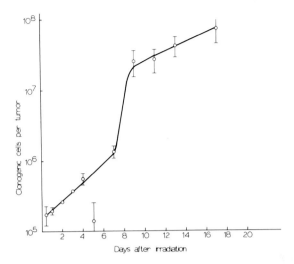

F$_{IG}$. 7. Changes in the total numbers of clonogenic cells in H-4-II-E after 1500 rads.

with increasing time interval from day 0. The degree of hemorrhage present appeared to have no correlation with treatment or time of evaluation. During day 3 after treatment, lymphocytes and plasma cells accumulated in the capsule surrounding the tumor and superficial parenchymal infiltration of the tumor by lymphocytes was noted. On day 5 the lymphocytic infiltrate became more prominent, penetrating deeply into the parenchyma via small lymphatic channels, and was associated with focal cell necrosis. The lymphocytic infiltrate became less prominent on day 9 and by day 11 only scattered lymphocytes were noted in the parenchyma.

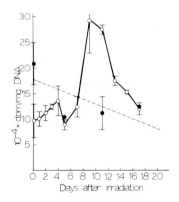

F$_{IG}$. 8. DNA specific activity of H-4-II-E tumors at intervals after 1500 rads (○) or no treatment (●). [³H]Thymidine was given 1 hour prior to killing the rat.

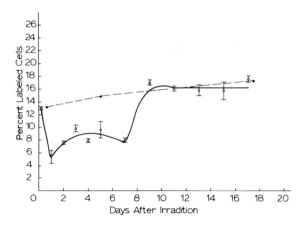

FIG. 9.   [³H]Thymidine labeling index in H-4-II-E tumors after 1500 rads (○) or no treatment (●).

Capsular lymphocytes and plasma cells were in evidence throughout the duration of this experiment (through day 17).

As has been suggested earlier (Kovacs *et al.*, 1977; Rowley *et al.*, 1980), tumor volume changes and regrowth delay may not be related solely to cell kill. Tumor regression and regrowth does not necessarily represent a simple product of interrupted and reestablished tumor cell repopulation and cell clearance. Both structural and vascular architecture (Thomlinson and Gray, 1955) as well as vascular supply (Denekamp, 1972) are known to contribute to the radiation response of tumors. Furthermore, there is evidence that a slower rate of removal of radiation-

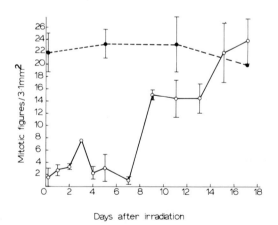

FIG. 10.   Number of mitotic figures per unit area of H-4-II-E tumor sections from tumors given 1500 rads (○) or no treatment (●).

sterilized tumor tissue occurs when it is adjacent to connective tissue (Thomlinson, 1973).

Nevertheless, the basis for defining tumor radiosensitivity and radioresistance, while highly influenced both by macro- and microenvironmental conditions, still lies in the response of individual tumor cells *in situ* to radiation. Many attempts have been made to relate changes in tumor growth parameters with changes in tumor cell survival following radiation. However, McNally (1973), based on observations of oxygenation effects on cell kill and growth delay, has proposed that "the use of *in vitro* techniques predicting detailed radiobiological responses *in vivo* may not be valid." Twentyman (1977) has also suggested that unless either "potentially lethal damage" or proliferation of survivors can be inhibited, there is no time at which the absolute value of "surviving fraction" can be measured and that the time at which "surviving fraction" determinations are made is largely arbitrary.

The relationship between cell kill assayed *in vitro* and the tumor growth delay of H-4-II-E following a series of radiation doses has been determined (Rowley *et al.*, 1980). Assuming a direct relationship between cell kill and growth delay, the theoretical semilog curve describing the corre-

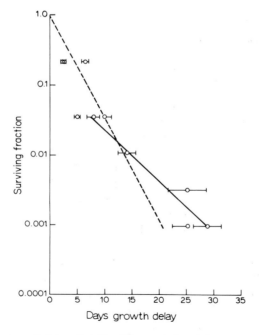

Fig. 11. Tumor growth delays (results of four experiments) versus surviving fraction of tumor cells assayed *in vitro* 1 hour after radiation *in vivo*.

lation between these two parameters would pass through the origin (Fig. 11). Instead, the correlation appears to be biphasic, diverging from the theoretical curve at doses above 2000 rads. Assuming that within a tumor the degree of cellular oxygenation represents a spectrum of magnitudes, the biphasic response could be explained by a "dose-dependent proliferative delay of radioresistant cells" or by a delay in recruitment of chronically hypoxic cells. Alternatively, a "tumor bed effect" may be at least partly responsible for the longer growth delay observed for H-4-II-E tumors at the higher radiation doses. Urano and Suit (1971) found that growth of C3H mammary carcinoma was slowed when transplanted into previously irradiated tissues. In any event, it is clear from these and other data (McNally, 1973; Stephens and Steel, 1980) that tumor growth delay cannot simply depend upon the fraction of cells that has retained the capacity for unlimited proliferation.

III. Chemotherapy

A. INTRODUCTION

The proper scheduling of cancer chemotherapeutic agents is dependent upon an understanding of dose–time relationships in expression of the deleterious effects of these agents on the critical host organs. The time of administration of the second series of chemotherapeutic agents is governed by the kinetics of recovery. The gastrointestinal epithelium and the bone marrow usually present the most life-threatening toxic reactions during cancer chemotherapy because of high rates of cell renewal normally occurring at these sites and the critical functions which these organs perform. We have determined that the gastrointestinal mucosa in the rat recovers in 4 to 5 days following one single, approximately LD_{10} dose of 5-fluorouracil (5-FU), adriamycin, or cyclophosphamide (Hopkins et al., 1976; Hopkins and Looney, 1978). The bone marrow recovers in 10 to 11 days. Since the gastrointestinal mucosa recovers in less than one-half the time necessary for the recovery of bone marrow, it is evident that bone marrow recovery, rather than gastrointestinal tract recovery, is the primary factor in determining the time for sequential treatment.

Hepatoma 3924A is a fast-growing, poorly differentiated tumor. The parenchymal tumor cells are hypotetraploid, having 73 chromosomes, 10 of which are abnormal. Repeated cell kinetic and growth studies over the past 10 years have shown hepatoma 3924A to be stable and reproducible.

The kinetics of cell proliferation and tumor growth are as follows: the actual volume doubling time for 3924A is 104 hours; potential volume doubling time is 42 hours. Cell cycle time is 27.4 hours. The different phases of the cycle are T_{G_1}, 14 hours; T_S, 9.3 hours; T_{G_2}, 3.7 hours; and T_M, 0.4 hour. The 1-hour thymidine labeling index is 17.6, growth fraction is 0.65, and cell loss factor is 0.60 (Looney *et al.*, 1978).

B. CYCLOPHOSPHAMIDE

1. Effects of Cyclophosphamide on Tumor Growth

Changes in mean tumor volumes for five groups of animals with 3924A given 50, 100, 150, 200, and 250 mg/kg cyclophosphamide are shown in Fig. 12. Average tumor volume increased for a period of 2 to 4 days following administration of cyclophosphamide. This was followed by reduction of tumor volume which, for intermediate doses, reached a nadir 8 to 10 days after treatment. Tumor volumes are compared in Fig. 13 at 8 and 25 days following treatment. Volumes of treated tumors were 2, 4, 4, 7, and 18% of controls on day 8 following 250, 200, 150, 100, and 50 mg/kg cyclophosphamide, respectively. Examination on day 25, when all tumor growth rates in the treated group had returned to rates comparable to control growth rates, revealed that the volume reduction which occurred following treatment was retained throughout the course of the study (Fig. 13). Growth delays and OTE for these treatment groups are given in Table II. The greatest change in both tumor growth delay and OTE occurred as the cyclophosphamide dose was increased from 50 to 150 mg/kg. Growth rates were extracted from the tumor volume curves as follows. Tumor volumes were normalized to the volume on day of treatment and plotted on a semilogarithmic scale for each animal. The result is a series of graphs of

$$\ln \frac{V(t)}{V_0}$$

versus time where $V(t)$ is the tumor volume at time t and V_0 is the volume at time of treatment. These tumor volume growth curves are then fitted by the method of least squares with a polynomial of degree N whose functional form is

$$\ln \frac{V(t)}{V_0} = a_0 + a_1 t + a_2 t^2 + \cdots a_N t^N \tag{1}$$

where N values of up to 6 are necessary for a proper fit. A "proper fit" is one whose χ^2 probability $[p(\chi^2)]$ falls between 5 and 95%, with the best case being a $p(\chi^2)$ of around 50%. Polynomials are fit to the volume curves for each animal. Specific instantaneous tumor growth rate at any time can

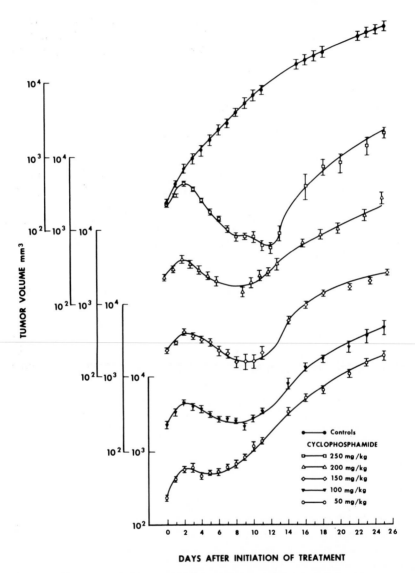

Fig. 12. Mean tumor volume ± SE after treatment of 3924A with 50 to 250 mg/kg cyclophosphamide.

then be determined by taking the first derivative of the polynomial with respect to time. Equation (1) then becomes

$$\frac{d}{dt} \ln \frac{V(t)}{V_0} = a_1 + 2a_2t + 3a_3t^2 + \cdots + Na_Nt^{N-1}$$

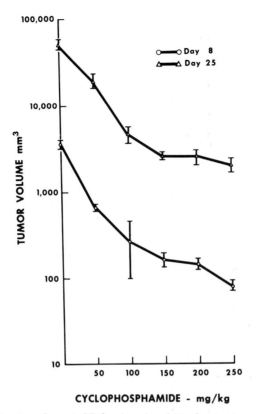

FIG. 13.   Mean tumor volume ± SE for days 8 and 25 after treatment with 50 to 250 mg/kg cyclophosphamide.

The value of the instantaneous growth rate on certain days is then found for each animal. The average value (± SE) of these measurements for the group is reported graphically. Alternatively, the maximum growth rates after the first regression for all of the individual tumors are averaged and the data reported in tabular form.

   The period during which the growth rates of treated tumors were above control levels was examined in the following manner. First, the average position (T_{max}) and magnitude (tumor growth rate at T_{max}) of the growth rate peak resulting from a particular treatment were obtained. This is possible since each animal in the treated group is fitted with its own individual growth rate curve, which has a particular value for the exact time of post-treatment growth rate maximum. Second, the duration of the period of accelerated growth rate was determined from the width of the growth rate curve obtained by averaging individual tumor growth rates for particular

TABLE II

CHANGES IN TUMOR VOLUME AND TUMOR GROWTH RATES FOLLOWING
INCREASING DOSES OF CYCLOPHOSPHAMIDE[a]

Treatment (mg/kg)	Tumor growth delay (days)	OTE ± SE[b]	T_{min} (days)	T_{max} (days)	Tumor growth rate[c] (day^{-1}) at T_{max}	FWHM (days)
250	17.5 ± 1.39[b]	2.67 ± 0.16	9.86 ± 0.40[b]	15.75 ± 0.16[b]	0.383 ± 0.023	8.8
200	16.3 ± 0.92	2.32 ± 0.20	8.40 ± 0.43	13.40 ± 0.37	0.254 ± 0.021	8.0
150	12.8 ± 0.49	2.37 ± 0.23	8.50 ± 0.22	14.33 ± 0.16	0.349 ± 0.030	7.5
100	10.7 ± 0.41	1.76 ± 0.21	8.10 ± 0.88	14.00 ± 0.49	0.350 ± 0.024	6.6
50	5.8 ± 0.54	1.33 ± 0.08	5.00 ± 0.33	13.10 ± 0.96	0.289 ± 0.019	—

[a] Tumor growth delay, increase in time (days) required for treated tumors to reach a volume of 1000 mm^3. Tumors of control group reached 1000 mm^3 in 4.1 ± 0.69 days. OTE (overall treatment efficiency), a term to quantitatively describe tumor volume changes following various forms of treatment. T_{min}, time of minimum tumor volume. T_{max}, time of maximum tumor growth. FWHM, full width of growth curve at one-half maximum of growth peak height.

[b] Standard error of the mean.

[c] Growth rates for untreated tumors at these times were 0.171 ± 0.012, 0.161 ± 0.011, 0.156 ± 0.011, 0.167 ± 0.011, and 0.128 ± 0.014 at T_{max} for 50, 100, 150, 200, and 250 mg/kg cyclophosphamide, respectively.

days. In order to characterize the width of the peak without ambiguity, we used the full width at half maximum peak height.

For the five groups of animals used to determine the effects of increasing doses of cyclophosphamide on tumor growth (Fig. 12), the time for maximum tumor growth rate (T_{max}) increased from 13 days following 50 mg/kg to 16 days following 250 mg/kg (Table II). The time of minimum tumor volume (T_{min}) was 8 to 10 days, except for 50 mg/kg which was 5 days. Although the growth rate peak following 50 mg/kg was not well defined and it was not possible to determine the full width at half maximum peak height, the growth rate of this group exceeded control rates. Well-defined growth rate peaks were present following 100, 150, 200, and 250 mg/kg. The full width at half maximum peak height (FWHM), an index for the duration of the accelerated growth, increased from 6.6 days after 100 mg/kg to 8.8 days after 250 mg/kg (Table II).

The magnitude of the tumor growth rate at T_{max} increased with increased doses of cyclophosphamide, from 0.289 ± 0.019 day^{-1} after 50 mg/kg to 0.383 ± 0.023 day^{-1} after 250 mg/kg. At the time of T_{max} for the 250 mg/kg group, the growth rate was over three times control growth rate of 0.128 ± 0.014 day^{-1}. During the period of growth rate maximum, the growth rate of treated tumors was significantly greater than that of time matched controls, and was similar to that of 0.298 day^{-1} for controls at the beginning of the experiment.

Changes in tumor growth rate following a single 150 mg/kg dose of cyclophosphamide are shown in Fig. 14. There was a marked depression in growth of the treated group, which reached a nadir 5 days after treatment, then a marked increase in growth rate, which reached a maximum on day 14. The growth rate at T_{max} on day 14.33 ± 0.16 was 0.349 ± 0.030 day^{-1}, over twice that for controls of 0.156 ± 0.011 day^{-1}. A second reduction in growth rate occurred following T_{max}. The gradual reduction in growth rate of control tumors is a reflection of the slowing of tumor growth with increasing tumor size. Tumor volume data on other experiments conducted for longer periods of time indicate that volume changes and, thus, growth rates for treated tumors eventually parallel those of control tumors.

At the time of maximum growth rate of treated tumors, we are comparing growth rates of control and treated tumors of markedly different size. The fact remains, however, that there is a significant increase in the growth rate of tumors following treatment with cyclophosphamide. Furthermore, growth rates of some of the treated tumors on day 14 are greater than those of control tumors at the beginning of treatment, 0.298 ± 0.026 day^{-1} on day 2. Our finding of accelerated tumor growth differs from Steel's (1977, p. 287) general conclusion that experimental tumors mostly have shown a smooth transition from regression to re-

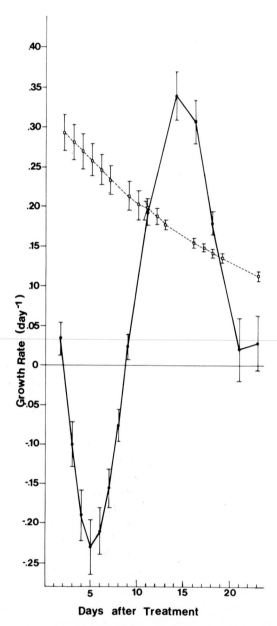

FIG. 14. Changes in tumor growth rate after a single, 150 mg/kg, dose of cyclophosphamide. Points are means of the instantaneous growth rates for 10 3924A tumors on the indicated day posttreatment. ●, Cyclophosphamide; □, controls.

growth, without a steep rise in tumor volume after treatment. Possibly, the frequent volume measurements and criteria for fit in our experiments now allow the accelerated growth after treatment to be recognized.

Tumor DNA content has been used as an index for tumor cell loss. The concentration of tumor DNA (milligram of DNA per gram of tumor) was reduced to approximately two-thirds of control values over the first 5 days after therapy (Fig. 15). DNA concentration remained depressed until day 9 and then rapidly returned to control values by day 11. Thus, the rapid increase in tumor DNA concentration after day 9 paralleled the rapid increase in tumor volume between days 9 and 12.

Tumor DNA specific activity has been utilized in previous studies as an index of tumor cell proliferation following treatment. Tumor DNA specific activity was depressed 12 hours after 150 mg/kg cyclophosphamide (Fig. 16) and reached a nadir 3 to 4 days after treatment. Recovery began on day 5. DNA specific activity reached a maximum on day 11, at which time it exceeded initial control values. The change in tumor DNA specific activity preceded the change in tumor growth rate. The nadir for negative tumor growth rate occurred on day 5, 1 to 2 days after the nadir for tumor DNA specific activity. Maximum tumor DNA specific activity on day 11 preceded the maximum in tumor growth rate on day 14.

Parallel studies on cellular changes in 3924A following cyclophosphamide and 5-FU have been carried out by Moore *et al.* (1980). The cellular response of rat hepatoma 3924A to a single ip injection of 150 mg/kg 5-FU has been measured in respect to the spatial relationship of the cells to tumor microvasculature. In this tumor the parenchyma is arranged in

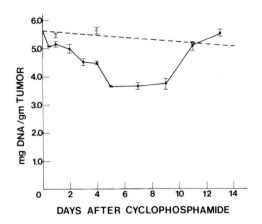

FIG. 15.   Effect of 150 mg/kg cyclophosphamide on DNA concentration of 3924A. ●, Cyclophosphamide; ○, controls.

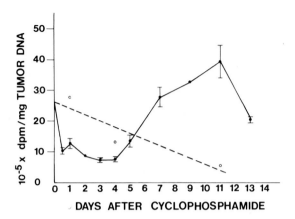

FIG. 16. Effect of 150 mg/kg cyclophosphamide on [³H]thymidine incorporation into DNA of 3924A. ●, Cyclophosphamide; ○, controls.

cords approximately 150 μm thick around central capillaries. For untreated tumors, those cells at distances less than 80 μm from the capillary had a mean, [³H]thymidine labeling index of 39% and a mitotic index of 2.1%, while for those cells more than 80 μm away the values were 14 and 0.8%, respectively. Two days after 150 mg/kg 5-FU, mean cord thickness was reduced by 25% and did not recover to control level until 11 days after treatment. This was also true for the mitotic index. Recovery of the labeling index was complete 2 days earlier. Although absolute values of parameters were different in the populations adjacent to and remote from the capillary, the time course of recovery was similar, with a "growth spurt" 7 to 9 days after treatment. The patterns of response to 5-FU and cyclophosphamide were different when measured in terms of cell density and cord radius. With 5-FU the cords shrank promptly but cell density was little altered, whereas with cyclophosphamide the cords remained at control size for at least 9 days but cell density declined sharply by 3 days. Recovery curves for labeling index and tumor DNA specific activity during recovery varied in a qualitatively similar manner.

If it is assumed that the magnitude of tumor growth rate can be related to the effectiveness of chemotherapy, it would be expected that proliferation-dependent agents such as 5-FU and cyclophosphamide would have their maximum effectiveness at the time of maximum tumor growth rate. Cyclophosphamide and 5-FU are Class III agents, defined by Bruce *et al.* (1966) as agents which kill cells in all or most portions of the generation cycle and for which sensitivity of the cell population depends strongly on the fraction in the proliferative state. It remains to be determined if sequential administration of chemotherapeutic agents at T_{max} would be more effective than if given at other times (such as T_{min}). It should be

noted that increased DNA synthesis in the tumor after cyclophosphamide, as measured by [³H]thymidine incorporation, substantiates changes
in growth rate taken from tumor volume measurements. Increased DNA
synthetic rate precedes increased tumor cell proliferation which, in turn,
increases tumor volume. Thus, biochemical studies demonstrating increased cellular proliferation confirm the accelerated tumor growth following treatment.

The full width at half maximum growth peak height of 7 to 9 days over
the 100 to 250 mg/kg cyclophosphamide dose range would provide flexibility for the sequential administration of chemotherapeutic agents once
T_{max} is established. Studies are in progress to determine the actual magnitude of therapeutic gain which could be realized by sequential administration of cyclophosphamide based on the magnitude and duration of T_{max}
induced by previous treatment.

2. Hematological Findings following Cyclophosphamide

Specific activity of the bone marrow DNA reached a nadir 2 days after
administration of 150 mg/kg cyclophosphamide (Fig. 17). This was followed by a rapid and pronounced increase which reached a maximum on
day 6. The DNA specific activity rapidly decreased by day 8 to 10, but
remained slightly above control values throughout the remaining 21 days
of the experiment.

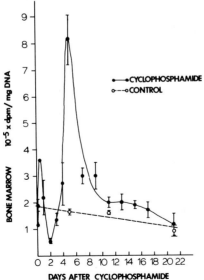

Fig. 17.   [³H]Thymidine incorporation into tibial bone marrow DNA after 150 mg/kg cyclophosphamide. ●, Cyclophosphamide; ○, controls.

Total DNA of the tibial marrow has been used in these and previous experiments as an index of bone marrow reserve. It provides a quantitative measure of cell loss from bone marrow following radiotherapy and chemotherapy since total DNA of the tibial bone marrow can be correlated with the total number of nucleated cells in the tibia. There was an immediate and rapid decline of total tibial bone marrow DNA following cyclophosphamide, which reached a nadir 4 days after initiation of treatment (Fig. 18). This was followed by a rapid recovery to 80% of control values by day 9, and a further gradual increase in total tibial bone marrow DNA to day 21, at which time values in treated animals were comparable to controls. The marked loss of total tibial bone marrow DNA was accompanied by a marked depletion of peripheral white blood cell counts (Table III). The WBC on day 5 was 127 ± 57 (mm^3). Recovery of the WBC lagged behind that of the bone marrow as measured by total tibial marrow DNA. Circulating lymphocytes declined rapidly and reached a nadir of 110 ± 51 on day 5. There was a similar decline of polymorphonuclear leukocytes. A nadir of 11 ± 5 was reached on day 4. Recovery of both lymphocytes and leukocytes was similar to recovery of the WBC; however, fluctuations were present in all three determinations during the recovery period.

Hemoglobin and hematocrit values were depressed by treatment with 150 mg/kg cyclophosphamide, however, this depression generally did not exceed 15%. Thus, the marked changes found in bone marrow and peripheral white counts were not accompanied by changes in either hemoglobin or hematocrit. Qualitative evaluation of platelet number showed no variation from control rats, with both showing approximately 100 to 140 platelets per high power field on the stained peripheral smears.

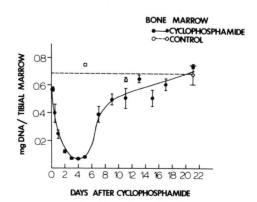

Fig. 18. Total tibial bone marrow DNA after 150 mg/kg cyclophosphamide. ●, Cyclophosphamide; ○, controls.

TABLE III

HEMATOLOGICAL CHANGES IN PERIPHERAL BLOOD AFTER CYCLOPHOSPHAMIDE
(150 mg/kg) ADMINISTRATION

Time after cyclophosphamide	White blood counts (mm³)	Absolute lymphocyte number	Absolute polymorphonuclear leukocyte number	Hemoglobin	Hematocrit
1 hour	3841 ± 364[a]	2719 ± 363	828 ± 22	14.2 ± 0.2	42.0 ± 0.5
1 day	1806 ± 185	507 ± 37	1247 ± 166	12.9 ± 0.3	37.4 ± 0.5
2 days	1154 ± 351	357 ± 206	756 ± 227	13.0 ± 0.4	38.0 ± 0.9
3 days	588 ± 81	136 ± 22	451 ± 61	12.6 ± 0.3	36.5 ± 0.9
4 days	128 ± 34	113 ± 31	11 ± 5	12.6 ± 0.3	37.0 ± 0.9
5 days	127 ± 57	110 ± 51	16 ± 6	12.2 ± 0.2	36.0 ± 0.3
7 days	477 ± 134	303 ± 84	170 ± 58	11.5 ± 0.4	34.0 ± 1.3
9 days	1939 ± 483	510 ± 64	1405 ± 482	12.6 ± 0.1	38.0 ± 0.3
11 days	1247 ± 343	302 ± 65	927 ± 281	12.4 ± 0.3	37.0 ± 0.8
13 days	5054 ± 1920	1471 ± 476	3570 ± 1596	12.8 ± 0.4	38.0 ± 1.7
15 days	1972 ± 972	1010 ± 120	1430 ± 953	12.4 ± 0.2	37.0 ± 0.8
17 days	3030 ± 601	585 ± 143	2353 ± 574	13.3 ± 0.4	40.0 ± 1.5
Controls					
1 hour	5553 ± 891[a]	4299 ± 556	995 ± 170	14.4 ± 0.1	43.0 ± 0.8
5 days	5392 ± 395	3378 ± 319	1942 ± 183	14.4 ± 0.1	42.0 ± 0.6
11 days	5482 ± 739	3324 ± 588	2080 ± 420	15.0 ± 0.2	45.0 ± 0.6
21 days	12000 ± 1058	4898 ± 399	6683 ± 890	14.1 ± 1.0	43.0 ± 2.9

[a] Mean ± SE: four animals were used in each control group and three animals were used in each treated group.

3. "Split Dose" Cyclophosphamide Survival Studies

One dose of cyclophosphamide (150 mg/kg) was given on day 0 and a second dose of 150 mg/kg was given at successively longer time intervals to groups of 10 rats (Fig. 19). A single dose of 300 mg/kg given on day 0 resulted in a 22% survival rate. However, when 150 mg/kg was given on day 0 and another 150 mg/kg on days 3 or 5, all animals died. There was marked recovery from the first dose after this time. Fifty-five percent of the animals survived when the second dose of 150 mg/kg was given 7 days after the first, and survival was equal to or greater than the single 150 mg/kg dose of cyclophosphamide when the second dose was given 9, 11, and 13 days after the first. The rapid increase in survival between days 5 and 9 parallels recovery in the bone marrow.

4. Animal Lethality with Increasing Doses of Cyclophosphamide

Ten animals were used in the control and treated groups. No animals were lost in the control and 50 mg/kg groups. There were 1, 2, 2, 4, and 6 animals lost in the 100, 150, 200, 250, and 300 mg/kg groups, respectively.

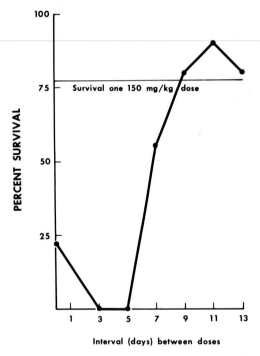

FIG. 19. Survival of rats as a function of the interval between two, 150 mg/kg doses of cyclophosphamide, the first being given on day 0.

IV. Interaction of Chemotherapy and Radiotherapy

A. Comparison of the Effects of Radiation Alone with Cyclophosphamide Alone

Comparison of the effects of 1500 rads radiation and 150 mg/kg cyclophosphamide on tumor growth was made in a second series of experiments. A plateau of the growth curve resulted during the first week after radiation treatment, whereas regression occurred following cyclophosphamide (Fig. 20). Mean tumor volume was 2 to 3% of control following cyclophosphamide and 14% of control following radiation at both 8 and 25 days after initiation of treatment. Within 1 hour of irradiation with 3750 rads, both the [³H]thymidine labeling index (LI) and the mitotic index (MI) were significantly depressed. Thereafter, the short-lived synchrony induced by irradiation resulted in a marked rise in LI at 12 hours and MI at 24 hours after irradiation (Kovacs *et al.*, 1976). After reaching maximal values, both the LI and MI remained depressed over the remaining 17-day

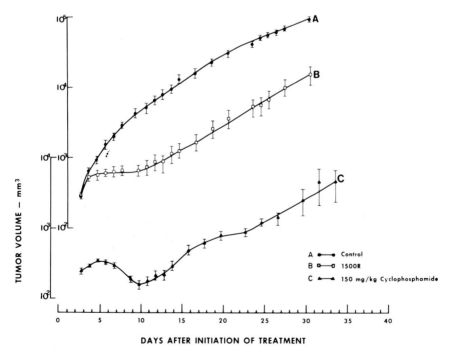

FIG. 20. Effect of 1500 rads radiation and 150 mg/kg cyclophosphamide on tumor growth of 3924A. (A) ●, Controls; (B) □, 1500 rads; (C) ▲, 150 mg/kg cyclophosphamide.

interval, although both showed signs of increasing, probably due to those tumors that were to initiate regrowth. Data for [³H]thymidine incorporation into tumor DNA (dpm per mg DNA) were similar to that for LI.

For the lower dose of irradiation (1500 rads), which we have used in combination with chemotherapy, [³H]thymidine incorporation into tumor DNA was similar to that observed after 3750 rads, except recovery to control or higher levels was observed after day 9 (Fig. 21). At 1 hour after 3750 rads, 80% of the mitotic cells demonstrated severe aberration. The percentage of damaged mitosis dropped sharply between days 4 and 8 and returned to unirradiated levels after day 12. A significant decrease in cell density (cell number per field) occurred within 12 hours after irradiation and approached 50% of control by day 8. Although observed microscopically, this decrease was also demonstrated by DNA analysis. By day 9 (after 3750 rads) the mg DNA/gm tumor was 70% of control, which was maintained as tumor regression proceeded during the next 10 days. At a dose of 1500 rads, DNA concentration in the tumor was similarly depressed but was restored to control levels by day 11 after treatment (Fig. 22). These changes in DNA/gm tumor and in [³H]thymidine incorporation into tumor DNA after radiation are similar to those occurring after cyclophosphamide which are shown in Figs. 15 and 16 in Section III. Recovery of DNA concentration to control levels occurs 11 days after either treatment and recovery at 11 days is accompanied by increased [³H]thymidine incorporation.

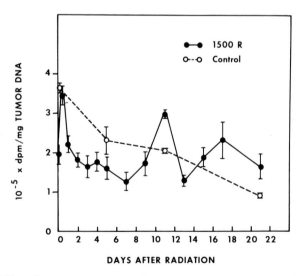

FIG. 21. Effect of 1500 rads radiation on [³H]thymidine incorporation into DNA of hepatoma 3924A.

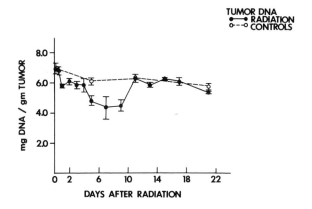

Fig. 22.   DNA concentration of 3924A after 1500 rads radiation.

B. Comparison of the Effects of Giving Radiation before and after Cyclophosphamide

In order to determine the time sequence for effective interaction of cyclophosphamide and radiation, the same radiation dose (1500 rads) was given 15, 11, 7 and 4 days before cyclophosphamide (150 mg/kg) and 4, 7, 11, and 15 days after cyclophosphamide. The relative effectiveness of giving radiation before or after cyclophosphamide has been evaluated by tumor growth delay. This is the additional time necessary for the treated tumor to reach a specific volume (1000 mm³ in these studies) in excess of the time needed for controls to reach this volume (Thomlinson and Craddock, 1967). The time for control tumor volumes to reach 1000 mm³ in this experiment was 5.72 ± 0.58 days. Radiation given within 7 days of the cyclophosphamide (either before or after) produced the largest growth delays (Fig. 23). Effectiveness was reduced when the interval between cyclophosphamide and radiation was increased to 11 or 15 days. Growth delays of 7.8 ± 1.87 days for radiation alone and 12.8 ± 0.49 days for cyclophosphamide alone have been obtained in previous studies. These results therefore demonstrate that more than additive effects of the two modalities can be obtained by giving radiation and cyclophosphamide within 7 days of each other. The ability to effectively interact the two modalities over a 7-day period has two therapeutic implications: it provides a 7-day interval for host recovery prior to giving the second modality, and it indicates that effective interaction of the two modalities does not depend upon which agent is given first.

Changes in tumor growth rates for these treatment groups have been

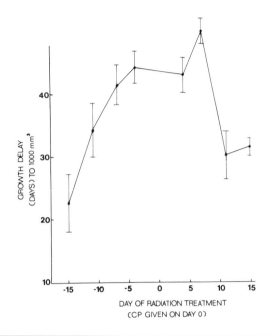

FIG. 23. Tumor growth delay of 3924A following combined treatment with 1500 rads radiation and 150 mg/kg cyclophosphamide. Treatments were separated by varying intervals of time as indicated.

obtained in the following manner. Initially, the tumor volumes for each animal were normalized and log-scaled to produce a series of curves with

$$\ln \frac{V(t)}{V_0}$$

versus time where $V(t)$ is the tumor volume at time t and V_0 is the volume at the beginning of treatment. Local error was then reduced by smoothing each of the curves with a variable point averaging filter in which a moving average of each point and a number of its neighbors (usually one on each side) is taken in both fractional volume and time. The derivatives of these smoothed curves were obtained via a standard, discrete, central-difference method of the form:

$$GR(T) = \frac{V_{j+1} - V_{j-1}}{\tau_{j+1} - \tau_{j-1}}$$

where j is a measurement point within the experimental period corresponding to a smoothed, log-scaled, fractional volume, V, τ is the adjusted time, and GR is the growth rate associated with time T, taken midway between τ_{j+1} and τ_{j-1}. The individual central difference curves, i.e., growth rates for each of the animals, were ensemble averaged to provide a mean growth curve unique for the treatment protocol used within the group.

This procedure presents several advantages over tumor volume averaging techniques since the resulting growth rates are relatively insensitive to changes in the number of animals used in the mean at different points along the final curve. These differences can occur when tumor volumes regress beyond the point at which they are palpable. Excluding these cures from the volume average or averaging in very small dummy volumes results in gross discontinuities in the resulting growth rate curve. Similar effects may be seen if complete responders regrow or where group size is reduced due to animal death at the end of an experiment. Since, at a given point during treatment, tumors that may not have equal volumes nevertheless usually have similar growth rates, cures may be excluded in a mean growth rate curve (as opposed to the growth rate of a mean volume curve) without fear of the discontinuities mentioned. The current procedure, therefore, allows conservative estimation of growth rate at points where many of the animals in a group are either cured or dead. Because of this unique property of derivative averaging, studies involving the integration of the final growth rate curve to provide a tumor volume curve also insensitive to animal number are being pursued.

The changes in growth rates for both treated and control groups are shown in Fig. 24. Radiation given 15, 11, 7, and 4 days before cyclophosphamide are groups O, N, M, and L, respectively. Radiation given 15, 11, 7, and 4 days after cyclophosphamide are groups H, I, J, and K, respectively. There are two distinct perturbations when the two modalities are given either at $\pm$ 15 days (O and H) or $\pm$ 11 days (N and I). When cyclophosphamide is given 15 or 11 days before radiation (H and I) the period and magnitude of negative growth is greater than if radiation is given first. When radiation and cyclophosphamide are given within 7 days of each other (groups M and J), negative growth continues for 20 days. The magnitude and duration of negative growth are greatest when each modality is given within 4 days of each other (groups L and K). There is some indication that accelerated growth occurs prior to growth stabilization, however, this is minor compared to the accelerated growth rate at day 14 after a single dose of cyclophosphamide alone (Fig. 14) or radiation alone.

One of the most significant differences in the growth rates after single and combined modality therapy is the stabilization of tumor growth rates for periods in excess of 1 month after termination of treatment. These findings indicate that greater flexibility in giving sequential therapy is possible because of this long period of diminished growth following combined modality therapy.

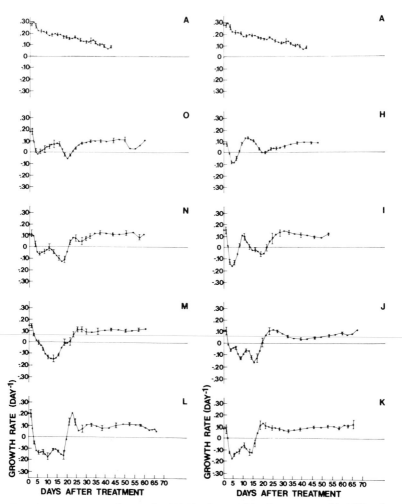

FIG. 24.   Tumor growth rates for 3924A after combined treatment with 1500 rads radiation and 150 mg/kg cyclophosphamide. With radiation given first, the intervals between radiation and cyclophosphamide were group O, 15 days; group N, 11 days; group M, 7 days; and group L, 4 days. With cyclophosphamide given first, the intervals were group H, 15 days; group I, 11 days; group J, 7 days; and group K, 4 days. Group A was untreated.

C. Changes in Tumor Growth Rates after Radiotherapy and Chemotherapy in Different Species

Numerous clinical studies have been carried out on primary and metastatic tumor volume changes in the lung because of the ability to measure changes in tumor volume from serial chest radiographs (Breur, 1966;

Courdi *et al.*, 1980; Dutreix *et al.*, 1971; Israel and Chahinian, 1976; Malaise *et al.*, 1972; Muggia and Rozencweig, 1979; Tubiana, 1971, 1977; Tubiana *et al.*, 1975; Tubiana and Malaise, 1979; Van Peperzeel, 1972). Other studies have evaluated changes in tumor size at different organ sites. Welin (1963) evaluated the rates and patterns of growth of 375 tumors of the large intestine and rectum by using serial double contrast media. More recently Order and his associates (1980) have employed CAT scanning techniques to evaluate tumor volume changes in the liver. Newer methods of quantitatively determining tumor volume changes following cancer treatment should provide the means for more accurate assessment of tumor response to therapy.

Van Peperzeel (1972) made a detailed evaluation of changes in lung tumor volumes before, during, and after radiotherapy. She found that the nadir for tumor volume reduction (T_{min}) for 11 patients with primary and metastatic lung tumors following radiation was 5.7 ± 0.45 days (range 3 to 7 days). This close range for T_{min} occurred in a variety of tumors with volume doubling times which varied by a factor of 13 (17 to 228 days). In addition to primary squamous cell and anaplastic carcinoma of the bronchus, metastatic tumors of the testicles, as well as liposarcomas and fibrosarcomas were included in the study. The T_{min} in dogs with pulmonary metastases was 5 days; volume doubling time was 27 days. The volume doubling times in the two experimental solid tumors in the rat used in our studies were 4 and 2 days, respectively, for 3924A and H-4-II-E. Even though the volume doubling time varied by a factor of 2, T_{min} was similar in both tumors following chemotherapy and radiotherapy (Table IV). Over a wide dose range for both radiation and chemotherapy (5-FU, adriamycin, and cyclophosphamide), T_{min} was 5 to 11 days after treatment. Previous biochemical and histological studies in both 3924A and H-4-II-E have shown that this time course for tumor volume reduction is related to tumor cell destruction and removal following chemotherapy and radiotherapy. Therefore, the temporal events leading to T_{min} in man, dogs, and rats are similar for a wide variation of tumors with markedly different growth rates. One possible explanation is that the time for clearance of the dead tumor cells by the hosts is similar for the three species. The similarity of occurrence of these events in man, dogs, and rats does not apply in all species, T_{min} for mice being much less at approximately ≈ 2 days.

Accelerated tumor growth following radiotherapy and chemotherapy is a phenomenon which has been found in our studies on two experimental solid tumors in rats. This phenomenon is not unique to this species since comparable accelerated tumor growth rates following radiotherapy have been observed in dogs and man by Van Peperzeel (1972) and Malaise *et*

TABLE IV

The Time for Minimum Tumor Volume (T_{min}) and Maximum
Tumor Growth Rates (T_{max}) in Man and Experimental Animals
after Radiotherapy and Chemotherapy

	3924A		H-4-II-E	
Treatment	T_{min} (days)[a]	T_{max} (days)[b]	T_{min} (days)	T_{max} (days)
I. Primary Solid tumors				
A. Rats				
5-FU				
(50–200) mg/kg	6–9	9–14	≈8	≈15
Adriamycin				
(5, 7.5, 10) mg/kg	6–11	14–16	5–9	12–17
Cyclophosphamide				
(50–250) mg/kg	5–10	14–16	7–8	11–14
Single dose radiation				
(750–4000) rads	7–11	13–23	5–9	9–16

	T_{min} (days)	T_{acc} (days)[c]
II. Primary and metastatic lung tumors[d]		
B. Man		
(300–700) rads		
single dose	5–10	8–40
C. Dogs		
(150–300) rads		
single dose	5–6	5–15
D. Mice		
210 rads single dose	≈2	≈3

[a] T_{min}, time of tumor volume minimum posttreatment (days).
[b] T_{max}, time of tumor growth rate maximum immediately following T_{min} (days) (Part I).
[c] T_{acc}, time interval of accelerated growth following T_{min} (days) (Part II).
[d] H. A. Van Peperzeel (1972).

al. (1972). The time of maximum tumor growth, which occurs approximately 2 weeks after treatment with both modalities in two tumors in rats in our studies, also has a temporal counterpart in dogs and man. Accelerated tumor growth rates were found in 10 of 11 patients treated with radiation by Van Peperzeel (see Table I). Tumor volume changes were determined by Malaise *et al.* (1972) in 27 patients with lung metastases from a variety of primary tumors before and after 1000 rads radiation as a single dose or two doses of 500 rads given 3 hours apart. The growth rate of lung metastases following radiation was 3 to 5 times faster than the rate before radiation. The close temporal relationship of accelerated growth following treatment in the three species suggests that host response may play a more important role on this phenomenon than had previously been realized.

The effects of treatment on the tumor result in cell loss with a reduction in tumor size. Our studies and many others on solid tumors have shown that growth rate decreases with increasing tumor size. Our results have shown that the growth rate at T_{max}, 14 days after 150 mg/kg cyclophosphamide, was greater (0.35 day^{-1}) than control tumor growth rate at initiation of the experiment (0.30 day^{-1}) and over twice that of the control tumor (0.15 day^{-1}) at the time of T_{max} on day 14.

One of the most logical explanations for the increased growth rate of treated tumors is that smaller tumors grow faster. In this case they are growing at rates comparable to tumors 14 days younger. The fact that the growth rate of treated tumors at T_{max} is greater than the growth rate of control tumors at V_0 raises a much less likely but intriguing question: are the growth rates of the tumors accelerated following therapeutic insult in a manner similar to the accelerated proliferation of host organs such as bone marrow and gut to therapeutic insult? If this is the case then it would suggest that the tumors are reacting similarly as normal tissue does to therapeutic insults. It would also suggest that the tumor is more responsive to host control mechanisms than previously realized. It is evident that additional information is needed on the interrelation between host and tumor and the changes in growth rates that occur following treatment to determine if these changes can be more effectively exploited therapeutically.

V. Sequential (Radiotherapy–Chemotherapy) Treatment

A. Introduction

Clinical experience has shown that sequential therapy is the most effective approach in treating patients with solid tumors, and the proper sequencing of one or more treatment modalities is a promising area for improving patient management. Many protocols in clinical use have been empirically designed. There is increasing evidence that human neoplasms are responsive to combined modality therapy, however, delineation of some of the parameters relevant to such therapy can be accomplished only in animal models. Much of the experimental information available pertains to the effects of either chemotherapy alone or radiotherapy alone; therefore, we have given priority to developing experimental protocols for sequential combined chemotherapy–radiotherapy. Proper scheduling of cancer chemotherapeutic agents is dependent upon an understanding for the dose–time relationships of the deleterious effects of these agents on critical host organs. The time of administration of a second series of chemotherapeutic agents is governed by recovery kinetics: scheduling for optimal destruction of tumor cells must be within constraints imposed by vulnerable host organs.

Studies on the effects of sequential administration of 5-FU and radiation have been shown to be successful if the 5-FU (150 mg/kg) and radiation (1500 rads) were given (1) after recovery of host and critical host organs from the previous treatment series, and (2) when tumor growth was accelerated after the previous series: (1) and (2) were satisfied with radiation and 5-FU given every 11 days. The salient features of our initial therapeutic strategy for the utilization of sequential chemotherapy with radiotherapy include the following.

1. The First Treatment Series

The administration of chemotherapy at the time of maximum tumor cell synchronization from radiotherapy, or radiotherapy at a time of maximum synchronization from chemotherapy.

2. The Second and Subsequent Treatment Series

1. Recovery of host and critical host organs from the previous treatment series.

2. The administration of the second and subsequent treatment series at times of maximum tumor proliferation after the previous series.

3. The sequential utilization of radiotherapy–chemotherapy for control of the primary tumor, and chemotherapy to control metastatic spread of the primary tumor.

One of the greatest difficulties to overcome in the more effective clinical utilization of combined modality therapy is increased toxicity. Parallel recovery of bone marrow with increasing animal survival in "split dose" cyclophosphamide toxicity studies (as with 5-FU) indicates that bone marrow is the critical organ with regard to sequential chemotherapy. Recovery of intestinal mucosa following cyclophosphamide (and 5-FU) occurs earlier than recovery of bone marrow. Results of experimental studies to date suggest that sequential combined modality therapy may be given at a time of maximum tumor growth rate that occurs following the previous treatment series. Since the time of maximum tumor growth rate occurs after recovery of the bone marrow from the previous treatment series, combined chemotherapy–radiotherapy schedules of this type should permit sequential administration of chemotherapeutic agents, such as 5-FU and cyclophosphamide, at a time of enhanced tumor sensitivity and

diminished host toxicity. Recovery of bone marrow and peripheral leukocytes from a 150 mg/kg (0.9 gm/m²) dose of cyclophosphamide after 9 to
12 days in the rat is comparable to the hematological recovery from either
a 1.0 or 1.5 mg/m² single dose after 17 to 21 days in humans (Bergsagel *et
al.*, 1968). Thus, frequency and dosage of cyclophosphamide or 5-FU
used with radiation in our experimental studies are within clinically feasible doses, and proper scheduling can produce cure rates ≧ 50%.

We have used our experimental systems to address three major clinical
problems in the utilization of sequential chemotherapy–radiotherapy: (1)
to effect tumor cures, (2) to control tumor growth, and (3) to increase life
expectancy.

B. Effects of 150 mg/kg Cyclophosphamide Every 11 Days on Tumor Growth Rates and Tumor Control

The sequential administration of 150 mg/kg cyclophosphamide every 11
days for 4 doses controlled tumor growth over the first 33 days of the
study (Fig. 25). There was a slight upward trend in treated tumor volumes
which accelerated after termination of treatment on day 33. Mean day of
death for controls was 30 ± 1.4 days, and for treated animals was 44 ± 7
days. Thus, treatment resulted in a 46% increased life span. One rat died
after each of the first two cyclophosphamide treatments and two after

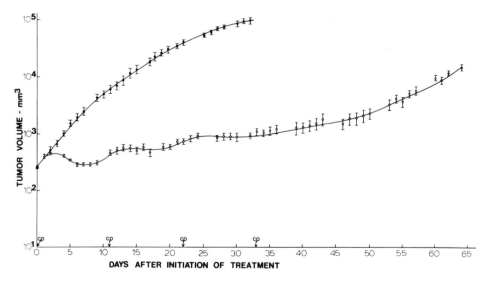

Fig. 25.   Mean tumor volume ± SE of 3924A after sequential administration of 150
mg/kg cyclophosphamide every 11 days, ○, Treated; ●, controls.

each of the next two treatments. The remaining four rats died with large tumors near termination of the experiment.

The time at which minimum tumor volume occurred (T_{min}) was 7 days after administration of each of the first three doses of cyclophosphamide and 5 days after the last dose of cyclophosphamide was given on day 33. T_{max} occurred 10, 11, and 15 days after administration of cyclophosphamide on days 0, 11, and 22, respectively, and 26 days after administration of the fourth and final dose on day 33. Tumor growth rate was 0.197 ± 0.003 day^{-1} at the time of T_{max} (9.75 ± 0.17 days) following the first cyclophosphamide dose. Tumor growth rates at T_{max} were successively smaller following administration of second and third doses of cyclophosphamide on days 11 and 22, being 0.116 ± 0.002 and 0.087 ± 0.002 day^{-1}, respectively. Growth rate at T_{max} (26 days after the fourth dose and 59 days after the first) was 0.195 ± 0.003. The cyclic nature of these growth rate changes is shown in Fig. 26, where individual growth rates have been averaged for particular days after treatment.

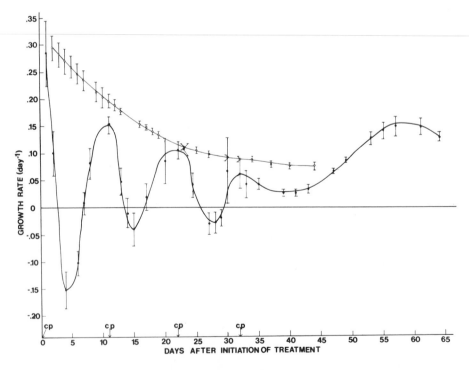

FIG. 26. Tumor growth rate changes $\pm$ SE for tumors in Fig. 25. ●, Treated; □, controls.

C. EFFECTS OF 1500 RADS RADIATION EVERY 11 DAYS ON TUMOR GROWTH RATES AND TUMOR CONTROL

The sequential administration of 1500 rads of local tumor radiation every 11 days is shown in Fig. 27. As with cyclophosphamide, there is also an upward trend of mean tumor volumes during the first 3 weeks. Reduction in mean tumor volume on day 26 and the increasing value of the standard errors are the result of an increasing heterogeneity of response of the tumors to radiation treatment. Two of the 10 tumors became nonpalpable 34 days after initiation of treatment for a cure rate of 20%. In a repeat of this experiment, a cure rate of 40% was realized.

D. EFFECTS OF 1500 RADS RADIATION AND 150 mg/kg CYCLOPHOSPHAMIDE 11 DAYS LATER

Changes in mean tumor volume following administration of four series of sequential combined modality therapy (1500 rads radiation and 150 mg/kg cyclophosphamide) at 11-day intervals are shown in Fig. 28. There was a reduction in tumor volume from 248 ± 14 mm^3 on day 0 to 97 ± 42 mm^3 on day 20, and a further 1 log reduction in tumor volume between days 20 and 60. Mean tumor volume on day 60 was 11 ± 10 mm^3. Tumor volumes changed little from day 60 until termination of the experiment on day 88.

Changes in tumor growth rates are shown in Fig. 29. The nadir for negative growth rate following radiation on day 0 and cyclophosphamide on day 11 occurred at day 14. Growth rate became positive only once, between days 22 and 24. Further fluctuations occurred between a second radiation dose on day 22 and a cyclophosphamide dose on day 33; however, growth rates continued to be negative during that time.

There was complete response in six of the nine animals given radiotherapy and chemotherapy alternately since they regressed to a point where no tumor mass could be detected at some point during the course of the experiment. There was a cure rate of 56% since one of the six tumors regrew. Mean time from initiation of treatment until the tumors became nonpalpable was 38 ± 4.8 days. Partial response occurred in two of the eight tumors (Table V).

Another experiment is shown in Fig. 30, where the initial radiation–cyclophosphamide series (radiation given on day 0 and cyclophosphamide on day 11) was the same as in the preceding experiment, but the interval between the first and second combined radiation–cyclophosphamide series was increased by a factor of approximately 4 (42 days versus 11 days). Average tumor volume was 1522 ± 196 mm^3 60 days after initiation

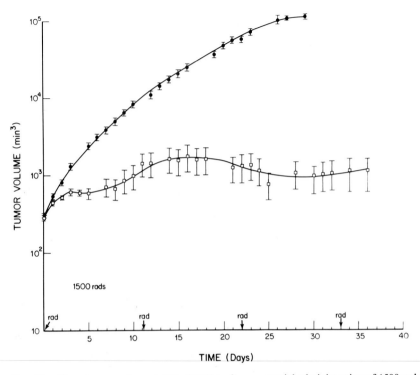

Fig. 27. Mean tumor volume ± SE of 3924A after sequential administration of 1500 rads radiation every 11 days. ○, Treated; ●, controls.

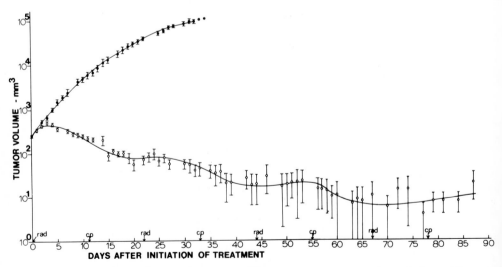

Fig. 28. Mean tumor volume ± SE of 3924A treated alternately with radiation (1500 rads) and cyclophosphamide (150 mg/kg) every 11 days. ○, Treated; ●, controls.

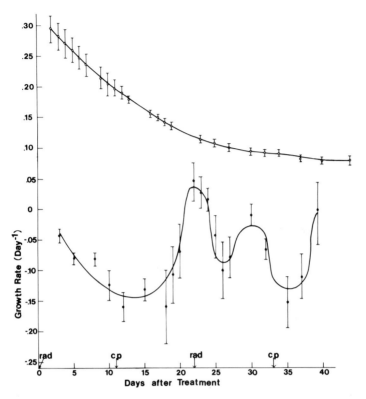

FIG. 29.   Mean tumor growth rate changes ± SE for tumors in Fig. 28. ●, Treated; ○, controls.

of the experiment. There were no complete or partial responses in this experiment.

Changes in mean growth rates of both treated and control tumors are shown in Fig. 31. These decreased in treated animals, reaching a nadir on day 11, then increased until they were comparable to growth rates of controls on day 25, and subsequently fell slightly below 0 by day 55. There was a positive growth rate in treated animals throughout the remainder of the experiment which was reflected in a gradual increase in mean tumor volumes (Fig. 30). All animals were living at termination of the experiment on day 88, representing at least a 3-fold increase in life span compared with the mean life span of controls of 30 ± 1 days.

Comparison was then made between this sequentially administered cyclophosphamide treatment, treatment at 11-day intervals with 1500 rads radiation, and treatment with both radiation and cyclophosphamide alternated at 11-day intervals. Neither cyclophosphamide nor radiation given

TABLE V

EFFECTIVENESS OF SEQUENTIAL COMBINED (RADIATION–CYCLOPHOSPHAMIDE) THERAPY IN PROVIDING COMPLETE RESPONSE, PARTIAL RESPONSE, AND TUMOR CURES (3924A)

Series	Treatment day RAD (1500 rads)	Treatment day CP (150 mg/kg)	Days between RAD and CP	Days between treatment series	Days between last CP and next RAD	Mean time to complete response	Complete response[a]	Partial response[b]	Regrew	Total tumors cured
1	0	7	7	—	—	30.7 ± 3.0	9	1	3	6
2	14	21	7	14	7					
3	28	35	7	14	7					
1	0	7	7	—	—		1	3	0	1
2	32	39	7	32	25					
3	63	70	7	31	24					
1	0	7	7	—	—		0	3	0	0
2	40	47	7	40	33					
1	0	11	11	—	—	38.3 ± 4.8	6	2	1	5
2	22	33	11	22	11					
3	44	55	11	22	11					
4	67	78	11	23	11					
1	0	11	11	—	—		0	0	0	0
2	42	53	11	42	31					
1	0	1	1	—	—	24.8 ± 1.7	9	0	0	5
2	16	17	1	15	15					
3	32	33	1	17	15					
4	48	49	1	18	15					
1	0	1	1	—	—		1	7	1	0
2	21	22	1	21	20					
3	42	43	1	21	20					
1	0	1	1	—	—		0	3	0	0
2	37	38	1	37	30					

[a] The term "complete response" has been used in its clinical context to denote no detectable evidence of remaining tumor (i.e., tumor non-palpable).

[b] Partial response has also been used in its clinical context to denote a greater than 50% reduction in tumor volume as compared with the initial volume.

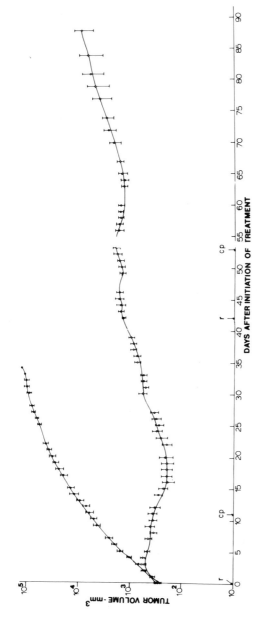

FIG. 30. Mean tumor volume ± SE of 3924A after two series of combined modality (1500 rads radiation and 150 mg/kg cyclophosphamide) therapy. First series, radiation day 0 and cyclophosphamide day 11; second series, radiation day 42 and cyclophosphamide day 53. ○, Treated; ●, controls.

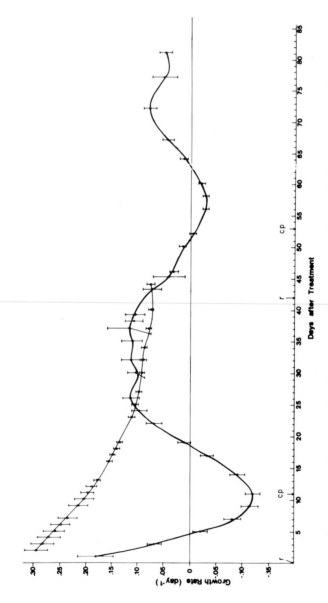

Fig. 31. Mean tumor growth rate changes ± SE for tumors in Fig. 30. ●, Treated; □, controls.

at 11-day intervals was as effective as alternating the two treatments in controlling growth of all the primary tumors. Comparing the three regimens where a treatment was given every 11 days, the number of animals with nonpalpable primary tumors was 0 of 10 for cyclophosphamide, 2 of 10 for radiation, and 5 of 9 for the alternating regimen.

Further studies are needed to elucidate the mechanism by which increased effectiveness occurs when radiation and cyclophosphamide are alternated at 11-day intervals. It would seem that the alternated treatment is no more intensive than the individual modalities alone since frequency of treatment is the same. The fact that this schedule is uniformly more effective in controlling tumor growth indicates that the two treatments do not act on exactly the same population of cells or that the kinetic and metabolic consequences of one treatment increase the effectiveness of the subsequent treatment. Since these observations have implications with regard to clinical cancer treatment, they should be verified in other experimental tumor systems.

E. Sequential Radiation and Cyclophosphamide Given on Days 0 and 7, Respectively

Tumor growth delay was 1.2 times greater than the additive effects of either agent given alone when radiation was given 7 days before cyclophosphamide. Cyclophosphamide administered at intervals of greater than 11 days permits recovery of both the GI tract and bone marrow. When three series of treatments with 1500 rads radiation and 150 mg/kg cyclophosphamide were given such that the radiation–drug intertreatment time was 7 days and the drug–drug intertreatment time was 14 days, the result was a cure rate of 60%. Changes in mean tumor volume following administration of the three series of sequential combined modality therapy given 7 days apart are shown in Fig. 32.

Mean tumor growth rate is plotted in Fig. 33 for these rats treated at 7-day intervals. Growth rate was negative throughout the experiment, reaching a nadir on day 22 of -0.34 ± 0.09 day^{-1}. By day 36, due to the relatively high number of cures, average growth rate was essentially zero. There was complete response for 9 of the 10 rats treated and partial response for one tumor. This alternate scheduling of radiotherapy with chemotherapy every 7 days resulted in a cure rate of 60% since three of the nine tumors regrew following treatment. Mean time for complete tumor response to occur was 30.7 ± 3.0 days after initiation of treatment. The first two series of combined radiation and cyclophosphamide are of primary importance in producing complete response and tumor cures. Mean day of death for control animals was 30 ± 1 days and for the six

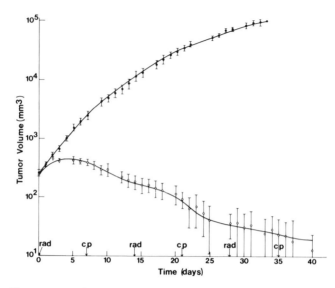

FIG. 32. Mean tumor volume ± SE of 3924A given three series of combined modality radiation (1500 rads) and cyclophosphamide (150 mg/kg) therapy. First series, radiation day 0 and cyclophosphamide day 7; second series, radiation day 14 and cyclophosphamide day 21; third series, radiation day 28 and cyclophosphamide day 35. ○, Treated; ●, controls.

treated animals which died it was 50 ± 3, representing a 66% increase in life span (Looney *et al.*, 1981a).

The cure rate was reduced to 10% when initiation of the second series of combined radiation–cyclophosphamide was increased from 14 to 32 days; however, effective control of tumor growth was realized. There were only three partial responses in this group. Increasing the time for the second treatment series for the second experiment from 14 to 32 days (days 0 and 7, 32 and 39, 63 and 70) omitted the critical treatment interval between 2 and 4 weeks and resulted in reduction in cure rate from 60 to 10%. However, increasing the treatment intervals over a 70-day period resulted in excellent control of tumor growth (Fig. 34).

Growth rate for treated tumors fluctuated over the course of treatment. Negative growth was demonstrated during the intervals of days 4–19, 36–51, and 69–79 (Fig. 35). Each interval of negative growth followed the beginning of a sequential combined modality treatment series by 4 to 6 days. During the periods of positive growth (days 20–35 and 52–68), treated tumors exhibited growth rates comparable to control tumors in the later stages of growth. The greatest negative growth rate of -0.16 ± 0.03 day^{-1} on day 11 occurred following the first treatment series.

An evaluation of the hematological status of the animals was made on days 84 to 86 after cyclophosphamide (150 mg/kg) was given on days 7,

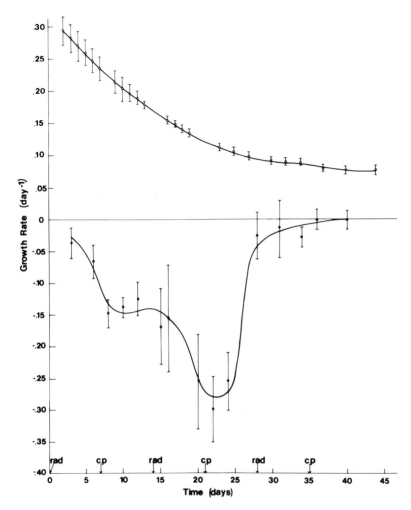

FIG. 33.   Mean tumor growth rate changes ± SE for tumors in Fig. 32. ●, Treated; ○, controls.

21, and 35 in one experiment, on days 7, 39, and 70 in a second, and on days 7 and 47 in a third experiment. Mean peripheral white blood counts were 4175 ± 620, 4100 ± 1071, and 6000 ± 1132 per mm³ for the first, second, and third experiments, respectively. Mean hemoglobins were 14.45 ± 0.35, 13.92 ± 0.39, and 16.40 ± 0.44 gm per 100 ml of blood, and mean hematocrits were 46.00 ± 1.08, 43.50 ± 0.99, and 52.38 ± 1.65, respectively. Thus, recovery from the acute effects of cyclophosphamide treatment continued to occur following each intermittent administration

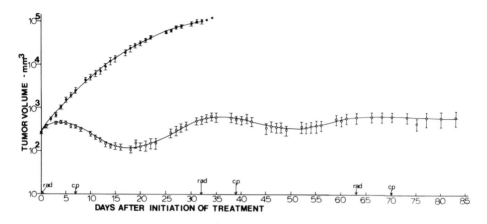

FIG. 34.   Mean tumor volume ± SE of 3924A given three series of combined radiation (1500 rads) and cyclophosphamide (150 mg/kg) therapy. First series, radiation day 0 and cyclophosphamide day 7; second series, radiation day 32 and cyclophosphamide day 39; third series, radiation day 63 and cyclophosphamide day 70. ○, Treated; ●, controls.

of cyclophosphamide (150 mg/kg) separated by sufficiently long time intervals to allow for bone marrow recovery.

F. Sequential Combined Radiation and Cyclophosphamide Given on Days 0 and 1, Respectively

This series of experiments was carried out to determine the effectiveness of giving radiation within 1 day of cyclophosphamide and lengthening the time between successive series of radiation combined with cyclophosphamide. The study was also made to compare the effectiveness of combined radiation and cyclophosphamide with the alternation of radiation and cyclophosphamide on day 7 and 11-day intervals used in the two previous series of experiments.

Radiation was given 1 day before cyclophosphamide for a series of four combined modality treatments every 16 days over a 48-day period. This resulted in a cure rate of 50% (Table V). The first two treatment series of combined radiation–cyclophosphamide given on days 0 and 1 and 16 and 17 were of primary importance in producing complete responses. In a second experiment, tumor growth rates became positive after both the first treatment series on days 0 and 1 as well as the second series on days 21 and 22. Thus, the time between treatments (21 versus 16 days for the previous experiment) was too long to keep the tumors in continuous negative growth. However, giving combined radiation–cyclophosphamide every 21 days for three series over a 42-day period was successful in preventing

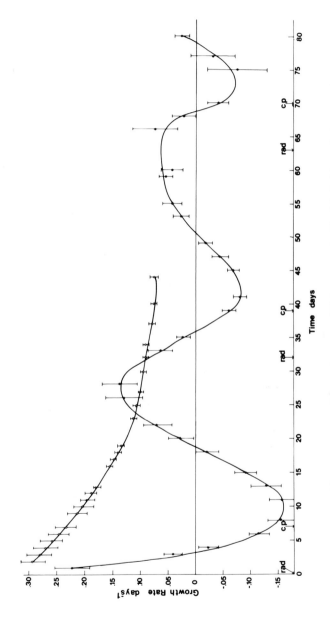

Fig. 35. Mean tumor growth rate changes ± SE for tumors in Fig. 34. ●, Treated; ○, controls.

increases in tumor volume above the original volume throughout the 87 days of the experiment. No tumors were cured in a third experiment when the time between the combined radiation–cyclophosphamide treatment series was further increased to 37 days (Table V). In addition, extending time between treatment series to 37 days was unsuccessful in preventing tumor volumes from increasing above the original volume, but did result in a 3-fold increase in life span over the 30-day life span of controls.

Tumor cure rates $\geq 50\%$ have been realized by the administration of three and four series of combined therapy using 1500 rads radiation and 150 mg/kg cyclophosphamide fractions separated by 1, 7, or 11 days. Increasing the time between treatment modalities from 1 to 7 and 11 days provided a 2- and 3-week recovery period for each treatment modality without causing a reduction in cure rates (Table V). The first and second treatment series given within the first 2 weeks are of primary importance in providing complete tumor responses and cure rates of 50% or greater. For example, giving the second series of radiation and cyclophosphamide on days 16 and 17 resulted in a cure rate of 50%. Increasing this interval to 21 to 22 days for the second series resulted in no cures. The results of giving each modality alone at 11-day intervals have been compared with results of alternating administration of the two modalities at 11-day intervals. Comparing the three regimens where a treatment was given every 11 days, the number of animals with cures was 0 of 10 for cyclophosphamide alone, 2 of 10 for radiation alone, and 5 of 9 for alternation of the two treatments. Well-defined periods of accelerated growth occur between 10 and 20 days after administration of either radiation or cyclophosphamide. The time between the last cyclophosphamide dose and the next radiation dose in the groups with more than 50% cures ranged from 1 to 2 weeks. If this was increased to 3 weeks or longer, essentially no cures occurred. The duration of accelerated tumor growth following the first treatment series is also 1 to 2 weeks. Therefore, sequential treatment, given near the times of maximum tumor specific activities and tumor growth rates induced by the previous treatment, was successful in curing over 50% of the tumors. The results imply that success or failure in tumor cure rates is dependent upon the rather well-defined temporal relationship between the first and second treatment series.

VI. The Evaluation of Dose–Response Surface of Cyclophosphamide and Radiation Given Sequentially

This method has the potential to determine the dose–response surfaces from which optimal treatment schedules for radiotherapy and chemotherapy can be obtained. Four series of combined radiation–cyclophosphamide therapy were given and the doses held constant as in previous experiments utilizing the two modalities in sequential therapy. In this experiment treatment consisted of a fixed dose of radiation (1500 rads) and a fixed dose of cyclophosphamide (150 mg/kg). The variables were T_1, the time between the radiation treatment and the chemotherapy, and T_2, the time between successive radiation treatments. It is of interest to determine the optimal values of these two variables since for small values of T_1 and T_2 severe toxicity is likely and no treatment effect is a possibility if the therapy is given over too wide a time interval. By using statistical modeling techniques developed by Carter *et al.* (1977, 1979) and Wampler *et al.* (1978), it is possible to estimate the treatment response surface as a function of T_1 and T_2 for both the tumor response and toxicity. From these surfaces it will then be possible to determine the most effective treatment for a tumor response and the least toxic treatment. Unfortunately it is not likely that the least toxic treatment will be associated with a desirable tumor response. Thus, as in the clinical situation, a certain amount of toxicity will have to be tolerated in order to achieve a desirable effect on the tumor. Once an acceptable level of toxicity has been specified it is possible to analyze the treatment response surfaces in such a manner as to determine the optimal values of T_1 and T_2 with respect to tumor response while not exceeding the toxicity constraint (Carter *et al.*, 1981).

Consider first the estimation of the relationship between T_1, T_2, and the tumor response. An acceptable tumor response was defined to have occurred if the tumor volume was ever reduced to less than or equal to 10 mm³. For this part of the analysis the logistic regression model was used. This model permits the estimation of the probability of the tumor volume becoming $\leq$ 10 mm³ as a function of T_1 and T_2. Specifically

Prob [Tumor volume $\leq$ 10 mm]
$$= [1 + \exp - (\beta_0 + \beta_1 T_1 + \beta_2 T_2 + \beta_{11} T_1^2 + \beta_{22} T_2^2 + \beta_{12} T_1 T_2)]^{-1}$$

where $\beta_0, \beta_1, \beta_2, \beta_{11}, \beta_{22}$, and β_{12} are unknown constants, which parameterize the model. They must be estimated from experimental data. These parameters are such that β_0 is an intercept term, β_1 is associated with the effect of T_1, β_2 is associated with the effect of T_2, β_{11} and β_{22} are terms which permit the model to account for the fact that as T_1 and T_2 go from small to large values the probability of the tumor volume ever becoming $\leq$ 10 mm³ must increase from a low value (since small T_1 and T_2 are likely associated with death before tumor volume reaches 10 mm³) through a maximum and then decline since large T_1 and T_2 are likely to be associated with ineffective treatment, and β_{12} is associated with the interaction between T_1 and T_2.

The model parameters were estimated from the experimental data contained in the first three columns of Table VI by the method of maximum

TABLE VI

T_1 (days)	T_2 (days)	Observed number of tumors $\leqq 10$ mm³	Predicted number of tumors $\leqq 10$ mm³	Survival times (days)
4	8	1	3.55	10,19,20,24,35,43
6	8	5	1.98	29,30,34,37,40,48
8	8	1	0.75	15,16,16,18,23,38
4	12	4	4.25	15,22,34,41,43,47
6	12	4	3.40	36,39,51,54,71,83
8	12	1	2.25	17,46,47,48,71,124[a]
10	12	1	1.15	17,21,25,29,78,149[a]
12	12	0	0.45	19,44,56,59,66,137
4	16	4	3.66	14,28,31,43,52,92
6	16	6	3.42	39,45,65,65,71,148[a]
8	16	1	2.94	18,26,30,54,59,62
10	16	2	2.25	21,66,71,73,73,73
12	16	1	1.46	20,67,68,69,72,105
14	16	1	0.77	22,40,48,55,70,71
16	16	0	0.33	21,24,32[a],55,66,79
4	20	2	1.66	13,14,14,15,67,147[a]
6	20	2	2.03	54,58,64,73,73,78
8	20	1	2.22	17,24,40[a],68,74,75
10	20	2	2.20	17,17,60,64,78,147[a]
12	20	3	1.97	22,59,60,60,62,99
14	20	3	1.57	46,60,60,66,74,83
16	20	1	1.08	27,45,63,64,68,147[a]
4	24	0	0.21	14,36,83,84,87,132
6	24	0	0.42	14,14,40,40,63,80
8	24	1	0.72	18,18,63,86,96,143
10	24	2	1.06	44,72,76,86,90,146[a]
12	24	1	1.33	50,65,66,93,93,145[a]
14	24	0	1.47	84,94,95,96,102,120[a]
16	24	2	1.45	24,75,102,142,145[a],145

[a] Animal alive at last day of observation.

likelihood. The predictive ability of the estimated model is illustrated in the third and fourth columns of the same table. Column three indicates the actual number of animals in each treatment group of six animals whose tumor was ever $\leqq 10$ mm³ while column 4 gives the predicted number of animals whose tumor was $\leqq 10$ mm³ as a result of the estimated relationship. The agreement between corresponding elements in these two columns appears reasonable. The χ^2 goodness of fit test was used to assess statistically the quality of prediction. It yielded a χ^2 value of 29.08 with 23 degrees of freedom and the p value associated with it is 0.18. Thus there is no evidence of statistically significant model inadequacy.

The estimated values of the model parameters are given in Table VII along with their standard errors and the p value associated with the significance of each considered individually. From this table it can be seen that the intercept, β_1, and β_2, the coefficient of T_2, do not differ significantly from zero. The practical importance of this result is that the effect of the time between successive irradiations is not as important in achieving a tumor volume ≤ 10 mm^3 as the time between irradiation and chemotherapy for the range of values of T_1 and T_2 used in this experiment. Although some of the individual parameters cannot be said to differ from zero, collectively they are important. The value of χ^2 for the model, i.e., for the parameters considered as a group, is 28.05 with 5 degrees of freedom and the associated p value is < 0.0001.

From considering the model equation it can be seen that the values of T_1 and T_2 associated with maximum probability of reducing the tumor volume to ≤ 10 mm^3 are such that $\beta_0 + \beta_1 T_1 + \beta_2 T_2 + \beta_{11} T_1^2 + \beta_{22} T_2^2 + \beta_{12} T_1 T_2$ is maximized. Using the parameter estimates it is possible to estimate the optimal values of T_1 and T_2. These values are

$$T_1 = 4 \text{ days}$$

$$T_2 = 12 \text{ days}$$

From considering Table VI this result appears reasonable.

Perhaps a better indication of the relationship between T_1 and T_2 and the chance of reducing the tumor volume to ≤ 10 mm^3 can be obtained from Fig. 36. This is a density plot of that relationship in which darker shading is associated with values of T_1 and T_2 for which the estimated probability of reducing the tumor volume to ≤ 10 mm^3 is increased. Thus, for example, the treatment for which $T_1 = 6$ days and $T_2 = 15$ days has a greater chance of reducing the tumor volume to ≤ 10 mm^3 than a treatment for which $T_1 = 15$ days and $T_2 = 15$ days. Actually from the figure's legend it can be seen that the estimated probability of such a desirable outcome for the former treatment is between 0.50 and 0.611 while for the latter treatment the probability is estimated to be between 0.00 and 0.05.

TABLE VII

Parameter	Estimated value	Standard error	p value
β_0	-0.0337	2.0542	0.9869
β_1	-0.8042	0.3075	0.0089
β_2	0.5032	0.2488	0.0431
β_{11}	-0.0192	0.0163	0.2367
β_{22}	-0.0301	0.0094	0.0013
β_{12}	0.0571	0.0166	0.0006

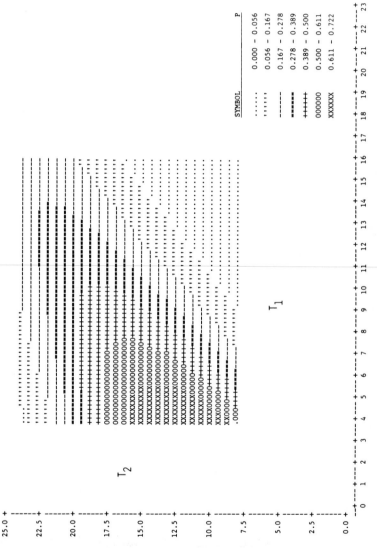

FIG. 36. Contour plot of the relationship between time interval between radiation and cyclophosphamide (T_1), and interval between radiation and radiation (T_2) in reducing tumor volume to $\leqq 10$ mm^3.

It is also informative to relate the levels of T_1 and T_2 to the survival times of the experimental animals. (The survival times are listed in the last column of Table VI.) This can be done through use of Cox's proportional hazards model as described by Carter *et al.* (1979). In this approach the instantaneous risk of failure or hazard function, $\lambda(t)$, at time t is taken to be of the form

$$\lambda(t) = \lambda_0(t) \exp (\beta_1 T_1 + \beta_2 T_2 + \beta_{11} T_1^2 + \beta_{22} T_2^2 + \beta_{12} T_1 T_2)$$

where $\lambda_0(t)$ is the underlying hazard function, the form of which does not need to be specified, and β_1 is an unknown constant associated with the effect of T_1, β_2 is an unknown constant associated with the effect of T_2, β_{11} and β_{22} are unknown constants which give the model sufficient flexibility to account for a quadratic relationship between the hazard function and the treatment variables. Such a relationship is possible since for small T_1 and T_2 the risk of failure is likely to be high due to treatment toxicity. As T_1 and T_2 increase the risk of failure is likely to decrease through a minimum and then increase due to inadequate treatment and hence increased risk of death from disease, and β_{12} is an unknown constant associated with the interaction between T_1 and T_2.

The method of maximum likelihood was used to estimate the model parameters. The estimates, their standard errors, and p values associated with the individual tests of significance appear in Table VIII. While individually some of the parameters cannot be said to differ from zero, the test of their importance as a group is highly significant ($p < 0.0001$). It is difficult to assess directly the fit of the proportional hazards model because the independent variable, hazard, is unobservable. This is in direct contrast to the situation with the logistic model where the dependent variable is the probability or proportion of animals experiencing a favorable outcome. However, an indication of the strength of the relationship between T_1 and T_2 and the survival times can be obtained by calculating and testing the significance of Spearman's correlation coefficient between the ranks of the estimated relative hazard [$\exp (\beta_1 T_1 + \beta_2 T_2 + \beta_{11} T_1^2 + \beta_{22} T_2^2 + \beta_{12} T_1 T_2)$] and the ranks of the median survival times of the various treatment groups. The estimated relative hazards and median survival

TABLE VIII

Parameter	Estimated value	Standard error	p value
β_1	−0.1451	0.1343	0.28
β_2	−0.2014	0.1183	0.09
β_{11}	0.0078	0.0063	0.21
β_{22}	0.0040	0.0038	0.29
β_{12}	−0.0030	0.0051	0.56

TABLE IX

T_1 (days)	T_2 (days)	Estimated relative hazard	Median survival time (days)
4	8	0.1488	22.0
6	8	0.1242	35.5
8	8	0.1103	17.0
4	12	0.0873	37.5
6	12	0.0711	52.5
8	12	0.0617	47.5
10	12	0.0570	27.0
12	12	0.0561	57.5
4	16	0.0582	37.0
6	16	0.0463	65.0
8	16	0.0393	42.0
10	16	0.0354	72.0
12	16	0.0340	68.5
14	16	0.0348	51.5
16	16	0.0379	43.5
4	20	0.0442	14.2
6	20	0.0343	68.5
8	20	0.0284	54.0
10	20	0.0250	62.0
12	20	0.0234	60.0
14	20	0.0234	63.0
16	20	0.0249	63.5
4	24	0.0380	83.5
6	24	0.0289	40.0
8	24	0.0233	75.5
10	24	0.0201	81.0
12	24	0.0184	79.5
14	24	0.0179	95.5
16	24	0.0186	122.0

times for the treatment groups appear in Table IX. The correlation coefficient is calculated to be -0.7585 with a p value of 0.0001. This indicates a significant relationship between the treatment levels and the survival times of the experimental animals.

Since there is no indication of model inadequacy further analysis is appropriate. With the proportional hazards model the treatment for which at any time t the animals are at minimum estimated risk of failing can be found by minimizing with respect to T_1 and T_2 the natural logarithm of the estimated relative hazard function, i.e., minimizing with respect to T_1 and T_2 the function

$$\hat{\beta}_1 T_1 + \hat{\beta}_2 T_2 + \hat{\beta}_{11} T_1{}^2 + \hat{\beta}_{22} T_2{}^2 + \hat{\beta}_{12} T_1 T_2$$

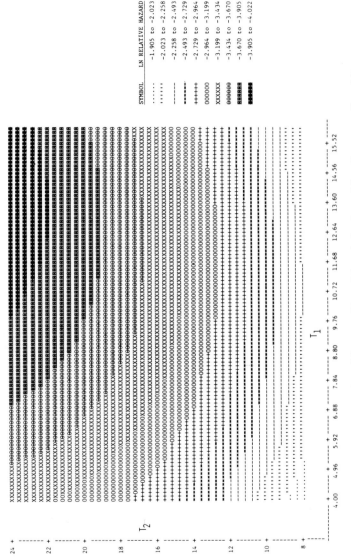

FIG. 37. Contour plot of the natural log of the relative hazard function versus T_1 and T_2.

where a circumflex above a parameter is used to denote its estimated value. In this case the estimated optimum treatment levels are

$$T_1 = 13.8 \text{ days}$$

$$T_2 = 24.0 \text{ days}$$

As with the logistic analysis it is more informative to consider a contour plot of the treatment–response relationship. Figure 37 is a contour plot of the natural logarithm of the relative hazard function versus T_1 and T_2. As in Fig. 36 the darker shadings are associated with the better treatments, i.e., those with lower estimated risk of failure. The relationship among shadings in Fig. 37 is not as apparent as that in the logistic analysis. However it is possible to estimate the risk of treatment in one region of shading relative to that associated treatments associated with a different shading. For example, the risk associated with treatments shaded with $+$ relative to that associated with θ, $\lambda(t) + /\lambda(t)_\theta$, is determined as follows:

1. From the legend of Fig. 37 the average value of ln relative risk associated with $+$ is $(-2.729 - 2.964)/2 \simeq -2.847$ while that associated with θ is -3.502.

2. From the form of the proportional hazards model we can write

$$\ln (\lambda(t) + /\lambda(t)_\theta) = \ln \left(\frac{\lambda(t) +}{\lambda_0(t)}\right) - \ln \left(\frac{\lambda(t)_\theta}{\lambda_0(t)}\right) = 3.502 - 2.847 = 0.655$$

Hence $\lambda(t) + /\lambda(t)_\theta = e^{0.655} = 1.925$. Thus, from this analysis it appears that the animals receiving treatments shaded with $+$ are 1.925 times as likely to fail as those treated with levels of T_1 and T_2 shaded with θ.

It is of interest to compare the results of the two analyses. From the figures it is apparent that the treatments associated with high probability of reducing the tumor volume to $\leq 10 \text{ mm}^3$ are also associated with high risk of failure. In fact the animals receiving the optimal treatment from a volume reduction viewpoint are estimated to be 4.9 times as likely to fail as those treated with the optimal treatment from a survival viewpoint. Conversely, the probability of reducing the tumor value to $\leq 10 \text{ mm}^3$ for the optimal treatment from the survival viewpoint is between 0.167 and 0.278 whereas the optimal treatment when considering tumor volume has an estimated probability 0.709 of a successful result.

It appears from the results of these analyses that it is not possible to determine values of T_1 and T_2 which simultaneously minimize the risk of failure and maximize the probability of reducing the tumor volume to $\leq 10 \text{ mm}^3$. In such a situation meaningful values of T_1 and T_2 may be found by considering constraints on the treatment. That is, it may be of

TABLE X

T_1 (days)	T_2 (days)	Constrained value of $\ln \lambda(t)/\lambda_0(t)$	Probability of tumor volume $\leq$ 10 mm^3
12.5	22.1	−3.9050	0.2925
10.1	19.7	−3.7437	0.3744
8.2	18.0	−3.4340	0.4536
6.3	17.1	−3.1990	0.5226
5.4	15.6	−2.9640	0.6022
4.3	14.4	−2.7290	0.6687
4.0	12.5	−2.4934	0.7083
4.0	12.1	−2.2580	0.7089
4.0	12.1	−2.4552	0.7089
4.0	12.1	−1.9050	0.7089

interest to find the levels of T_1 and T_2 which maximize the probability of reducing the tumor volume to $\leq$ 10 mm^3 subject to the constraint that the risk of failure does not exceed a specified value. Without the knowledge of $\lambda_0(t)$ it is not possible to specify the value of the constraint. In some situations it is possible to estimate $\lambda_0(t)$.

It is informative to consider values of $\ln \lambda(t)/\lambda_0(t)$ as constraints. Table X lists the optimum treatment levels subject to the constraint that $\ln \lambda(t)/\lambda_0(t)$ is that associated with the various contours in Fig. 37 and also gives the probability of a favorable tumor volume reduction associated with that treatment. For example, the first row of the table gives the values of T_1 and T_2 which maximize the probability of reducing the tumor volume to $\leq$ 10 mm^3 subject to $\ln \lambda(t)/\lambda_0(t) \leq 3.9050$. The last entry in the first row indicates that the probability of a favorable volume reduction is 0.2925.

This table illustrates that the probability of a favorable volume reduction rises with the natural logarithm of the relative risk of treatment. It also illustrates the difficulty associated with interpreting $\ln \lambda(t)/\lambda_0(t)$ when $\lambda_0(t)$ is not known. However, if a standard treatment is known, it is possible to determine the risk of other treatments relative to the standard as was done earlier in this discussion. For example, suppose that the treatment represented by $T_1 = 10$ days and $T_2 = 16$ days is an accepted standard. For this treatment it can be determined from Fig. 37 (or alternatively the model and the parameter estimates) that

$$\ln \frac{\lambda(t)}{\lambda_0(t)} \simeq -3.317$$

For the treatment represented by $T_1 = 5.4$ days and $T_2 = 15.6$ days it can be determined in the same manner that

$$\ln \frac{\lambda(t)}{\lambda_0(t)} \simeq -2.964$$

Thus, relative to the standard therapy the animals treated with $T_1 = 5.4$ days and $T_2 = 15.6$ days are 1.4233 times as likely to fail. However, the new treatment has probability 0.6022 associated with a favorable tumor reduction while the probability associated with the standard therapy is estimated from Fig. 1 (or from the logistic model with the parameter estimates) to be 0.38. In other words, the new therapy is 1.6 times as likely as the standard to be associated with a favorable tumor volume reduction.

This type of analysis will be used to evaluate our current experiments as well as future ones with the objective of devising optimum treatment schedules for sequential combined chemotherapy–radiotherapy. One of the potentials of this method of analysis is that it provides the means for determining estimated optimum dose and schedule interactions for fractionated and hyperfractionated radiation alone or in combination with chemotherapy. Results of the experiment presented in the next section, showing increased effectiveness of hyperfractionated radiation schedules with cyclophosphamide, are now being analyzed by this method. The ability to determine the significance of drug interactions with different radiation time–dose combinations to estimate optimum treatment levels provides a powerful tool in reaching our objectives. For different fractionated, hyperfractionated, and radiation dose schedules alone, the analysis would complement those now in use in radiotherapy (such as the Ellis formula) to relate total radiation dose and overall treatment time to normal tissue reaction and tumor cures. The analyses of experiments using biochemical and cell survival methods, along with adopting response surface methodology and other biomathematical methods, constitute continuing attempts to better understand the effective interaction of chemotherapy and radiotherapy.

VII. Fractionated and Hyperfractionated Radiation Dose Schedules Alone or in Combination with Cyclophosphamide

Extensive experimental radiation and chemotherapeutic dose fractionation studies have been carried out on both normal tissue and tumors (Fowler et al., 1974; Suit et al., 1977; Withers, 1975; Schabel et al., 1979; Barendsen and Broerse, 1970; Fischer and Reinhold, 1972). The four major parameters of radiation response which are considered to be major determinants of the reaction of tissue to fractionated radiation are (1) repair of radiation damage, (2) repopulation, (3) shifts in age density distribution, and (4) changes in distribution of p_{O_2} levels (reoxygenation) (Suit *et al.*, 1977; Withers, 1975).

The results of 16 clinical studies using varying daily hyperfractionated radiation dose schedules and varying radiation dose per fraction (100–320 rads) have recently been reported by Kotalik (1981). Clinical studies comparing different weekly radiation dose schedules have been reported. The sixth interim progress report of the British Institute of Radiology, in a study of three versus five fractions per week, showed no difference in the two regimens in the treatment of 687 patients with cancer of the laryngopharynx (Wiernik *et al.*, 1978). Recent data of Ellis and Goldson (1977) indicated that radiation given to 35 patients once a week was as effective as four to five fractions per week based on measured regression of the treated lesion. In reviewing the development of fractionated schedules in radiation oncology, Ellis and Goldson pointed out that early German practice advocated a large single dose of radiation, which contrasted with the French practice of small fractions of the total dose over several weeks. Various modifications of these two approaches still exist because neither clinical nor experimental results have provided the necessary information to conclude that one approach is superior to the other. Giving different fractionated and hyperfractionated radiation doses alone or with cyclophosphamide enables us to obtain information relevant to three clinical problems: (1) the hyperfractionated radiation schedule which will most effectively interact with chemotherapy, (2) the relative effectiveness of different hyperfractionated radiation dose schedules alone, and (3) the basis for attempts to determine the relative contribution of each modality.

Radiation totaling 4500 rads and cyclophosphamide totaling 450 mg/kg, or 2.7 gm/m², were given in three series at 11-day intervals over a treatment period of 23 days. Each series of fractionated or hyperfractionated radiation was followed next day by cyclophosphamide (150 mg/kg). Holding the total radiation and cyclophosphamide doses constant and giving cyclophosphamide as three 150 mg/kg doses in all groups permitted direct comparison of the effectiveness of different radiation fractionation schedules with and without cyclophosphamide on tumor cure rates, tumor control, animal survival rates, and normal tissue toxicity. The fractions delivered ranged in size from 1500 rads at 11-day intervals to 188 rads four times daily at 2-hour intervals for 2 days, repeated at 11-day intervals (Looney *et al.*, 1981b).

As summarized in Table XI, three radiation doses of 1500 rads given on days 0, 11, and 22 resulted in complete responses 23 ± 3 days after initiation of treatment for 7 of 10 tumors, and partial response in 1 tumor. The complete and partial response rate was reduced as the radiation dose per

TABLE XI

The Effect of Fractionated and Hyperfractionated Radiation Dose Schedules Alone or in Combination with Cyclophosphamide on Partial Response, Complete Response, Tumor Cure Rates, and Animal Survival

Group	Treatment day Rads[a]	Rads[a]	CP[b] 150 mg/kg	Rads per fraction[a]	Rets[c]	Rens[d]	Mean time (days) to complete response	Complete response[e]	Partial response[f]	Tumor cures	Mean day of death[g]	Survival day 260	Lung metastases	Skin reaction (42 days)
B	1500 / 0, 11, 22			1500	2461	3457	23 ± 3	7	1	4	165 ± 21	40%	1/10	1.94 ± 0.06
D	750 / 0, 11, 22	750 / 1, 12, 23		750 Days 0,1, etc.	2073	2927	50	1	5	1	99 ± 13	10%	8/10	0.89 ± 0.16
C	500 × 3 / 0, 11, 22			500 at 8 AM, 12,4 PM Days 0,11,22	1890	2656	38	1	3	0	105 ± 12	0%	9/10	0.65 ± 0.15
E	250 × 3 / 0, 11, 22	250 × 3 / 1, 12, 23		250 at 8 AM, 12,4 PM Days 0,1, etc.	1593	2249		0	0	0	73 ± 2	0%	9/10	0.72 ± 0.22
F	1500 / 0, 11, 22		1, 12, 23	1500	2461	3457	26 ± 5	8	0	8	38 ± 10	0%	0/10	1.50

I	750 0 11 22	750 1 12 23	750 Days 0,1, etc.	2073	2927	43 ± 6	8	2	8	59 ± 11	50%	0/10	1.25 ± 0.09
G	500 × 3 0 11 22	1 12 23	500 at 8 AM, 12,4 PM Days 0,11,22	1890	2656	54 ± 9	8	2	8	99 ± 41	60%	0/10	0.88 ± 0.12
J	375 × 4 0 11 22	1 12 23	375 at 8,10 AM, 12,2 PM Days 0,11, etc.	1764	2479	57 ± 9	10		7	82 ± 20	60%	0/10	1.00 ± 0.13
H	250 × 3 0 11 22	1 12 23	250 at 8 AM, 12,4 PM Days 0,1,etc.	1593	2249	54 ± 8	7	3	6	58 ± 15	70%	0/10	0.50
K	188 × 4 0 11 22	1 12 23	188 at 8,10 AM, 12,2 PM Days 0,1, etc.	1487	2099	65 ± 7	6	3	5	± 3	40%	0/10	0.50

[a] The total radiation dose to the tumor was held constant at 4500 rads for all groups.
[b] The total cyclophosphamide dose was held constant and given as three 150 mg/kg doses at 11-day intervals.
[c] rets, Rad equivalent therapy units = total dose $\times F^{-0.24} \times T^{-0.11}$ (Ellis, 1968).
[d] rens, Rad equivalent neoplasm units = total dose $\times F^{-0.24} \times T^{-0.11}$ (Ellis, 1971) where F = number of fractions and T = total treatment in days.
[e] The term "complete response" has been used in its clinical context to denote no detectable evidence of remaining tumor (i.e., tumor nonpalpable).
[f] Partial response has also been used in its clinical context to denote a greater than 50% reduction in tumor volume as compared with the initial volume.
[g] Anesthetic deaths were excluded.

fraction was reduced. One tumor in 10 had complete response with 750 rads (group D) or 500 rads (group C) per fraction, but no complete responses occurred when the dose per fraction was reduced to 250 rads (group E). Partial responses observed were 5 of 10 tumors for 750 rad fractions, 3 of 10 for 500 rad fractions, and none for 250 rad fractions. Fractionation or hyperfractionation of 1500 rads on days 0 and 1, 11 and 12, and 22 and 23 resulted in a survival of 40% for the 1500 rad per fraction groups, 10% for the 750 rad per fraction group, and 0% for the 500 and 250 rad per fraction groups. Lung metastases were found in only one animal in the 1500 rad per fraction group. However, the incidence of lung metastases was 80, 90, and 90% for the 750, 500, and 250 rad per fraction groups, respectively. Deaths in these three groups of animals occurred on days 99 ± 13, 105 ± 12, and 73 ± 2 days, respectively. These deaths were attributed to the failure of the fractionated and hyperfractionated radiation dose schedules alone to control either the growth of the primary tumor or its metastatic dissemination.

The effectiveness of the interaction of cyclophosphamide given 1 day after radiation was determined in the remaining groups of animals in the experiment of Table XI. There was complete response in 8 of 10 tumors 26 ± 5 days after initiation of treatment in the 1500 rad per fraction group combined with cyclophosphamide. However, combination of the two modalities was less effective therapeutically than radiation alone since increased toxicity resulted in major loss of animals in which complete response had occurred. For the 750, 500, 375, 250, and 188 rad per fraction

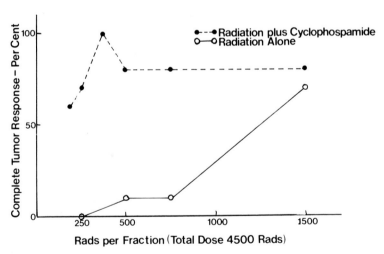

Fig. 38.   Complete tumor response. Radiation alone, ○; radiation and cyclophosphamide, ●.

groups given cyclophosphamide, tumor cure rates and complete tumor responses were $\geq 50\%$ (Fig. 38). Tumor cures in Table XI include animals which died with no detectable tumor. Survival on day 260 accounts for deaths related to both uncontrolled tumor and treatment toxicity.

Previous studies have shown that 150 mg/kg cyclophosphamide alone every 11 days produces no tumor cures. For combined radiotherapy–chemotherapy the mean time for complete response increased from 26 ± 5 days for the 1500 rad per fraction group to 65 ± 7 days for the 188 rad per fraction group. This indicates that the rate of tumor regression is directly related to the size of the dose per fraction. The smaller hyperfractionated radiation doses are less effective in terms of the rate at which complete tumor response occurs when combined with cyclophosphamide as well as in producing tumor cures when given alone. However, the addition of the cyclophosphamide did control metastatic dissemination even for the small radiation dose fractions. None of the fractionated or hyperfractionated groups given cyclophosphamide had pulmonary metastases compared to an incidence of 80 to 90% for the 750, 500, and 250 rad per fraction groups given only radiation.

Tumor regrowth after complete response occurred in 2 of 10 tumors in the 1500 rad per fraction group and in 1 of 10 tumors in the 500 rad per fraction group. Regrowth also occurred in 2 of 10 tumors given 375 rads per fraction with cyclophosphamide, and in 1 of 10 tumors given 250 or 188 rads per fraction with cyclophosphamide. Time to reappearance from initiation of treatment ranged from 29 to 174 days. The complete response rate in 750, 500, 375, and 250 rad per fraction groups with cyclophosphamide was 70 to 100%, and the cure rate 50 to 70%. Animal survival at 260 days varied from 40 to 70% and mean day of death was 60 to 100 days after initiation of treatment. No pulmonary metastases were found in these groups and no significant long-term hematological changes have been found following three doses of cyclophosphamide (150 mg/kg) given at 11-day intervals. There are no specific reasons to account for the animals dying in which the primary tumor has been controlled or eradicated. These animals do reduce their food intake, and are completely devoid of body fat at autopsy. It is possible that they go into negative nutritional balance as is seen in patients (DeWys, 1980). The cachexia that develops appears to be the result of a number of interrelated effects of the cancer and cancer treatment on the patient. The most plausible explanation for these deaths is therefore related to these processes.

We have calculated the nominal standard dose (NSD) equivalent for the different dose fractionations using the Ellis equations given at the bottom of Table XI. The rad equivalent therapy units (rets) and rad equivalent neoplasm units (rens) were determined for each dose fractionation schedule. Ellis has indicated that a radiation dose corresponding to 34 fractions of 200 rads given 5 times weekly is approximately the level of normal tissue tolerance in patients, although 37 fractions of 200 rads is necessary for curing larger tumors even though the risk of necrosis is greater. The total clinical radiation dose of 6800 rads given in 34, 200 rad fractions calculates as 1905 rets. In our experimental studies 2461 rets for the 1500 rad per fraction schedule, and 2073 rets for the 750 rad per fraction schedule were both above this accepted value for clinical practice, but the hyperfractionated experimental schedules employing 500, 375, 250, and 188 rads per fraction have calculated rets below the clinical value (1890, 1764, 1593, and 1487, respectively).

Acute skin reaction on day 42 for single, fractionated, or hyperfractionated doses ending on day 23 is tabulated in Table XI and shown in Figs. 39, 40, and 41. Day 42 was chosen since this was in the period of the acute skin reaction after completion of radiation on day 23. The reaction was evaluated by a slight modification of the method of Fowler and associates (1972). Their procedure has been modified slightly for this experiment since we irradiated the skin on the tumor over the abdominal flank of the rat, whereas Fowler irradiated the foot of the mouse. Scoring of skin reaction in these experiments is as follows: 0.0, no detectable damage; 0.5, discoloration but no dryness; 1.0, slightly scaly; 1.5, scaly appearance;

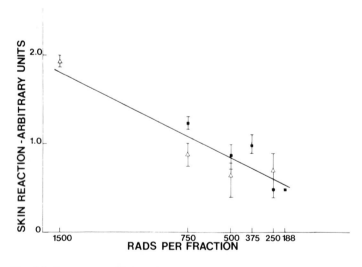

FIG. 39. Maximum acute skin reaction, day 42, after termination of radiation on day 23. The coefficient of determination for the linear regression analysis was 0.93. Radiation alone, △; radiation and cyclophosphamide, ■.

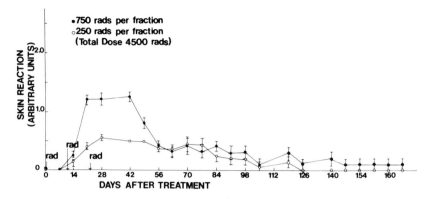

FIG. 40. Skin reaction during and after radiation in the groups given 750 rads per fraction plus cyclophosphamide, ●; and 250 rads per fraction plus cyclophosphamide, ○.

2.0, dry scab; 2.5, moist scab. There was a consistent reduction in acute skin reaction as the rads per fraction were reduced from 1500 to 750, 500, 375, 250, and 188 (Fig. 39). The recovery of skin between 56 and 105 days after termination of radiation on day 23 (Figs. 40 and 41), which left almost no residual injury, offers the further possibility of using more hyper-fractionated radiation if given intermittently 2 to 4 months after the initial series. It is planned to extend these studies to determine the radiation dose schedules which will result in tumor cure rates of $\geq$ 50% with the least effect on normal tissue reaction when the hyperfractionated radiation is given in 1 to 2 days time and repeated intermittently over longer time intervals (7 to 11 days).

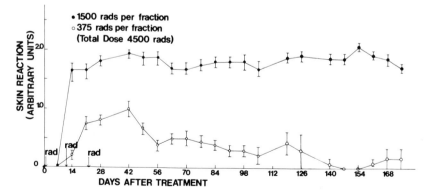

FIG. 41. Skin reaction during and after radiation in the groups given 375 rads per fraction plus cyclophosphamide, ○; and 1500 rads per fraction without cyclophosphamide, ●. Toxic deaths prevented the use of the 1500 rads per fraction plus cyclophosphamide group.

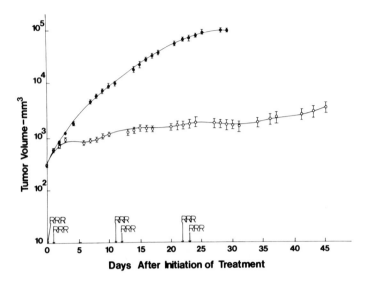

FIG. 42.   Changes in mean tumor volumes (± standard error of the mean) in the group given 250 rads per fraction at 8 AM, 12 noon, and 4 PM on days 0 and 1, 11 and 12, and 22 and 23 (total radiation dose, 4500 rads). Controls, ●; treated, ○.

Results of the 250 rad per fraction groups alone and combined with cyclophosphamide summarized below demonstrate the major increase in effectiveness of interacting hyperfractionated radiation dose schedules with cyclophosphamide. This hyperfractionated radiation dose schedule of 250 rads per fraction alone resulted in no complete or partial tumor responses and no tumor cures (group E, Table XI). There was a slight increase in mean tumor volume throughout the period of treatment with radiation

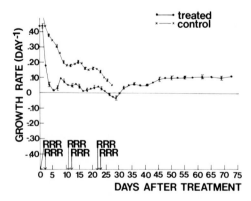

FIG. 43.   Changes in mean tumor growth rates (± standard error of the mean) for the treated, ●, and control, X, tumors shown in Fig. 42.

alone (Fig. 42), however, life expectancy was increased by more than 2. Mean day of death was 69 ± 3 days, over twice that for untreated controls of 28 ± 1 days. Rate of tumor growth was diminished by the radiation, but was slightly positive throughout the 45-day period for which growth rates were determined (Fig. 43).

The mean volume of radiation treated tumors on day 42 is comparable to the mean volume of untreated controls on day 6. The growth rate of controls on day 6 was 0.3 day^{-1}. Mean growth rate of treated animals of 0.05 day^{-1} on day 90 is comparable to the growth rates at the end of treatment on day 23 (Fig. 43). Treated tumors on day 90 have growth rates one-sixth that of untreated tumors of comparable volume 2 months after termination of treatment on day 23. This long duration of major reductions in growth rate after sequential therapy is in contrast to well-defined changes in growth rates found in this solid tumor line after single doses of either cyclophosphamide or radiation. There is marked reduction in growth rate after a single dose of 150 mg/kg cyclophosphamide, which reaches a nadir of -0.23 day^{-1} on day 5 after treatment, followed by a marked acceleration in growth rate, reaching a maximum of $+0.35$ day^{-1} on day 14 (see Fig. 14, Section III).

Combined use of cyclophosphamide with 250 rads per fraction (group H, Table XI) resulted in complete tumor response in 7 of 10 tumors 54 ± 8 days after initiation of treatment, and partial response of the re-

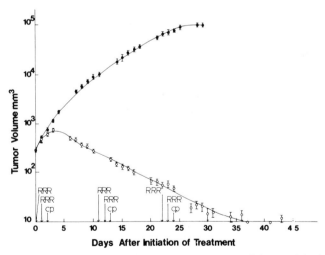

FIG. 44. Changes in mean tumor volumes ($\pm$ standard error of the mean) in the 250 rads per fraction plus cyclophosphamide group. The 250 rad fractions were administered at 8 AM, 12 noon, and 4 PM on days 0 and 1, 11 and 12, and 22 and 23; plus cyclophosphamide (150 mg/kg) on days 2, 13, and 24 (total radiation dose, 4500 rads). Controls, ●; treated, ○.

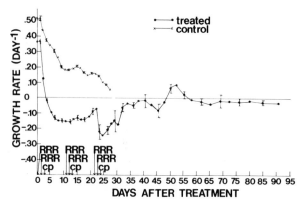

FIG. 45. Changes in mean tumor growth rates (± standard error of the mean) for the treated, ●, and control, X, tumors shown in Fig. 44.

maining 3 tumors 19 ± 1 days after treatment. One tumor regrew for a cure rate of 60%. The addition of cyclophosphamide to these hyperfractionated radiation dose schedules resulted in a constant reduction in mean tumor volume during the 23 days of treatment which continued after the end of treatment (Fig. 44). A rapid decrease in tumor growth rate occurred during the first few days after treatment; then the growth rate became negative (Fig. 45). The long duration of negative growth of 90 days (67 days after termination of treatment on day 23) demonstrates the greater effectiveness of the combined use of cyclophosphamide with hyperfractionated radiation dose schedules compared to radiation alone in controlling tumor growth. It also demonstrates a 67-day "therapeutic window" with stabilized tumor growth rate. With combined modality treatment the continued negative growth rate throughout the 67-day period will allow time to institute sequential adjuvant therapy to prevent metastatic dissemination and recurrence of the primary.

VIII. Long-Term Functional and Morphologic Studies in Host and Tumor

The successful strategy for interacting radiotherapy and chemotherapy sequentially to cure the primary tumor has been based on (1) the effective interaction of chemotherapy and radiotherapy in the first treatment series, and (2) the recovery of the host and critical host organs prior to administration of the second and subsequent series. Treatment after recovery of bone marrow and gut has permitted delivery of two to three series of cyclophosphamide–radiation to produce tumor cure rates ≥ 50%. In our continuing efforts to further improve sequential therapy, treatment for much longer periods of time necessitates the study of other vital organs such as heart, lungs, liver, spleen, kidneys, and bladder. The successful utilization of sequential therapy for primary as well as adjuvant therapy will be dependent to a large degree upon being able to give combined treatment to minimize the cumulative and long-term effects on these organs as well as on bone marrow and gut.

Diagrammatic representation of the time sequence of tumor response to sequential combined chemotherapy–radiotherapy and recurrence of the primary tumor and pulmonary metastases is presented in Fig. 46. The recovery of critical organs of the host to radiotherapy and chemotherapy is also presented. This time sequence of host recovery provides initial information for the development of protocols designed to further improve treatment of the primary as well as for adjuvant therapy.

We have previously determined the scheduling necessary to avoid mortality from acute toxicity to gut or marrow, with marrow being the limiting organ for sequential therapy since its recovery is after that of gut in the rat. The LD_{10} for a single dose of cyclophosphamide in the ACI rat is approximately 150 mg/kg. Three doses of cyclophosphamide (150 mg/kg

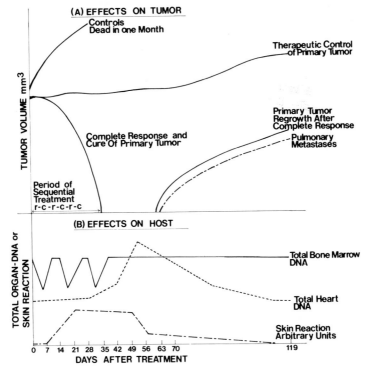

FIG. 46. Diagrammatic representation of tumor and host responses to sequential combined chemotherapy–radiotherapy.

each) were given at 2-week intervals, with sacrifices scheduled 4 and 14 days after each individual treatment to examine acute recovery, and at 5-week intervals thereafter for 1 year. These doses and scheduling of cyclophosphamide were selected since it has been shown that three series of cyclophosphamide given with radiation 11 or 14 days apart will result in cure rates $\geq 50\%$. The organ weight, DNA content, collagen content, and [³H]TdR incorporation into DNA were determined in liver, gut, kidney, bone marrow, spleen, heart, lung, thymus, and bladder. WBC, Hgb, and Hct values were obtained in peripheral blood. The following serum determinations were made: glucose, potassium, sodium, CO_2, chloride, calcium, phosphorus, BUN, creatinine, albumin, total billirubin, alkaline phosphatase, SGPT, SGOT, LDH, and cholesterol. Sections were taken for pathologic evaluation to correlate organ dysfunction with organ damage if or when it develops (Hopkins *et al.*, 1981).

We are currently to day 127 in evaluation of long-term cyclophosphamide toxicity. Data obtained for heart are shown in Fig. 47. Heart weight did not change during the period of treatment but began to increase on completion of three courses of treatment, and was almost double that of untreated controls on day 56. This increase in weight was paralleled by an increase in total heart DNA, signifying an increase in the number of nucleated cells. Pathologic evaluation of these hearts revealed that a prominent influx of lymphocytes is the likely explanation for the DNA changes. It is of interest that [³H]TdR incorporation into total DNA increases shortly after the onset of cyclophosphamide treatment and continues at approximately the same rate during the period of DNA accumulation. Both weight and DNA content of the heart have returned to control levels on day 127.

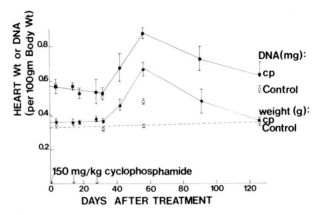

FIG. 47. Effect of sequential treatment of ACI rats with three, 150 mg/kg doses of cyclophosphamide at 14-day intervals on heart weight (●, ○) and DNA content (■, □). Treated, ●, ■; controls, ○, □.

Morphologic evaluation of the heart in animals receiving cyclophospha-mide demonstrates striking abnormalities at 56 days. These include marked myocytic vacuolar degeneration, mild interstitial hemorrhage, de-generative vascular changes involving predominantly small arteries and arterioles, and a prominent focal lymphocytic infiltrate surrounding those areas of vacuolar change. Myocardial changes were focal. Intervening tis-sue appeared normal, for the most part, at the light microscopic level. Such changes have been seen in human cardiac tissues after cyclophos-phamide treatment (Slaven *et al.*, 1975). In tissues examined at 90 and 127 days, microscopic abnormalities were also present; the extent of disease was milder than at 56 days. Vessels manifested more chronic changes (vascular sclerosis) and the myocardium also demonstrated chronic ef-fects of tissue damage, e.g., focal calcification and cartilaginous metapla-sia. The lungs manifested significant changes in the 56-day samples. These changes consisted of vascular sclerosis (predominantly small ar-teries and arterioles), focal intraalveolar hemorrhage with histiocyte re-sponse, focal chronic inflammatory infiltrate, pneumocyte atypia, and in one case a giant cell response. These changes were present but less re-markable at 90 and 127 days. Incorporation of [^{3}H]TdR is elevated in lung as a result of treatment with cyclophosphamide, and this effect is still pre-sent on day 56 after initiation of treatment. The amount of collagen in the lung, as assessed by hydroxyproline determinations, is increased on day 56, suggesting that damage to the lung has resulted in fibrosis, at least to that point in time. The kidneys manifested sporatic vacuolar change of the proximal convoluted tubules. This could not with certainty be attributed to drug effect. There was no evidence of coagulation defects in capillaries of small renal arteries. As cyclophosphamide and other can-cer chemotherapeutic agents are successfully employed in combined mo-dality therapy, the long-term toxicities associated with their use become more important. Animal systems such as the ones we use may be em-ployed not only to identify some of these limiting long-term toxicities but also to discover modifications of treatment protocols which can minimize these effects.

IX. Adjuvant Therapy

A. Sudies on Primary and Metastatic Tumor Cell Populations

While some tumors regrow and the volumes then become stabilized fol-lowing sequential combined chemotherapy–radiotherapy, others regrow and establish growth rates comparable to control tumors. These marked differences in growth rates are illustrated for three different tumors in Fig. 48. Complete response occurred approximately 1 month after two series of cyclophosphamide and radiation were given on days 0 and 7 and days 14 and 21. Regrowth of these tumors occurred approximately 2 months after treatment began. The tumor from rat 44 regrew at growth rates comparable to controls whereas for rat 43 tumor growth rate was stabilized. Tumor growth rate for rat 45 was intermediate between those of rats 44 and 43.

The possibility was considered that the clonogenic potential of the tumor cells is greatly diminished or even lost after repeated insults of radiotherapy and chemotherapy. Reinoculation of tumor cells from treated tumors with stabilized or reduced growth rates into untreated animals resulted in growth rates comparable to untreated control tumors. Figure 49 shows the tumor volume changes of tumor J99 over the 55 days of treatment and the following 47 days in which no further treatment was given. Three doses of 1500 rads radiation were given on days 0, 22, and 44, and three doses of cyclophosphamide (150 mg/kg) on days 11, 33, and 55. There was a gradual decrease in volume which reached a nadir on day 65, followed by some increase in volume which reached a plateau on day 80 and remained stable until tumor excision on day 102. The volume never returned to original volume (V_0) at any time before or after treatment. On

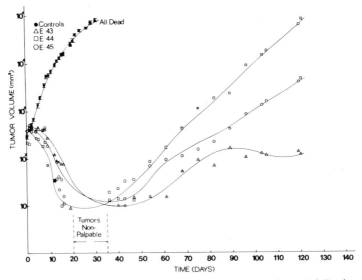

FIG. 48. Tumor volume changes in three different tumors during and following two series of radiation (1500 rads) and cyclophosphamide (150 mg/kg) given on days 0 and 7, and 14 and 21.

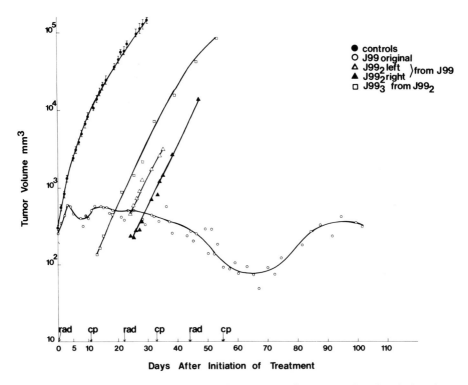

FIG. 49. Tumor volume changes in a primary tumor after three series of cyclophospha-mide and radiation given 11 days apart. Regrowth of the treated primary tumors removed on day 102 and reinoculated into normal rats is shown for three different tumors.

day 102 cells from the treated tumor were transplanted into each side of another normal rat. The growth rates of both left and right tumors ($J99_2$) taken from the original tumor (J99) were comparable to the mean value of untreated control tumors as shown on the left side of the figure. Cells were again taken from the first transplant generation ($J99_2$) of the original tumor (J99) and inoculated into another normal animal. This second trans-plant generation tumor ($J99_2$) also grew at rates comparable to untreated controls. these results indicate that the clonogenic potential of the tumor cells is retained even though treatment has reduced or stopped tumor growth.

Studies have recently been initiated in order to determine if significant cytogenetic changes occur in tumor cell populations following sequential combined radiotherapy–chemotherapy. G banding and Q banding tech-niques have been carried out on five different groups of tumors: (1) con-trols, (2) tumors given sequential cyclophosphamide–radiation therapy,

(3) treated tumors retransplanted into normal hosts, (4) metastatic lung tumors, and (5) metastatic lung tumors retransplanted into normal hosts. Of the five categories of tumors analyzed cytogenetically, all, as evidenced by the marker and general karyotypic features, were clearly derived from 3924A. Variations in chromosomal number and some new markers were observed. These variations, however, are also characteristic features of 3924A (Kovi and Morris, 1976; Wyandt et al., 1981).

The most significant finding in the cytogenetic studies to date is the lack of major changes in primary tumor cells subjected to repeated doses of two mutagenic agents. The markers of 3924A, in spite of prolonged treatment, appear to be stable; newly arisen markers appear less so. Insufficient number of cells have been analyzed from the various lines to know if certain markers are more susceptible to treatment than others. Sections from each of the five categories of tumors analyzed cytogenetically have been evaluated. The pathology of all five tumor categories is identical, confirming that the pulmonary metastases are from the primary tumors. The cytogenetic and pathologic results rule out the possibility of therapeutically induced pulmonary tumors.

These studies will provide useful information for the evaluation of changes which may occur following both single and combined modality therapy in either the host or the tumor cell population, as well as differences in the therapeutic sensitivities of the primary tumor, the regrowing primary, or the pulmonary metastases. These studies should be particularly useful in the evaluation of therapeutic resistance which may develop.

B. IMMUNOLOGICAL RAMIFICATIONS OF CHEMOTHERAPY AND RADIOTHERAPY

Chemotherapy and radiotherapy have the potential to inhibit immune responses in man and in experimental animals (Mukherji and Mukhopadhyay, 1980; Stewart and Perez, 1976; Meyer, 1970). It is clear, for example, that ionizing irradiation does decrease absolute T- and B-cell counts in peripheral blood and spleen, and that significant leukopenia may occur even with limited-field irradiation. Further, in many cases, the functional integrity of the remaining lymphoid cells may be impaired, as demonstrated by a reduction in treated animals of capacity to synthesize antibodies (Mukherji and Mukhopadyay, 1980; DeMacedo and Catty, 1977; Zaalberg et al., 1973). Chemotherapy with cyclophosphamide also has potent immunosuppressive activity, depending on the dose of the agent used in therapy, and the time course of the treatment. High-dose cyclophosphamide therapy in humans has been reported to have more severe and longer lasting effects on B cells than on T cells, thus causing a reduction in circulating immunoglobulin titers (LaGrange *et al.*, 1974; Lerman and Weidanz, 1970). Cyclophosphamide at low doses (20–50 mg/kg) appears to selectively eliminate T-suppressor cell precursors (Mitsuoka *et al.*, 1976; Man-San *et al.*, 1979; Lando *et al.*, 1979), which can result in increases in both antibody production as well as immune T-cell responses, such as delayed hypersensitivity reactions and cytotoxic activity.

To see if tumor-specific immunity had developed in animals with cured primary tumors, three groups of three cured animals each were reinoculated with 3924A tumors. Mean time between cure of the first primary and reinoculation of the second tumor was 282 ± 22, 107 ± 0.7, and 19.5 ± 17.5 days for the three groups. Tumors grew in all three groups and tumor growth rates were comparable to those in animals growing their first tumor. Any immune response that occurs as a result of the first tumor has little or no effect on subsequent growth or "tumor takes" of reinoculated 3924A tumor cells. This may also apply to tumor regrowth at the primary site following complete response as well as to growth of pulmonary metastases following cure of the primary, although this point needs to be established with small numbers of cells.

Wepsic *et al.* (1976) have reported data indicating that 3924A is weakly antigenic, in that animals repeatedly immunized with 3924A irradiated tumor cells resisted challenge with 1×10^5 tumor cells but not 1×10^6 cells. The low incidence of pulmonary metastases in animals with im or sc 3924A tumors, suggesting that the tumor line was immunogenic, is now believed to be a consequence of rapid growth of the primary tumor with death occurring before metastases are apparent. Death in untreated animals occurs at approximately 30 days after implanting tumor cells and metastases appear at approximately 60 days in animals in which tumor growth has been slowed by effective therapy or, in a preliminary experiment, where surgical excision of the tumor has been done.

Localized irradiation of tumors may have unanticipated effects on the immune response, based on evidence from a number of studies that a large number of important lymphoid effector cells with cytolytic potential do infiltrate many (if not most) recognizable solid tumors. It is possible that the *in situ* functions of these infiltrating lymphoid cells may bring about not only cytolysis and cytostasis of the tumor cells in the immediate environment, but such effector cells may also serve two other extremely useful functions. First, such effectors may recruit other immunologic effector cells to the tumor site by releasing soluble chemotactic factors which disperse to surrounding tissue; second, following an *in situ* sojourn, some of these effectors may migrate out to the peripheral circulation to act as immunologic memory cells which would be capable of rapid immunologic destruction of new tumor cells when encountered at a later time. A significant number of these infiltrating lymphoid cells have characteristics of natural killer (NK) cells (Gerson *et al.*, 1980), which are large granular lymphocytes ("non-T, non-B") currently believed to be the primary cellular defense system against developing, incipient tumors in humans, as well as in such animal models as mice and rats (Herberman and Holden, 1978; Roder and Haliotis, 1980). NK cells are also believed to be the critical effector cells which suppress circulating tumor emboli (Hanna and Fidler, 1980), as well as pulmonary emboli (Puccetti *et al.*, 1980; Ricardi *et al.*, 1980).

The cytolytic function of NK cells, which are critically dependent on an intact bone marrow for maintenance of antitumor cytotoxic potential (Kurmar *et al.*, 1979), is also sensitive to exposure to high doses of cyclophosphamide (>200 mg/kg, ip). At the doses used in the present studies (150 mg/kg), however, it is not certain that the natural defenses by NK cells were suppressed. Because there is high correlation in mice between innate levels of NK cell activity and ability to resist transplantable tumors, it would be useful in future studies in the rat hepatoma model to monitor for the effects of radiotherapy and chemotherapy on NK cell activity *in vitro*.

The curative role of radiation and of chemotherapy for certain types of cancer is well established. Whether the last few neoplastic cells in these instances are killed by the treatments or by a recovered immunologic host defense mechanism has not been established. It is clear that the immunosuppressive properties of radiation and chemotherapy are not necessarily a deterrent against their use in cancer management. However, a better understanding of the kinetics of recovery from therapy-induced immunosuppression and the role of host immune mechanisms against minimal neoplastic disease may permit scheduling of therapy to potentiate neoplastic cell killing by immunologic means. A greater understanding of the immunological changes following chemotherapy and radiotherapy will be helpful in minimizing deleterious effects of the interaction of the three treatment modalities on the host.

C. DEVELOPMENT OF A STRATEGY FOR ADJUVANT THERAPY

Many tumors have a high incidence of recurrence following therapy of 'curative intent', such as surgery, radiation therapy, or chemotherapy. The most accepted explanation is that after treatment, microscopic foci of malignant cells (micrometastases) remain in the body and eventually lead to the recurrence of the malignant process. Adjuvant therapy is intended to help eradicate these micrometastases and to prevent the subsequent recurrence of disease (Sarna, 1980, p. 32).

Primary tumors which regrow, and pulmonary metastases which develop in 3924A after the initial series of sequential combined chemotherapy–radiotherapy, provide an experimental solid tumor system for development of adjuvant therapy. In Section VII it was shown that sequential chemotherapy combined with radiotherapy could effectively control metastatic dissemination and cure the primary tumor since no pulmonary metastases developed. It was also shown that fractionated and hyperfractionated radiation alone would not control metastatic dissemination since lung metastases occurred in 70, 80, and 90% of the animals treated with 750, 500, and 250 rads per fraction. Deaths in these groups occurred 99, 97, and 72 days after initiation of treatment and approximately 2 to 2.5 months after termination of treatment on day 23.

Removal of the primary tumor either by surgery or radiation during the first 3 weeks after implantation will therefore provide a solid tumor system for studies designed to treat metastatic dissemination of solid tumors. Growth rates of pulmonary metastases in Lewis lung tumor were greater than for the primary tumors (Simpson-Herren, 1974). However, more recent studies have shown that growth rates of metastases to the lungs from mammary adenocarcinoma 16/c are less than for the primary tumor. Thus, the sensitivity of pulmonary metastases to therapy may be greater or less than for the primary tumor. Little experimental information is available on the relative sensitivities of the primary tumor and its metastases to combined modality therapy. Our studies on successful treatment of the primary tumor therefore provide an excellent solid tumor system to study the effects of adjuvant therapy designed to prevent metastatic dissemination and primary regrowth, and to treat the pulmonary metastases following cure of the primary tumor either by surgical removal or local tumor radiation.

Diagrammatic representation of the tumor response time sequence to combined chemotherapy–radiotherapy is presented in Fig. 46. Recovery of host critical organs to both radiotherapy and chemotherapy is also presented. This time sequence of host recovery provides information for developing a treatment strategy for adjuvant therapy. The time sequence for the recurrence of the primary tumor and pulmonary metastases is included. These results provide basic information for the development of a therapeutic strategy for adjuvant therapy to prevent regrowth of the primary and dissemination of the primary after the initial phase of "curative therapy" is complete.

Three series of sequential hyperfractionated radiation–cyclophosphamide therapy result in continued negative growth rates for at least 67 days (to day 90) beyond termination of treatment on day 23 (Fig. 45). Tumors of this group still have not regrown at 160 days after initiation of treatment. The long period of continued control of tumor growth after completion of the induction and consolidation therapy over the first 23 days of treatment provides flexibility in beginning adjuvant therapy to prevent regrowth of the primary and pulmonary metastases.

ACKNOWLEDGMENTS

The authors wish to thank the following persons for their contributions to this manuscript.

Dr. W. H. Carter, Jr., Department of Biostatistics, Medical College of Virginia, Richmond, Virginia, for preparation of Section VI; Dr. H. David Kay, Department of Internal Medicine, Division of Rheumatology, University of Virginia School of Medicine, for preparation of Section IX,B; Dr. W. L. Betsill, Jr., Department of Pathology, Medical University of South Carolina, Charleston, South Carolina; Dr. John Savory and Mrs. Ann S. Hobson of the Department of Pathology, University of Virginia School of Medicine, for collaborative studies in Section VIII; Dr. H. E. Wyandt and Dr. Harshad Shah, Department of Pediatrics, Division of Medical Genetics, University of Virginia School of Medicine for collaborative studies in Section IX,A.

Pathologic evaluation of primary and metastatic tumors was through the courtesy of Dr. Robert Fechner, Head of the Division of Surgical Pathology, University of Virginia School of Medicine.

The authors also thank Dr. Harold P. Morris and Mrs. Charity M. Jackson, Howard University, Washington, D.C., for tumor transplants of hepatoma 3924A.

Excellent technical assistance has been provided by Shirley T. Mays, Martha S. MacLeod, John H. Key, Jr., and Karen S. Lotts of this Division. Dr. Roy Rowley performed the clonogenic assays.

Computer analysis of data was by Mark B. Longerbeam and Dr. E. Russell Ritenour, also of the Division of Radiobiology and Biophysics.

Supported in part by a U.S. Public Health Service Research Emphasis Grant (CREG) CA20516 on Experimental Combined Modality (Radiotherapy–Chemotherapy) Studies (ECMRC) from the National Cancer Institute.

REFERENCES

Barendsen, G. W., and Broerse, J. J. (1970). *Eur. J. Cancer* **6**, 89.

Bergsagel, D. E., Robertson, G. L., and Hasselback, R. (1968). *Can. Med. Assoc. J.* **98**, 532.

Breur, K. (1966). *Eur. J. Cancer* **2**, 157.

Bruce, W. R., Meeker, B. E., and Valeriote, F. A. (1966). *J. Natl. Cancer Inst.* **37**, 233.

Carter, W. H., Jr., Wampler, G. L., Crews, S. L., and Howells, R. (1977). *Cancer Treat. Rep.* **61**, 849.

Carter, W. H., Jr., Stablein, D. M., and Wampler, G. L. (1979). *Cancer Res.* **39**, 3446.

Carter, W. H., Jr., Looney, W. B., Hopkins, H. A., and Longerbeam, M. B. (1981). (In preparation).

Courdi, A., Tubiana, M., Chavaudra, N., and Malaise, E. P. (1980). *Int. J. Radiat. Oncol. Biol. Phys.* **6**, 1639.

DeMacedo, M. S., and Catty, D. (1977). *Immunology* **33**, 611.

Denekamp, J. (1972). *Eur. J. Cancer* **8**, 335.

DeWys, W. D. (1980). *J. Am. Med. Assoc.* **244**, 374.

Dutreix, J., Tubiana, M., Wambersie, A., and Malaise, E. (1971). *Eur. J. Cancer* **7**, 205.

Ellis, F. (1968). *Curr. Top. Radiat. Res.* **4,** 359.

Ellis, F. (1971). *Br. J. Radiat.* **44,** 101.

Ellis, F., and Goldson, A. L. (1977). *Int. J. Radiat. Oncol. Biol. Phys.* **2,** 537.

Evans, M. J., and Kovacs, C. J. (1977). *Cell Tissue Kinet.* **10,** 233.

Fischer, J. J., and Reinhold, H. S. (1972). *Radiology* **105,** 429.

Fowler, J. F., Denekamp, J., Page, A. L., Begg, A. C., Field, S. B., and Butler, K. (1972). *Br. J. Radiol.* **45,** 237.

Fowler, J. F., Denekamp, J., Sheldon, P. W., Smith, A. M., Begg, A. C., Harris, S. R., and Page, A. L. (1974). *Br. J. Radiol.* **47,** 781.

Gerson, J. M., Varesio, L., and Herberman, R. B. (1980). *J. Natl. Cancer Inst.* **65,** 905.

Hanna, N., and Fidler, I. J. (1980). *J. Natl. Cancer Inst.* **65,** 801.

Herberman, R. B., and Holden, H. T. (1978). *Adv. Cancer Res.* **27,** 305.

Hopkins, H. A., and Looney, W. B. (1978). *Antibiot. Chemother.* **23,** 135.

Hopkins, H. A., Kovacs, C. J., Looney, W. B., Wakefield, J. A., and Morris, H. P. (1976). *Cancer Biochem. Biophys.* **1,** 303.

Hopkins, H. A., Looney, W. B., Betsill, Jr., W. L., Wyandt, H., Shah, H., Shipe, J. R., Savory, J., and Hobson, A. S. (1981). *Int. J. Radiat. Oncol. Biol. Phys.,* in press.

Israel, L., and Chahinian, A. P., eds. (1976). ''Lung Cancer. Natural History, Prognosis, and Therapy.'' Academic Press, New York.

Isselbacher, K. L., Adams, R. D., Braunwald, E., Petersdorf, R. G., and Wilson, J. D., eds. (1980). ''Harrison's Principles of Internal Medicine,'' 9th Ed. McGraw-Hill, New York.

Kotalik, J. F. (1981). *Cancer Treat. Rev.* **8,** 127.

Kovacs, C. J., Hopkins, H. A., Evans, M. J., and Looney, W. B. (1976). *Int. J. Radiat. Biol.* **30,** 101.

Kovacks, C. J., Evans, M. J., and Hopkins, H. A. (1977). *Cell Tissue Kinet.* **10,** 245.

Kovi, E., and Morris, H. P. (1976). *Adv. Enzyme Regul.* **14,** 139.

Kurmar, V., Ben-Ezra, J., Bennett, M., and Sonnenfeld, G. (1979). *J. Immunol.* **123,** 1832.

LaGrange, P. H., Mackanesa, G. B., and Miller, T. E. (1974). *J. Exp. Med.* **139,** 1529.

Lando, Z., Teitelbaum, D., and Arnon, R. (1979). *J. Immunol.* **123,** 2156.

Lerman, S. P., and Weidanz, W. P. (1970). *J. Immunol.* **105,** 614.

Looney, W. B., Hopkins, H. A., and Trefil, J. S. (1978). *In* ''Advances in Expermental Medicine and Biology'' (H. P. Morris and W. E. Criss, eds.), Vol. 92, p. 677. Plenum, New York.

Looney, W. B., Ritenour, E. R., and Hopkins, H. A. (1980). *Cancer Res.* **40,** 2179.

Looney, W. B., Ritenour, E. R., and Hopkins, H. A. (1981a). *Cancer* **47,** 860.

Looney, W. B., Longerbeam, M. B., and Hopkins, H. A. (1981b). *Int. J. Radiat. Oncol. Biol. Phys.,* in press.

McNally, N. J. (1973). *Br. J. Radiol.* **46,** 450.

Malaise, E. P., Charbit, A., Chavaudra, N., Combes, P. F., Douchez, J., and Tubiana, M. (1972). *Br. J. Cancer* **26,** 43.

Man-San, S., Bach, B. A., Dohi, Y., Nisonoff, A., Benecreaff, B., and Greene, M. I. (1979). *J. Exp. Med.* **150,** 1216.

Meyer, K. K. (1970). *Arch. Surg.* **101,** 114.

Mitsuoka, A., Baba, M., and Morikawa. (1976). *Nature (London)* **262,** 77.

Moore, J. V., Hopkins, H. A., and Looney, W. B. (1980). *Cell Tissue Kinet.* **13,** 53.

Muggia, F. M., and Rozencweig, M., eds. (1979). ''Progress in Cancer Research and Therapy,'' Vol. 11. Raven, New York.

Mukherji, B., and Mukhopadhyay, M. (1980). *In* ''Radiation—Drug Interactions in the Treatment of Cancer'' (G. H. Sokal and R. P. Maickel, eds.), pp. 155–174. Wiley, New York.

Order, S. E., Klein, J. L., Ettinger, D., Alderson, P., Siegelman, S., and Leichner, P. (1980). *Int. J. Radiat. Oncol. Biol. Phys.* **6**, 703.

Puccetti, P., Santoni, A., Riccardi, C., and Herberman, R. B. (1980). *Int. J. Cancer* **25**, 153.

Riccardi, C., Santoni, A., Barlozzari, T., Puccetti, P., and Herberman, R. B. (1980). *Int. J. Cancer* **25**, 475.

Roder, J. C., and Haliotis, T. (1980). *Immunol. Today* **1**, 96.

Rowley, R., Hopkins, H. A., Betsill, W. L., Jr., Ritenour, E. R., and Looney, W. B. (1980). *Br. J. Cancer* **42**, 586.

Sarna, G., ed. (1980). "Practical Oncology." Houghton, Boston, Massachusetts.

Schabel, Jr., F. M., Griswold, Jr., D. P., Corbett, T. A., Laster, Jr., W. R., Mayo, J. G., and Lloyd, H. H. (1979). *In* "Methods in Cancer Research" (H. Busch and V. DeVita, Jr., eds.), Vol. 17, p. 3. Academic Press, New York.

Simpson-Herren, L., Sanford, A. H., and Holmquist, J. P. (1974). *Cell Tissue Kinet.* **7**, 349.

Slavin, R. E., Millan, J. C., and Mullins, G. M. (1975). *Human Pathol.* **6**, 693.

Steel, G. G. (1977). "Growth Kinetics of Tumors," p. 258. Oxford Univ. Press (Clarendon), London and New York.

Stephens, T. C., and Steel, G. G. (1980). *In* "Radiation Biology in Cancer Research" (Meyn and Withers, eds.), p. 385. Raven, New York.

Stewart, C. C., and Perez, C. A. (1976). *Radiology* **118**, 201.

Suit, H. D., Howes, A. E., and Hunter, N. (1977). *Radiat. Res.* **72**, 440.

Thomlinson, R. H. (1973). *Br. Med. Bull.* **29**, 29.

Thomlinson, R. H., and Craddock, E. A. (1967). *Br. J. Cancer* **21**, 108.

Thomlinson, R. H., and Gray, L. H. (1955). *Br. J. Cancer* **9**, 539.

Trefil, J. S., Schaffner, J. G., Looney, W. B., and Hopkins, H. A. (1978). *In* "Methods in Cancer Research" (H. Busch, ed.), Vol. XIV, Ch. VIII, p. 325. Academic Press, New York.

Tubiana, M. (1971). *Br. J. Radiol.* **44**, 325.

Tubiana, M. (1977). *In* "Recent Advances in Cancer Treatment" (H. J. Tagnon and M. J. Staquet, eds.), p. 69. Raven, New York.

Tubiana, M., and Malaise, E. P. (1979). *In* "Lung Cancer: Progress in Therapeutic Research" (F. Muggia and M. Rozencweig, eds.), p. 51. Raven, New York.

Tubiana, M., Richard, J. M., and Malaise, E. (1975). *Laryngoscope* **6**, 1039.

Twentyman, P. R. (1977). *Br. J. Cancer* **35**, 208.

Urano, M., and Suit, H. D. (1971). *Radiat. Res.* **45**, 41.

Van Peperzeel, H. A. (1972). *Eur. J. Cancer* **8**, 665.

Wampler, G. L., Carter, W. H., Jr., and Williams, V. R. (1978). *Cancer Treat. Rep.* **62**, 333.

Welin, S. (1963). *Am. J. Roentgenol. Radium Ther. Nucl. Med.* **90**, 673.

Wepsic, H. T., Nickel, R., and Alaimo, J. (1976). *Cancer Res.* **36**, 246.

Wiernik, G., Bleehen, N. M., Brindle, J., Bullimore, J., Churchill-Davidson, I. F. J., Davidson, J., Fowler, J. F., Francis, P., Hadden, R. C. M., Haybittle, J. L., Howard, N., Lansley, I. F., Lindup, R., Phillips, D. L., and Skeggs, D. (1978). *Br. J. Radiol.* **51**, 241.

Withers, H. R. (1975). *In* "Advances in Radiation Biology," Vol. V, p. 241. Academic Press, New York.

Wyandt, H., Shah, H., Hopkins, H. A., and Looney, W. B. (1981). (In preparation).

Zaalberg, O. B., van der Meul, V. A., and Rossi, G. (1973). *Eur. J. Immunol.* **3**, 698.

CHAPTER IX

IN VITRO IMMUNIZATION AS A METHOD FOR GENERATING CYTOTOXIC CELLS POTENTIALLY USEFUL IN ADOPTIVE IMMUNOTHERAPY

MARGALIT B. MOKYR AND SHELDON DRAY

I. Introduction

Over the past two decades several groups of investigators have clearly demonstrated the role of cell-mediated immunity in tumor rejection (as reviewed by Old and Boyse, 1964; Sjogren, 1965; Klein, 1966; Rosenberg and Terry, 1977). This stimulated attempts to employ tumor-immune lymphocytes in adoptive immunotherapeutic trials, but disappointingly these were only rarely successful in the therapy of established tumors and only when large numbers of lymphoid cells ($>1 \times 10^8$) from hyperimmune donors were used (Delorme and Alexander, 1964; Alexander and Delorme, 1971; Borberg *et al.*, 1972). Thus, methods to augment the therapeutic ability of lymphoid cells had to be developed if lymphoid cells were to be effective in adoptive immunotherapy of tumors. As a result, considerable interest has developed in evaluating the therapeutic potential of *in vitro* immunized lymphoid cells. The potential advantages of utilizing *in vitro* immunized cells rather than *in vivo* immunized cells for therapeutic purposes are as follows: (1) the level of cell-mediated tumor lysis produced is significantly higher (7- to 10-fold) (Berke *et al.*, 1971; Bernstein, 1977); (2) antigens which are weakly immunogenic *in vivo* can evoke high levels of cell-mediated tumor lysis upon *in vitro* immunization (Berke *et al.*, 1971); (3) the risks involved in immunizing hosts with malignant cells are eliminated; and (4) a more rapid generation of cytotoxicity occurs (5 days) (Burton *et al.*, 1975; Mokyr *et al.*, 1978).

Any approach aimed at utilizing *in vitro* immunized lymphoid cells for therapeutic purposes must be based on the use of proper methods for generation and evaluation of antitumor activity as well as the use of an appropriate source of responder lymphoid cells and stimulator tumor cells. Therefore, in this chapter we will review the following aspects: (1) the critical factors for the success of *in vitro* immunization; (2) the optimal source of responder and stimulator cells; (3) methods to potentiate the antitumor activity of *in vitro* immunized cells; (4) methods to screen *in vitro* immunized cells for their immunotherapeutic potential; and (5) the advantages of using *in vitro* immunized lymphoid cells as an adjunct to chemotherapy. For some other aspects of cell-mediated immunity induced *in vitro*, the reader is referred to a review by Kedar and Weiss (1982).

II. Description of the Method for *in Vitro* Immunization of Lymphoid Cells with Tumor Cells and the Critical Technical Factors for Its Success

The method for *in vitro* generation of cytotoxic lymphoid cells was first described in 1968 by Ginsburg for a xenogeneic system in which rat lymphocytes responded to stimulating mouse fibroblasts. Subsequently, Wunderlich and Canty (1970) reported the *in vitro* generation of allogeneic antitumor cytotoxicity. The method has since been modified and employed extensively for the generation of allogeneic (as reviewed by Feldman *et al.*, 1972; Wagner *et al.*, 1973; Engers and MacDonald, 1976) and syngeneic (Rollinghoff and Wagner, 1973; Burton *et al.*, 1975; Kedar *et al.*, 1976; Bernstein *et al.*, 1976) antitumor cytotoxicity. Several investigators have defined the optimal conditions for the generation of primary (Burton *et al.*, 1975; Kedar *et al.*, 1976) or secondary (Bernstein *et al.*, 1976; Cheever *et al.*, 1977) cellular antitumor responses. From these studies it became clear that the important factors for a successful *in vitro* immunization include the following: (1) the concentration of 2-mercaptoethanol (2-ME), (2) the percentage of macrophages, (3) the batch of fetal calf

TABLE I

EXPERIMENTAL CONDITIONS REQUIRED FOR GENERATION OF ANTITUMOR
CYTOTOXICITY FOLLOWING *in Vitro* IMMUNIZATION OF LYMPHOID
CELLS WITH TUMOR CELLS

Parameter	Experimental conditions
2-ME concentration	1×10^{-5} to 1×10^{-4} M
Marcophage percentage	At least 3%
FCS concentration	5 to 20%
Density of lymphoid cells	1×10^6/ml to 3×10^6/ml
R/S ratio	2.5/1 to 100/1
Duration of immunization	4 to 9 days

serum (FCS), (4) the ratio of responder lymphoid cells to stimulator tumor cells (R/S ratio), and (5) the duration of the immunization process.

In general, *in vitro* immunization is performed by cocultivating lymphoid cells with inactivated tumor cells in tissue culture flasks (Kedar *et al.*, 1976), tubes (Kedar *et al.*, 1976), trays (Burton *et al.*, 1975), or petri dishes (Schechter *et al.*, 1976) at 37°C in humidified atmosphere of 5% CO_2 in air. Various tissue culture media have been employed successfully including Eagle's minimal essential medium (Wagner *et al.*, 1973), Dulbecco's modified Eagle's medium (Burton *et al.*, 1975; Plata *et al.*, 1975), and Roswell Park Memorial Institute Medium 1640 (Bernstein *et al.*, 1976; Kedar *et al.*, 1976; Mokyr *et al.*, 1978). The tissue culture media used is supplemented by 1×10^{-5} to 1×10^{-4} M 2-ME and 5 to 20% FCS. In most of these studies, the tumor cells employed were (1) immunogenic leading to the generation of high levels of antitumor cytotoxicity without the need to modify them so as to augment their immunogenicity, and (2) susceptible to rapid *in vitro* lysis by cytotoxic cells thereby allowing the use of a 3 to 6 hour ^{51}Cr release assay for quantitation of the level of antitumor cytotoxicity obtained.

The experimental conditions required for successful *in vitro* immunization of rodent lymphoid cells are summarized in Table I. The concentration of 2-ME is critical for the generation of antitumor cytotoxicity, and cytotoxicity is not obtained when its concentration is higher than 1×10^{-3} or lower than 1×10^{-6} (Burton *et al.*, 1975; Kedar *et al.*, 1976). Pierce *et al.* (1974) attributed the activity of 2-ME to its ability to replace part of the function of macrophages in allowing for better survival of lymphocytes in culture. More recently Harris *et al.* (1976) showed that 2-ME increases the differentation of precursor cells into cytotoxic cells. The presence of 2-ME in the culture medium on the last day of the *in vitro* immunization led to the development of levels of cytotoxicity similar to that obtained in cultures containing 2-ME throughout the entire immunization period (Harris *et al.*, 1976). When 2-ME was added on the last day of the immunization, slight augmentation in the cytotoxic activity was obtained as early as 4 hours after its addition and did not require DNA synthesis but the major increase in cytotoxic activity was obtained 12 to 24 hours after its addition and required DNA synthesis. Nevertheless, only a minor increase in the total number of lymphoid cells was observed suggesting that the cell division induced by 2-ME is limited to only a few precursor cells (Harris et al., 1976).

Macrophages were found to be essential for the induction phase of allogeneic (Wagner et al., 1973) and syngeneic (Igarashi et al., 1979; Mokyr et al., 1979a; Ting et al., 1979) antitumor cytotoxicity. Depletion of macrophages from normal spleen cells by surface adherence resulted in diminished generation of cytotoxic activity (Wagner et al., 1973; Mokyr et al., 1979a). Subjection of spleen cells to both antimacrophage serum and depletion of glass-adherent cells resulted in total abolition of their capacity to generate antitumor cytotoxicity; however, restoration was achieved by addition of peripheral macrophages (Wagner et al., 1973). One of the functions attributed to macrophages in the in vitro immunization process is presentation of antigenic material to lymphocytes in an immunogenic form (Treves, 1978). Incubation of lymphocytes on a monolayer of tumor antigen fed macrophages, for at least 4 days, was shown to result in the generation of antitumor cytotoxicity (Treves et al., 1976b; Treves, 1978).

The presence of serum in the culture medium is essential for the in vitro generation of antitumor cytotoxicity (Burton et al., 1975; Kedar et al., 1976). Most frequently FCS is used although sera from other sources such as human or mouse (Engers and MacDonald, 1976) have also been used. The minimal concentration of FCS required may vary from one tumor system to another. For example, 5% FCS was required for the MOPC-11 (Burton et al., 1975) or MOPC-315 (Mokyr et al., 1978) plasmacytomas whereas 15 to 20% was required for the EL4 lymphoma (Kedar et al., 1976). Different batches of FCS might have varying effects on the level of cytotoxicity obtained and/or activate lymphoid cells nonspecifically in the absence of stimulator tumor cells. Thus, investigators might have to screen sera and select the "appropriate" ones (Wagner et al., 1973).

The density of lymphoid cells employed also affects the outcome of in vitro immunization. Although a high density tends to facilitate immunization, the density used is limited by the availability of nutrients. The density of lymphoid cells which has been used ranged between 1×10^6 and 3×10^6 cells per ml (Burton et al., 1975; Kedar et al., 1976; Mokyr et al., 1978), but should be determined for each experimental system. In most studies, stimulator cells are tumor cells that were inactivated either by X-irradiation or mitomycin C. The dose of radiation or drug used is selected so that it will render the stimulator cells unresponsive without interfering with its ability to stimulate the generation of cytotoxic cells. The relative effectiveness of irradiated or mitomycin C-treated cells might vary from one system to another and this might account for the conflicting results found in the literature (Hodes and Terry, 1974). The responder/stimulator cell ratio (R/S) is also critical for the achievement of optimal immunization and might vary with the tumor system. For example, the optimal R/S ratio for the generation of syngeneic antitumor cytotoxicity was 2.5/1 for the EL4 lymphoma (Kedar *et al.*, 1976), 30/1 for the Gross virus induced lymphoma (C58NT)D (Bernstein *et al.*, 1976) or the MOPC-315 plasmacytoma (Mokyr *et al.*, 1978), and 100/1 for the MOPC-11 plasmacytoma (Burton *et al.*, 1975) or mammary adenocarcinoma 13762A (Kuperman *et al.*, 1975a). The reason for these differences in the optimal R/S ratio in the various tumor systems is unknown. However, it might reflect differences in the density of surface tumor antigens, metabolism of these antigens, inhibitory factors released by the tumor cells, and/or differences in the ability of lymphoid cells from different animals to respond.

The optimal duration of the *in vitro* immunization process may vary from 4 days (Schechter *et al.*, 1976) to 8 days (Plata *et al.*, 1975) for the generation of primary or secondary syngeneic antitumor cytotoxicity. Increasing or decreasing the duration of the *in vitro* immunization even by 1 day can result in a sharp drop in the level of antitumor cytotoxicity obtained (Fig. 1).

Thus far we have discussed how to evaluate the optimal conditions for the generation of antitumor cytotoxicity. However, it should be emphasized that when *in vitro* immunizations are performed in the same tumor system, by the same investigators, and under the same optimal conditions they still might result in the generation of substantially different (up to 2-fold) levels of antitumor cytotoxicity (Burton *et al.*, 1975; Mokyr *et al.*, 1980). These fluctuations in the level of cytotoxicity obtained might be attributed in part to differences in the composition of the tumor cells em-

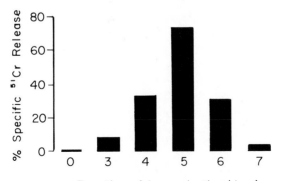

FIG. 1. The dependency of the level of antitumor cytotoxicity obtained on the duration of the *in vitro* immunization. Normal BALB/c spleen cells (75×10^6) were cultured for 3 to 7 days with mitomycin C-treated MOPC-315 tumor cells (2.5×10^6) at the end of which the spleen cells were evaluated for their anti-MOPC-315 cytotoxicity in the 4 hour ^{51}Cr release assay at an effector/target cell ratio of 100/1

ployed either as stimulator or as target cells [e.g., early vs late stages of tumor growth (Russell *et al.*, 1978), ratio of metastatic to nonmetastatic cells (Fogel *et al.*, 1979; Schirrmacher *et al.*, 1979), or ratio of adherent to nonadherent tumor cells (Fortner *et al.*, 1975)] as well as the composition of the lymphoid cells employed as responder cells [e.g., the relative number of macrophages (Igarashi *et al.*, 1979; Mokyr *et al.*, 1979a) or helper T cells (Pilarski, 1979)].

The method used in our laboratory for the *in vitro* immunization of spleen cells against syngeneic tumor cells is outlined below.

1. *Preparation of responder lymphoid cells.* Spleens from BALB/c mice are placed in petri dishes containing Eagle's minimal essential medium (MEM). Spleen cells suspensions are prepared by gently squeezing the spleens between the rough edges of two sterile glass slides, allowing clumps to settle. The cells are washed three times in MEM and the viability as determined by trypan blue dye (0.4%) always exceeds 95%.

2. *Preparation of stimulator tumor cells.* MOPC-315 plasmacytoma tumors are maintained by serial subcutaneous inoculations in syngeneic BALB/c mice. Single cell suspensions are prepared in RPMI-1640 medium by mechanical disruption between glass slides. The red blood cells are lysed by addition of a few (2–5) ml of water to the cell pellets followed by rapid addition of a large volume (~ 45 ml) of RPMI-1640. The viability of the tumor cells as determined by trypan blue dye (0.4%) always exceeds 85%. The tumor cells are inactivated by incubating 2×10^6 cells/ml with 50 μg/ml mitomycin C for 30 minutes at 37°C. At the end of the incubation period the cells are washed four times.

3. *Setting up immunization cultures.* Responder spleen cells (75×10^6) are mixed with stimulator tumor cells (2.5×10^6) in 250-ml tissue culture flasks in a final volume of 50 ml RPMI-1640 medium supplemented with 5% fetal calf serum, 1% nonessential amino acids, 50 U/ml penicillin, and 50 μg/ml streptomycin. Fresh medium is prepared on the day of the experiment and 2-mercaptoethanol is added to give a final concentration of 10^{-4} M prior to use. Cultures are incubated upright for 5 days at 37°C in humidified atmosphere of 5% CO_2 in air.

III. Potential Applicability of *in Vitro* Immunized Lymphoid Cells for Adoptive Immunotherapy

A. SELECTION OF THE OPTIMAL SOURCE OF RESPONDER LYMPHOID CELLS

In recent years, several investigators have employed the *in vitro* immunization technique to generate cytotoxicity in lymphoid cells against allogeneic (Kedar *et al.*, 1978c) or syngeneic (Rollinghoff and Wagner, 1973;

Burton and Warner, 1977; Kedar *et al.*, 1978c; Mokyr *et al.*, 1978) tumor cells with the hope of using these lymphoid cells in immunotherapeutic regimens. Although both allogeneic and syngeneic *in vitro* immunized lymphoid cells were effective in preventing tumor growth *in vivo* in the local adoptive transfer assay (Winn assay) (Winn, 1959), the use of allogeneic cells for therapy of tumor-bearing animals poses some problems. To produce a therapeutic effect, adoptively transferred cells must persist in the recipient for several days (Fefer, 1970; Fefer *et al.*, 1976). However, if the infused cells differ from the recipient at the major histocompatibility complex, they will be eliminated from the circulation and not be able to adoptively transfer immunity (Fefer, 1970; Kende *et al.*, 1975; Fefer *et al.*, 1976). Survival of allogeneic transferred cells can be extended by immunosuppression of the tumor-bearing recipient, resulting in graft-vs-host responses which are difficult to control (Elkins, 1971; Fefer *et al.*, 1976). The use of lymphoid cells from donors with close similarity of histocompatibility antigens with the recipient will reduce the severity of the graft-vs-host reaction and facilitate the survival of *in vitro* immunized infused cells. However, for potential application to humans, the use of cells with similarity of histocompatible antigens is severely limited by the availability of cells from closely matched donors.

Due to the limitations of employing *in vitro* immunized allogeneic lymphoid cells for adoptive immunotherapy, several investigators have evaluated the potential usefulness of *in vitro* immunized syngeneic lymphoid cells from normal (Rollinghoff and Wagner, 1973; Burton and Warner, 1977; Kedar *et al.*, 1978c; Mokyr *et al.*, 1978), tumor-immune (Bernstein *et al.*, 1976; Bernstein, 1977; Cheever *et al.*, 1977, 1978; Fernandez-Cruz *et al.*, 1979), or tumor-bearing (Treves *et al.*, 1975, 1976a; Mokyr *et al.*, 1978, 1979a) animals. These studies revealed that although *in vitro* immunized spleen cells from normal animals are able to suppress tumor growth *in vivo* in the local adoptive transfer assay, they have either no effect, or only marginal effect when administered systemically to animals just prior to (Bernstein, 1977), or shortly after (Burton and Warner, 1977; Kedar *et al.*, 1978c) the injection of tumor cells. On the other hand, *in vitro* immunized spleen cells from tumor-immune animals are able to suppress tumor growth both in the local adoptive transfer assay and when administered systemically to animals prior to the injection of tumor cells (Bernstein, 1977), 1 day following (Cheever *et al.*, 1977, 1978) the injection of tumor cells, or even later when the animals bore 1.0 to 1.5 cm tumors (Fernandez-Cruz *et al.*, 1979). Regardless of the systemic antitumor activity of *in vitro* immunized lymphoid cells from tumor-immune animals, such an approach is not applicable for human immunotherapy due to the unavailability of either normal or tumor-immune syngeneic donors of lymphoid cells. It seems, therefore, that the potential usefulness of the *in vitro* immunization technique for human immunotherapy would depend on the ability to successfully immunize the tumor bearer's own lymphoid cells.

Our efforts in the past 4 years were directed toward finding methods to augment the level of antitumor cytotoxicity exhibited by tumor-bearer spleen cells following *in vitro* immunization. Before we describe our main findings we would like to emphasize that other groups of investigators have subjected tumor-bearer lymphoid cells to *in vitro* immunization. However, the few studies that were successful in generating antitumor cytotoxicity employed spleen cells obtained from tumor bearers at early stages of tumor growth (Kuperman *et al.*, 1975b; Treves *et al.*, 1975, 1976a; Takei *et al.*, 1976; Schirrmacher *et al.*, 1979), whereas we and Mills and Paetkau (1980) were successful in obtaining high levels of antitumor cytotoxicity with spleen cells from terminal tumor bearers (Mokyr *et al.*, 1979a,b; Przepiorka *et al.*, 1980). We worked mainly on spleen cells from BALB/c mice bearing various sizes of MOPC-315 plasmacytomas. Mice were injected sc with 1×10^6 to 3.5×10^6 tumor cells, a dose which leads to progressively growing tumors that kill the mice in about 21 days. Spleen cells from MOPC-315 tumor-bearing mice are not cytotoxic at any stage of tumor growth. Following *in vitro* immunization, the tumor-bearer spleen cells can mount an antitumor cytotoxic response. The level of antitumor cytotoxicity exhibited by *in vitro* immunized tumor-bearer spleen cells is dependent on tumor size. *In vitro* immunized spleen cells from mice bearing small size tumors (up to 15 mm) exhibit similar levels of antitumor cytotoxicity as do *in vitro* immunized spleen cells from normal mice. On the other hand, *in vitro* immunized spleen cells from mice bearing larger size tumors (20 mm or more) exhibit reduced levels of antitumor cytotoxicity such that *in vitro* immunized spleen cells from mice at terminal stages of tumor growth are virtually noncytotoxic. This reduced ability of *in vitro* immunized spleen cells from terminal tumor-bearing mice to mount antitumor cytotoxicity is not due to an inappropriate R/S ratio (Mokyr *et al.*, 1979a), an inappropriate duration of *in vitro* immunization (Mokyr *et al.*, 1978), or altered culture conditions [such as depletion of nutrients or release of toxic substances by cultured cells (Mokyr *et al.*, 1979b)] but rather to the presence of suppressor elements in the spleen (Mokyr *et al.*, 1979a,b) that can inhibit the generation and/or the expression of antitumor cytotoxicity. Removal of the suppressor elements from suspensions of tumor-bearer spleen cells by depletion of glass-adherent cells enabled the remaining glass-nonadherent spleen cells to behave like tumor-immune cells in the generation of *in vitro* antitumor cytotoxicity upon *in vitro* immunization (Fig. 2). Thus far we have not evaluated the ability of *in vitro* immunized, glass-nonadherent spleen cells from terminal tumor-bearing mice to mediate systemic antitumor immunity. However, if these cells prove to be as effective as *in vitro* immunized

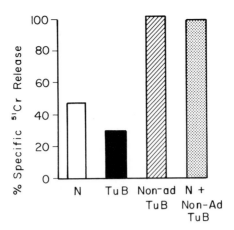

Fig. 2. Removal of suppressor cells from the spleens of tumor bearers enables the remaining cells to mount a secondary type antitumor cytotoxic response upon *in vitro* immunization. MOPC-315 tumor-bearer spleen cells were depleted of suppressor cells by fractionation on glass wool columns prior to their *in vitro* immunization for 5 days with MOPC-315 tumor cells. Seventy-five million normal (N), unfractionated (TuB), or glass-nonadherent (Non-ad TuB) tumor-bearer spleen cells as well as a mixture of N + Non-ad TuB at a ratio of 1/1 were immunized *in vitro* and subsequently tested for their anti-MOPC-315 cytotoxicity in the ^{51}Cr release assay at an effector/target cell ratio of 100/1. Depletion of glass-adherent cells from normal spleen cells reduced their ability to generate anti-MOPC-315 cytotoxicity upon *in vitro* immunization and resulted in 24% specific ^{51}Cr release.

spleen cells from tumor-immune animals in mediating systemic antitumor immunity, tumor-bearer spleen cells might be an ideal source of lymphoid cells for adoptive immunotherapy.

In the search for an optimal source of tumor-bearer lymphoid cells for use in therapy of tumor-bearing animals, we evaluated the ability of pooled lymph node cells to mount antitumor cytotoxicity following *in vitro* immunization. As seen with *in vitro* immunized spleen cells (Mokyr *et al.*, 1978), the level of antitumor cytotoxicity exhibited by *in vitro* immunized lymph node cells is also dependent on tumor size. At most stages of tumor growth tested, the level of antitumor cytotoxicity exhibited by *in vitro* immunized lymph node cells did not differ substantially from that exhibited by *in vitro* immunized spleen cells. Since it appears that tumor-bearer lymph node cells are similar to tumor-bearer spleen cells in their ability to generate antitumor cytotoxicity following *in vitro* immunization and since it is much less complicated to obtain a large number of spleen cells than of lymph node cells, spleen cells seem to be a better source of lymphoid cells for adoptive immunotherapy experiments at least in the MOPC 315 tumor system. It should be emphasized, however, that we evaluated the antitumor potential of pooled lymph node cells and not of cells obtained from lymph node(s) which are draining the site of the tumor as compared with cells from distant lymph nodes which might differ substantially.

Although *in vitro* immunized, autochthonous, lymphoid cells appear to be desirable for use in adoptive immunotherapy, they might not be available in sufficient numbers. This problem might be overcome by recently introduced methods to propagate large numbers of tumor-specific cytotoxic lymphocytes through the use of growth factors (interleukin 2) obtained from supernatants of mitogen stimulated spleen cells (Gillis and Smith 1977; Gillis *et al.*, 1978a,b; Nablholz *et al.*, 1978; Strausser and Rosenberg, 1978; Rosenberg *et al.*, 1978b). Gillis and Smith (1977) have shown that by addition of growth factors it is possible to propagate murine cytotoxic lymphocytes *in vitro* for periods of more than 4 months without the loss of cytotoxic activity. Continued proliferation of cytotoxic cells is dependent on the presence of growth factors since the cells die within 48 hours if switched to fresh medium not containing growth factors or to fresh medium supplemented with Con A (Gillis *et al.*, 1978b; Rosenberg *et al.*, 1978b). The cytotoxic cells can grow in culture about 10-fold every 5 to 7 days (Rosenberg *et al.*, 1978a,b). Thus, it might be useful to expand cytotoxic cells *in vitro* and administer them repeatedly in large numbers to tumor bearers thereby increasing the potential effectiveness of the adoptively transferred cells for immunotherapy. Thus far, there are limited reports in which long-term cytotoxic cells were used successfully in adoptive immunotherapy. Cheever *et al.* (1981) were able to prolong the survival of tumor-bearing mice when lymphoid cells cultured *in vitro* for 19 days were used as an adjunct to chemotherapy. These investigators did not test cells cultured for longer periods since a "crisis" occurs after 4 to 5 weeks (Watson, 1979) in which the growth rate falls off and many cells die, and although several weeks later the cells recover with the resumption of a rapid growth rate, a drift in the cell population might occur.

B. Selection of the Optimal Source of Stimulator Tumor Cells

One explanation for the limited success of *in vitro* immunized lymphoid cells in immunotherapy (Burton and Warner, 1977; Kedar *et al.*, 1978c) is that the primary tumor site might not be the optimal source of stimulator tumor cells for the *in vitro* generation of antitumor cytotoxicity since antigenic differences have been demonstrated between tumor cells obtained from primary tumor site and those obtained from metastatic deposits (Sugarbaker and Cohen, 1972; Faraci, 1974; Fogel *et al.*, 1979; Pimm and Baldwin, 1977; Schirrmacher *et al.*, 1979). The importance of this concept is nicely illustrated in the Lewis lung carcinoma (3LL) system (Fogel *et al.*, 1979). Lymphoid cells immunized *in vitro* against tumor cells from the local site of injection (L-3LL) were more cytotoxic *in vitro* to L-3LL target cells than to tumor cells from the metastatic site (M-3LL), whereas lymphocytes immunized against M-3LL were more cytotoxic to M-3LL than to L-3LL. More importantly, only lymphoid cells immunized against M-3LL were able to inhibit lung metastases after inoculation of either M-3LL or L-3LL in a local adoptive transfer assay (Fogel *et al.*, 1979).

IV. Effect of Responder Cell Composition on the Level of Antitumor Cytotoxicity Obtained upon *in Vitro* Immunization

A. T Lymphocytes

Many studies have illustrated the central requirement for T lymphocytes in the initiation and consummation of *in vitro* cellular antitumor responses (for review see Wagner *et al.*, 1973). Therefore, some attempts to augment the antitumor cytotoxicity generated upon *in vitro* immunization were aimed at heightening the frequency of (pre-)cytotoxic T lymphocytes. Such an approach has been tried successfully by Wagner *et al.* (1973) who found that splenic T cells purified by the method of Basten *et al.* (1972) as well as cortisone-resistant thymocytes (Wagner *et al.*, 1972) were enriched for precursors of cytotoxic lymphocytes; following *in vitro* immunization, these cells exhibited up to 20-fold greater antitumor cytotoxicity than that of *in vitro* immunized unfractionated spleen cells or *in vitro* immunized thymocytes from untreated hosts.

Another approach that might be useful in augmenting the antitumor potential of responder lymphoid cells is the removal of suppressor cells that might interfere with the generation and/or the expression of antitumor cytotoxicity. When suppressor T cells are present, one would not use antithymocyte serum and complement (C') to lyse them since the potentially cytotoxic cells are also T cells. Furthermore, in mice, both the suppressor and cytotoxic cells are Ly23 positive (Boyse and Cantor, 1977; Hardt *et al.*, 1980). Recently, some suppressor T cells were shown to possess surface markers recognized by anti-I-J (subregion of Ia) antiserum (Okumura *et al.*, 1976; Tada *et al.*, 1976; Levy *et al.*, 1979; and reviewed by Germain and Benacerraf, 1980). Elimination of suppressor T cells, while leaving the cytotoxic potential intact, was accomplished by absorption with anti-I-J or by treatment with anti-I-J and C' (Levy *et al.*, 1979).

An alternative method used successfully to separate suppressor and cytotoxic T cells present in the spleens of mice at late stages of Lewis lung carcinoma (3LL) growth is fractionation by velocity sedimentation (Small and Trainin, 1976). The suppressor cells were immature T cells whereas the cytotoxic ones were mature T cells. When these two subpopulations were mixed, only enhancement of tumor growth was manifested. Schechter *et al.* (1977) employing the same tumor system, were able to separate the two subpopulations of T cells by the use of affinity chromatography on histamine/rabbit serum albumin/Sepharose. The adherent fraction was enriched for enhancing activity, whereas the nonadherent fraction was depleted of enhancing activity and exhibited anti-3LL cytotoxicity.

The antitumor potential of responder lymphoid cells can also be augmented by treatment of the cell donors with cyclophosphamide (CY) (Bonavida, 1977b; Glaser, 1979; Hengst *et al.*, 1980, 1981). The timing of CY administration is critical for its success. Administration of CY prior to immunization with allogeneic (Bonavida, 1977b) or syngeneic (Glaser, 1979) tumor cells was shown to result in nonspecific elimination of suppressor T cells leading to the development of stronger antitumor responses than that exhibited by untreated, immunized counterparts. On the other hand, administration of CY to animals 2 to 6 days after immunization was shown to result in the elimination of antigen stimulated prekiller or killer cells or induction of suppressor cells thereby leading to the development of weaker antitumor responses than that exhibited by immunized, untreated counterparts. In these studies, the effect of administration of CY to animals later than 6 days after immunization was not evaluated. However, since CY kills dividing cells, it might be possible that its administration at later stages, when the cytotoxic potential is fully developed and is being reduced by actively proliferating suppressor cells, will result in elimination of suppressive activity while leaving the cytotoxic potential intact. Indeed, administration of (15 mg/kg) CY to mice bearing 20–25 mm MOPC-315 tumors resulted in elimination of suppressor elements in the spleens and following *in vitro* immunization of the spleen cells they developed a "secondary type" antitumor cytotoxic response (Hengst *et al.*, 1980).

B. MACROPHAGES

Studies concerning the regulation of immune responses have revealed that the balance between immunostimulation and immunosuppression can be subject to the action of macrophages (Allison, 1978). The nature of this regulation appears to be dependent on the ratio of macrophages to immunocompetent lymphocytes; low ratios augment the response of puri-fied lymphocytes while high ratios suppress their response (Mokyr and Mitchell, 1975; Pellis *et al.*, 1977; Wing and Remington, 1977).

It is relatively easy to eliminate suppression mediated by macrophages. However, one should be careful not to reduce the concentration of active macrophages below that needed for an effective *in vitro* immunization (Wagner *et al.*, 1973; Mokyr *et al.*, 1979a). If it happens, a low concentra-tion of normal macrophages should be added back to allow an effective *in vitro* immunization. The methods used to eliminate suppression mediated by macrophages are based on the adherence or phagocytic properties of the cells. Adherence to petri dishes was used extensively in the late 1960s and early 1970s to remove macrophages (Mosier, 1967). However, this method is not used much now since in order to deplete most of the macro-phages present in spleen cell suspensions, the spleen cells must undergo a few cycles of adherence (Mokyr and Mitchell, 1975). Instead, the adher-ent cells are usually depleted by fractionation on columns of glass beads (Yoshinaga *et al.*, 1972) or glass wool fibers (Kirchner *et al.*, 1974). By fractionation on glass wool columns, we reduced the percentage of mac-rophages present in the spleens of MOPC-315 tumor bearers from 23% to less than 4% (Mokyr *et al.*, 1979a). The yield of cells recovered from such columns is rather low and usually ranges between 15 and 30% (Yoshinaga *et al.*, 1972; Kirchner *et al.*, 1974; Mokyr *et al.*, 1979a). Fractionation by the aid of carbonyl iron and magnet (Kirchner *et al.*, 1974) is at least as effective as fractionation on glass columns in depleting macrophages from tumor-bearer spleen cells. The yield of recovered cells is much higher (70% with MOPC-315 tumor-bearer spleen cells). Elimination of sup-pression mediated by macrophages can also be accomplished by inactiva-tion of the cells either *in vivo* (by treating the donor of lymphoid cells) (Ting *et al.*, 1979), or *in vitro* (Kirchner *et al.*, 1975) prior to setting up *in vitro* immunization cultures. Selective inactivation of macrophages with-out obvious impairment of B or T lymphocyte functions can be achieved by the use of silica (Allison *et al.*, 1966), carrageenan (Kirchner *et al.*, 1975; Ting *et al.*, 1979) or trypan blue (Hibbs, 1975). Recently, macro-phages have been identified as the primary source of prostaglandins (Humes *et al.*, 1977), a family of membrane-derived hydroxylated fatty acids that can exert potent immunosuppressive effects on a variety of im-mune functions (Gordon *et al.*, 1976; Pelus and Strausser, 1977). There-fore, researchers attempted to abolish the suppressive activity of macro-phages by inhibiting prostaglandin synthesis. Inhibition of prostaglandin was accomplished by indomethacin and resulted in augmentation in the responsiveness of lymphocytes from mice bearing a variety of transplant-able tumors to mitogenic stimulation (Pelus and Strausser, 1976).

C. Metastatic Tumor Cells

If tumor cells have metastasized into the lymphoid organs, the intact tumor cells or free antigens shed by them into the culture may interfere with the generation and/or expression of antitumor cytotoxicity (Bonavida, 1974; Baldwin and Price, 1976; Mokyr *et al.*, 1979b). The method to be used to remove metastatic tumor cells depends on the nature of the cells. For glass-adherent tumor lines, the cells obtained from the lymphoid organ can be incubated on glass petri dishes for a few hours or overnight and then the nonadherent cells can be used for *in vitro* immunization. However, not all tumor cell lines are glass adherent in culture and other means for their removal should be sought. For example, although MOPC-315 tumor cells are not glass adherent, most tumor cells present in MOPC-315 tumor-bearer spleens can be removed by fractionation on glass wool columns (Mokyr *et al.*, 1979b). It is not clear whether the tumor cells are being removed because they are too big to pass through the glass wool fibers or because they bind to lymphoid cells which adhere to the glass wool. Another method to remove the MOPC-315 tumor cells from tumor-bearer spleen cell suspensions is fractionation on DNP–lysine–Sepharose since the tumor cells possess high affinity surface IgA with specificity for nitrophenyl compounds (Mokyr *et al.*, 1979b). Indeed, removal of most tumor cells from tumor-bearer spleens enabled the spleen cells to exhibit augmented levels of antitumor cytotoxicity following *in vitro* immunization (Mokyr *et al.*, 1979b).

D. Several Types of Suppressor Cells

In some tumor systems, more than one type of suppressor cell is present (Elgert and Farrar, 1978; Pope *et al.*, 1978; Mokyr *et al.*, 1979b,c). To reveal the full cytotoxic potential of lymphoid cells, elimination of all suppressor elements is required. For example, in the MOPC-315 tumor system, metastatic tumor cells, an increased percentage of macrophages, and possibly suppressor T cells are present in the spleens of terminal tumor-bearing mice and are responsible for the reduced ability of the spleen cells to mediate antitumor cytotoxicity following *in vitro* immunization. Partial recovery of antitumor potential of tumor-bearer spleen cells was achieved by depletion of either tumor cells, by fractionation on DNP–lysine–Sepharose, or macrophages, by carbonyl iron and magnet. Depletion of glass-adherent cells from tumor-bearer spleens included removal of most tumor cells and macrophages, and resulted in much greater antitumor potential than that of tumor-bearer spleen cells subjected to fractionation on DNP–lysine–Sepharose, carbonyl iron and magnet, or even carbonyl iron and magnet followed by fractionation on DNP–lysine–Sepharose. These results suggest that in addition to metastatic tumor cells and an increased percentage of macrophages, another type of glass-adherent suppressor cell operates in the spleens of terminal MOPC-315 tumor-bearing mice. In light of Folch and Waksman's (1973) observation that T cells, which inhibit the response of normal rat spleen cells to supraoptimal doses of mitogen are removed by glass adherence, it is possible that the additional type of suppressor cell in the MOPC-315 tumor system is a suppressor T cell. Fractionation on glass wool is presumed to be effective in removing three different types of suppressor cells from spleens of terminal MOPC-315 tumor-bearing mice thereby allowing the nonadherent cells to respond to *in vitro* immunization in a manner similar to a secondary response.

V. Potentiation of Antitumor Cytotoxicity Generated upon *in Vitro* Immunization

A. Administration of Immunomodulators to Spleen Cell Doners

The responsiveness of lymphoid cells can be increased by *in vivo* administration of nonspecific stimulants to lymphoid cells donors. One of such stimulants is Bacillus Calmette–Guérin (BCG) which was chosen by several investigators as a means for augmenting the level of antitumor cytotoxicity obtained by *in vitro* immunization since it is known to augment the *in vivo* generation of antitumor cytotoxicity (Hawrylko and Mackaness, 1973; Mitchell *et al.*, 1973; Hawrylko, 1977). Substantial augmentation of the level of antitumor cytotoxicity (as compared to that exhibited by *in vitro* immunized spleen cells from untreated donors) was observed by us (Braun *et al.*, 1978) when normal BALB/c mice were injected ip with 1×10^6 to 5×10^7 BCG Phipps strain prior to *in vitro* immunization of their spleen cells. On the other hand, suppression of antitumor cytotoxicity was observed by Bennett *et al.* (1978) and by Klimpel and Henney (1978), when C57BL/6 mice were injected iv with 2×10^7 BCG Tice strain or ip with 1×10^8 BCG Pasteur strain prior to *in vitro* immunization of their spleen cells with allogeneic P815 tumor cells. Joint studies by Bennett, Mitchell, and us (Mokyr *et al.*, 1980) revealed that the discrepancy in the effect of BCG pretreatment on the *in vitro* generation of antitumor cytotoxicity cannot be attributed to differences between the tumor systems used (syngeneic vs allogeneic) but rather to differences between BCG vaccines used. In addition, differences between the ability of different batches of the same strain of BCG to augment the antitumor potential of

spleen cells were found. These unpredictable effects of BCG clearly demonstrate the need for screening of the vaccines for augmenting capacity
before their injection into tumor-bearing hosts. Furthermore, when BCG
is injected into tumor-bearing hosts its effect on *in vivo* antitumor immunity should be monitored to find out whether it leads to inhibition or enhancement of tumor growth. If there is a correlation between the effect of
BCG on the *in vivo* and *in vitro* potential, the effect of BCG pretreatment
on the *in vitro* generation of antitumor cytotoxicity might also be a useful
method in screening vaccines for their potential in immunotherapy.

Employing an augmenting batch of BCG, we evaluated the effect of
BCG injection into mice bearing various sizes of MOPC-315 tumors on
the antitumor potential of their spleen cells (Fig. 3). The spleen cells were
obtained from the mice 14 days posttumor inoculation, at a stage when
following *in vitro* immunization spleen cells from untreated tumor-bearing
mice exhibit reduced levels of antitumor cytotoxicity as compared to the
level exhibited by *in vitro* immunized spleen cells from normal mice
(Mokyr *et al.*, 1978). Treatment of tumor-bearing mice with BCG on day 3
or 7 posttumor inoculation (day 11 or 7 prior to *in vitro* immunization) led
to greater augmentation than that obtained when mice were treated with
BCG at later stages of tumor growth (shorter intervals between BCG
treatment and *in vitro* immunization). Still, treatment of tumor-bearing
mice even 2 days prior to *in vitro* immunization, at a stage when the mice
were bearing 15–20 mm tumors, led to augmented levels of antitumor cytotoxicity. In addition, the cytotoxicity exhibited by *in vitro* immunized
spleen cells from BCG-treated tumor-bearing mice developed earlier and
persisted longer than that exhibited by *in vitro* immunized spleen cells
from untreated tumor-bearing mice.

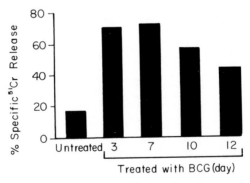

FIG. 3.   The effect of treating mice with BCG on various days posttumor inoculation on
the ability of their spleen cells to mount an *in vitro* antitumor cytotoxic response following *in
vitro* immunization. BALB/c mice were injected ip with 2×10^7 BCG Phipps strain on days
3, 7, 10, or 12 posttumor inoculation. Spleen cells were collected on day 14 posttumor inoculation and immunized *in vitro* with MOPC-315 tumor cells for 5 days.

B. ADDITION OF IMMUNOMODULATORS TO IMMUNIZATION
   CULTURES

BCG has been reported to exert immunostimulatory effects on lymphoid cells *in vitro* (Mokyr and Mitchell, 1975). Therefore, researchers were hopeful that addition of BCG to *in vitro* immunization cultures will lead to the generation of augmented levels of antitumor cytotoxicity. Indeed, Weiss' group was able to obtain augmented levels of antitumor cytotoxicity when a methanol-extraction residue of BCG Phipps strain (MER) was added to the immunization culture of C57BL/6 spleen cells and EL4 tumor cells (Weiss *et al.*, 1976; Kedar *et al.*, 1978a). However, not all batches of MER tested had an augmenting capacity (Kedar *et al.*, 1978a). This observation is not surprising in light of our findings that different batches of viable BCG Phipps strain might have opposite effects on the *in vitro* generation of syngeneic antitumor cytotoxicity (Mokyr *et al.*, 1980). Thus, it might be desirable to evaluate the augmenting capacity of the intact organism before extracting MER from it.

Another nonspecific stimulant that was employed successfully to augment the level of antitumor cytotoxicity generated *in vitro* is concanavalin A (Con A). Addition of suboptimal or optimal mitogenic concentration of Con A to immune lymphocytes and allogeneic stimulator tumor cells resulted in augmentation in the level of secondary antitumor responses (Bonavida, 1977a). Furthermore, addition of Con A to lymphocytes immune to allogeneic tumor cells led to the development of antitumor cytotoxicity with specificity for the priming antigens (Bonavida, 1977a). Con A activation of a secondary cytotoxic response resembles the activation of a specific secondary response by lymphocyte-defined antigens which does not require homology with the priming lymphocyte-defined antigens (Alter *et al.*, 1976). Thus far, the effect of Con A addition to *tumor-bearer* spleen cells on their antitumor response has not been evaluated. However, since tumor-bearer spleen cells are primed to tumor antigens, it might be possible to trigger a secondary response when Con A is added in the absence of additional stimulator cells or to augment the secondary response when Con A is added in the presence of stimulator cells. The possible need to remove suppressor elements from tumor-bearer spleens in order to see any effect with Con A should be considered.

There is a striking similarity between Con A activity for *tumor-immune* spleen cells and the activity of polyethylene glycol 6000 (PEG) for *tumor-bearer* spleen cells (Fig. 4) (Przepiorka *et al.*, 1980). Addition of 2% PEG to *in vitro* immunization cultures of MOPC-315 tumor-bearer spleen cells resulted in augmentation of specific antitumor cytotoxicity. Furthermore, addition of PEG to tumor-bearer spleen cells cultured in the absence of

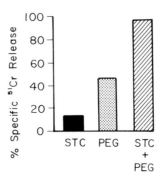

FIG. 4. Effect of addition of 2% PEG to MOPC-315 tumor-bearer spleen cells cultured in the presence or absence of MOPC-315 stimulator tumor cells (STC) on the level of *in vitro* antitumor cytotoxicity obtained.

added stimulator tumor cells resulted in the development of substantial levels of specific antitumor cytotoxicity. The exact mode of action of PEG is not known; however, it is not mediated via a direct toxic effect for suppressor elements present in tumor-bearer spleen cells (Przepiorka, Mokyr, and Dray, manuscript in preparation). The number of lymphocytes recovered from cultures of spleen cells in the presence of 2% PEG was about 2-fold greater than that recovered from cultures in its absence, probably due to better survival of splenic lymphocytes or to their proliferation. The increase in the number of lymphocytes might have resulted in a drop in the concentration of suppressive elements below suppressing levels, thus allowing the expression of existing antitumor cytotoxicity and the generation of cytotoxic activity in response to metastatic tumor cells.

Recently, Mills and Paetkau (1980) were able to augment the level of anti-P815 cytotoxicity generated by *in vitro* immunized spleen cells from DBA/2 mice bearing P815 tumors by addition of Con A induced interleukin 2 to the immunization culture. Augmentation was observed even at late stages of tumor growth (day 25 tumor bearers) when ~20% of the nucleated cells in the spleen were P815. The kinetics of generation of anti-P815 cytotoxicity by tumor-bearer spleen cells immunized *in vitro* with P815 tumor cells in the presence of interleukin 2 was similar to that exhibited by spleen cells from normal mice immunized under the same conditions; namely, it peaked at day 5 to 6 and declined rapidly thereafter. The level of cytotoxicity obtained by spleen cells from tumor-bearing mice was much higher (~10-fold) than that obtained by spleen cells from normal mice and was similar to that generated by DBA/2 spleen cells against allogeneic tumor cells. Such *in vitro* immunized tumor-bearer spleen cells were also effective in killing P815 tumor cells *in vivo* (Mills *et al.*, 1980).

The nonspecific stimulants discussed are by no means the only ones used to augment the *in vitro* generation of antitumor cytotoxicity. Other stimulants such as polysaccharides of the β (1–3) glucan type (Hamuro *et al.*, 1978) or supernatants from secondary mixed leucocyte cultures (Ryser *et al.*, 1979) have been used successfully. However, none of them has been evaluated for its effectiveness in augmenting the cytotoxicity generated *in vitro* by tumor-bearer spleen cells.

C. MODIFICATION OF STIMULATOR TUMOR CELLS

To heighten the immunogenicity of tumor cells, cells have been subjected to chemical or enzymatic modifications. Such modifications include (1) introduction of new haptenic groups (such as TNP) onto the cell surface resulting in either the appearance of completely new antigenic determinants or the formation of immunogenic self-modified groups (Shearer, 1974); (2) cleavage of terminal sialic acid residues by neuraminidase to unmask cryptic antigenic determinants (Ray and Simmons, 1973); (3) mild proteolytic digestion to expose hidden antigenic determinants (Tarro, 1973).

When modified tumor cells are employed as stimulator cells for the *in vitro* immunization process, it has to be established that the cytotoxicity generated is also effective against unmodified tumor cells. Kedar and Lupu (1978) modified mouse leukemia EL4 or RBL-5 of C57BL/6 origin as well as YAC of A origin with different agents that have the above effects. The modified tumor cells were superior to the unmodified cells when used as stimulator cells for the *in vitro* generation of antitumor cytotoxicity and led to the development of augmented levels of antitumor cytotoxicity against the unmodified tumor cells. The authors emphasized that the same modifying agent had markedly variable effects at different concentrations for different tumor cells; doses which were optimal for increasing the immunogenicity of one tumor were sometimes unsatisfactory for another, or even lowered their immunizing capacity. We used the same modifying agents as Kedar and Lupu (1978), namely, 2,4,6-trinitrobenzene sulfonic acid, iodoacetamide, neuraminidase, or trypsin to modify MOPC-315 plasmacytoma cells for use as stimulator cells. Although large ranges of concentrations were used for each agent, augmented levels of antitumor cytotoxicity were not obtained (Hengst, Mokyr, and Dray, unpublished observations). Thus, some modifying agents effective in some tumors may not be effective in others, probably due to differences in the immunogenicity of the unmodified cells.

VI. Methods to Screen *in Vitro* Immunized Lymphoid Cells for Their Immunotherapeutic Potential

Although many studies have demonstrated that immune lymphoid cells can inhibit tumor growth *in vivo* (for review see Rosenberg and Terry, 1977), a few studies have shown that under certain conditions immune lymphocytes can enhance tumor growth (Prehn, 1972; Jeejeebhoy, 1974; Small and Trainin, 1976; Pellis *et al.*, 1978). These observations illustrate the need for a reliable method to screen immune lymphoid cells for their *in vivo* antitumor potential since their administration to tumor-bearing hosts might not only be without therapeutic effect, but actually have a harmful effect by facilitating tumor growth. Much effort was focused on developing *in vitro* methods to evaluate the antitumor cytotoxicity of immune lymphoid cells which included both short (3 to 6 hour) and longer (24 to 72 hour) term assays. The commonly used 3 to 6 hour ^{51}Cr release assay (Brunner *et al.*, 1970) is applicable to tumor lines which (1) incorporate sufficient amount of ^{51}Cr, (2) exhibit low spontaneous release, and (3) exhibit high sensitivity to rapid lysis (Herberman, 1974). This assay measures the presence of cytotoxic T cells (Leclerc *et al.*, 1973) or natural killer cells (Silva *et al.*, 1980). The ^{51}Cr release assay is not reliable with target cells requiring at least overnight incubation since extensive spontaneous release occurs (Cerottini and Brunner, 1974). Thus, the ^{51}Cr release assay is not applicable to tumor lines which are more resistant to lysis, or lines which require longer periods of incubation to manifest lysis (Herberman, 1974). When such tumor lines are employed, other assays might be suitable to evaluate the antitumor cytotoxicity of immune lymphoid cells. These assays include visual (Takasugi and Klein, 1970) or isotope counting of the target cells remaining at the end of the assay. The latter technique utilizes target cells prelabeled with radioactive thymidine (Perlman and Holm, 1969; Jagarlamoody *et al.*, 1971), ^{125}IUdR (Cohen *et al.*, 1972), or radioactive amino acids such as [^{3}H]proline (Bean *et al.*, 1973). In addition, the terminal labeling technique was developed to enumerate the remaining viable target cells after incubation with cytotoxic lymphoid cells. In this technique, incorporation of labeled precursors usually correlated with cell count and is advantageous since changes in the rate of protein or DNA synthesis were recorded long before changes in cell number (Schechter *et al.*, 1976).

Once *in vitro* methods for evaluating antitumor cytotoxicity were established, investigators compared the *in vitro* cytotoxic activity of immune lymphoid cells with their *in vivo* activity in tumor rejection. The *in vivo* assay most commonly used was the local adoptive transfer assay (Winn, 1959), in which the immune lymphocytes were mixed with tumor cells and the mixture was injected into susceptible recipients. In a few studies, a good correlation between *in vitro* assays and the local adoptive transfer assay was found (Rouse *et al.*, 1972; 1973; Kedar *et al.*, 1978c). For example, Kedar *et al.*, (1978c) observed that allogeneic and syngeneic EL4-immune lymphoid cells which exhibited strong *in vitro* cytotoxicity also exhibited strong *in vivo* neutralizing activity in the local adoptive transfer assay, whereas lymphoid cells which exhibited poor *in vitro* cytotoxicity also exhibited poor *in vivo* activity. In most studies, such a correlation between *in vitro* and *in vivo* antitumor activity was not found (Howell *et al.*, 1974; Burton and Warner, 1977; Mokyr *et al.*, 1978). For example, Burton and Warner (1977) evaluated the antitumor activity of BALB/c spleen cells immunized *in vitro* against MPC-11 plasmacytoma cells and presented results of eight different experiments illustrating that "there was no situation" in which the *in vitro* cytotoxicity as measured in the ^{51}Cr release assay could be clearly correlated with *in vivo* neutralizing activity in the local adoptive transfer assay.

Most investigators also failed to establish a correlation between the *in vitro* antitumor activity of *in vitro* immunized lymphoid cells and the ability of the cells to transfer systemic antitumor immunity (Glaser *et al.*, 1976; Bernstein, 1977; Burton and Warner, 1977; Treves, 1978). For example, lymphoid cells which were highly cytotoxic *in vitro* were only marginally effective *in vivo* in conferring systemic immunity (Burton and Warner, 1977). On the other hand, in some experiments, lymphoid cells which were not cytotoxic *in vitro* were very effective in conferring systemic immunity (Bernstein, 1977; Treves, 1978). Thus, there is inconsistency between the ability of immune lymphoid cells to exhibit *in vitro* antitumor cytotoxicity and to transfer local or systemic antitumor immunity. Perhaps, different populations of cells are responsible for *in vitro* and for *in vivo* antitumor activity. In addition, the *in vivo* activity of adoptively transferred lymphoid cells might depend on their ability to recruit host cells which can then participate in the immune response. Indeed, the effectiveness of adoptively transferred cells in conferring antitumor immunity was shown to depend on the ability of the host to develop an immune response against tumor antigens (Alexander *et al.*, 1966; Cohen, 1973; Treves *et al.*, 1979).

Since it appears that the above *in vitro* assays cannot be used to screen lymphoid cells for their ability to confer immunity *in vivo*, investigators evaluated whether lymphoid cells which are capable of neutralizing tumor growth *in vivo* in the local adoptive transfer assay will also be effective in transferring systemic antitumor immunity. In some experiments, lymphoid cells with strong antitumor activity in the local adoptive transfer assay were only marginally effective in conferring systemic antitumor immunity (Burton and Warner, 1977; Kedar *et al.*, 1978c). These differences in the activity of lymphoid cells as measured by the two assays indicate that in order to transfer systemic antitumor immunity it is not enough to have cells capable of mediating local antitumor immunity. Perhaps, the cells also need to reach the tumor foci. Thus, evaluation of the migratory pattern of adoptively transferred lymphoid cells might aid in predicting their therapeutic potential. this can be done by labeling immune lymphoid cells free of erythrocytes with $Na_2[^{51}CrO_4]$ (^{51}Cr) and injecting the labeled cells iv into animals which received sc injections of tumor cells at least 24 hours earlier (Zatz and Lance, 1970). The distribution of ^{51}Cr-labeled cells was shown to provide a useful index for the assessment of recirculating lymphocytes in various lymphoid compartments (Zatz and Lance, 1970; Gillette and Bellanti, 1973). Furthermore, cells immune to a given antigen have the tendency to home to lymph nodes draining the same antigen but not to lymph nodes draining another antigen (Durkin and Thorbecke, 1972). However, in order to obtain a significant increase in the homing of immune lymphoid cells to lymph nodes draining the specific antigen, administration of the lymphoid cells has to be delayed for at least 24 hours to allow enough drainage of the antigen into the lymph nodes (Zatz, 1971). In spite of the apparent importance of the homing pattern of lymphoid cells to predict their therapeutic potential, such experiments have not been done. Therefore, it is necessary to determine whether lymphoid cells, which are both capable of mediating local antitumor immunity and show an increased tendency to home to lymph nodes draining the site of tumor injection, will consistently be effective in conferring systemic antitumor immunity.

Some disappointing results regarding the future of *in vitro* immunized lymphoid cells for immunotherapy were obtained when the rate of clearance of such adoptively transferred cells from the blood of normal recipients was evaluated. Normal lymphoid cells, which were cultured *in vitro* in the absence of stimulator tumor cells (Kedar *et al.*, 1978b) or immunized *in vitro* against allogeneic (Rouse and Wagner, 1973) or syngeneic (Burton and Warner, 1977; Kedar *et al.*, 1978b) tumor cells prior to their iv injection into recipient animals, were rapidly lost from the blood and 2 to 20 hours later two-thirds of the cells were found in the liver and lung as compared to one-third or less for freshly prepared lymphoid cells. The *in vitro* cultured lymphoid cells that were present in the liver did not recirculate and probably represented cells that were so altered by the *in vitro* culture conditions that they were destroyed (Rouse and Wagner, 1973). In spite of the fast elimination of a substantial portion of *in vitro* immunized lymphoid cells, several studies demonstrated that *in vitro* reimmunized tumor-immune lymphoid cells were quite effective in mediating systemic antitumor immunity (Bernstein, 1977; Cheever *et al.*, 1977, 1978; Fernandez-Cruz *et al.*, 1979) and in certain systems even *in vitro* immunized normal lymphoid cells exhibited some effectiveness (Treves *et al.*, 1975, 1976). It is possible therefore, that the remaining infused, *in vitro* immunized, lymphoid cells which are not cleared into the lung or liver are capable of reaching the tumor foci and mediating strong antitumor immunity.

VII. Advantages of Utilizing *in Vitro* Immunized Lymphoid Cells as an Adjunct to Cytostatic Therapy for the Eradication of Established Tumors

The effectiveness of adoptively transferred *in vitro* immunized cells for the therapy of tumor bearers is limited by its inability to cope with a large tumor load. In most studies even *in vitro* reimmunized tumor immune lymphoid cells were effective in mediating systemic antitumor immunity only when administered at most 1 day following inoculation of tumor cells (Bernstein, 1977; Cheever *et al.*, 1977). On the other hand, chemotherapy and radiation therapy can destroy a large tumor load but are limited by their nonspecific activity against the host's normal tissues and surgical therapy can be used to remove tumor from the primary site but not from metastatic sites. Therefore, adoptive immunotherapy might be beneficial as an adjunct to cytostatic therapy for specific eradication of residual tumor cells which otherwise might result in the host's death. Thus far only a few reported studies have employed *in vitro* immunized lymphoid cells in conjunction with cytostatic therapy. In these studies, the cytostatic therapy used was surgical removal of primary tumors in the 3LL system (Treves *et al.*, 1975, 1976) or cyclophosphamide (CY) administration to tumor bearers in the following tumor systems: FBL-3, Friend leukemia of C57BL/6 origin (Cheever *et al.*, 1977, 1978); EL4, a chemically induced lymphoma of C57BL/6 origin (Kedar *et al.*, 1978b); YAC, leukemia induced by Moloney virus in strain A mice (Kedar *et al.*, 1978b); and LSTRA, Moloney virus-induced leukemia of BALB/c origin (Cheever *et al.*, 1981). The timing of tumor excision (day 7 tumor bearers) by Treves *et al.* (1975, 1976) was such that it cured some of the mice (45%) while the others died of lung metastasis. When tumor excision was followed by administration of *in vitro* immunized normal spleen cells, a significantly larger proportion of the animals were cured (71%). The dose of CY used by Fefer's group (Cheever *et al.*, 1977, 1978) for treatment of mice inoculated 5 days earlier with FBL-3 was such that it extended the survival of the mice (from 14 days to 4–8 weeks), but was not curative. *In vitro* reimmunized immune spleen cells, when administered to tumor bearers 6 hours post CY therapy, were able to cure up to 73% (16/22) of the mice. Kedar *et al.* (1978b) confirmed Fefer's results in the EL4 and YAC tumor systems. Treatment of tumor-bearing mice (day 1 or 3 tumor bearers) with CY followed by administration of *in vitro* immunized spleen cells cured a significantly larger proportion of the mice (80–100%) than either CY or *in vitro* immunized cells alone (20–60 and 5–15%, respectively). More recently, Fefer's group (Cheever *et al.*, 1981) extended their observations with chemoimmunotherapy to the LSTRA tumor system. We evaluated the effectiveness of chemoimmunotherapy for treatment of MOPC-315 tumor-bearing mice. CY was employed since this drug (1) is known to exert potent antitumor effects in plasmacytoma tumor systems (Ogawa *et al.*, 1973; Lubet and Carlson, 1977); (2) might render the remaining tumor cells more susceptible to immune lysis (Borsos *et al.*, 1976); and (3) disappears from the plasma of mice within a few hours of its administration (Brock, 1976; Kline *et al.*, 1968), and therefore will not kill *in vitro* immunized cells administered several hours after drug treatment. Our initial experiments were designed to determine the dose of CY which extends the survival of tumor bearers but is not curative. Unlike the FBL-3 and LSTRA tumor systems, in which administration of 180 mg/kg of CY was required to extend the survival of day 5 tumor bearers (Cheever *et al.*, 1977, 1981), for the MOPC-315 tumor system administration of 35 mg/kg of CY substantially extended the survival of day 5 tumor bearers (from 21 days to 5–8 weeks). When CY therapy was followed by adoptive immunotherapy with *in vitro* immunized lymphoid cells, a substantial percentage of the mice (40%) were tumor-free 60 days after the initiation of the therapy (when the experiments were terminated).

Although *in vitro* immunized lymphoid cells facilitated the effectiveness of CY therapy for mice at early stages of tumor growth, they might not do so at advanced stages of tumor growth. Progression of tumor growth is associated with the appearance of suppressor elements which might block the infused *in vitro* immunized lymphoid cells from reaching the tumor foci or from inhibiting tumor growth. Therefore, before intervention with adoptive immunotherapy at late stages of tumor growth, it is necessary not only to reduce the tumor burden but also to eliminate suppressor elements. Initially the effect of CY therapy was evaluated on the survival time of mice bearing various sizes of MOPC-315 tumors (Fig. 5). Paradoxically, CY therapy is increasingly more effective with progression of tumor growth such that a dose of drug (15 mg/kg) which just extended the survival of mice bearing nonpalpable tumors (day 4 tumor bearers) was curative for most mice bearing 10 to 25 mm tumors (day 8 to 16 tumor bearers) (Hengst *et al.*, 1980). The ineffectiveness of CY therapy in curing mice bearing nonpalpable tumors was not due to tumor load but rather to

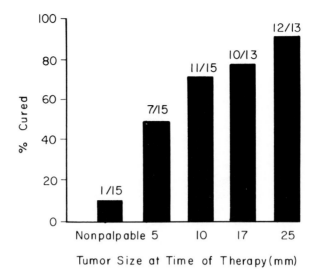

FIG. 5. Effectiveness of cyclophosphamide (15 mg/kg intraperitoneally) for curing BALB/c mice bearing various sizes of MOPC-315 tumors. Mice free of primary tumors 60 days posttherapy were considered to be cured. Numbers above bars represent number of mice cured per number of mice treated.

time interval between tumor inoculation and CY therapy. This was evident from experiments in which the time interval between tumor inoculation and CY therapy of mice bearing nonpalpable tumors was increased to 12 days by lowering the number of tumor cells used for inoculation from 3.5×10^6 to 0.1×10^6; the time interval of 12 days was required for the generation of optimal levels of anti-MOPC-315 cytotoxicity. During the course of CY therapy of mice bearing larger size MOPC-315 tumors, suppressor elements are eliminated allowing the expression of existing *in vivo* antitumor immunity (Fig. 6). Spleen cells obtained from such mice even 2 days following CY therapy responded *in vitro* to stimulator tumor cells in a manner similar to a secondary response. Furthermore, the antitumor potential of such spleen cells could not be augmented by subjecting them to glass wool fractionation prior to *in vitro* immunization, a procedure which was shown to be effective in eliminating suppressor cells from the spleen of untreated tumor-bearing mice (Mokyr *et al.*, 1979a,b). The antitumor immunity expressed by such CY-treated tumor-bearing mice can act synergistically with the CY cytotoxic effect in the eradication of tumor cells. The ability of an active antitumor response to facilitate the action of CY has been reported by others (Moore and Williams, 1973; Radov *et al.*, 1976; Chassoux *et al.*, 1978; Lubet and Carlson, 1978). CY was more effective when administered to tumor-bearing animals that ex-

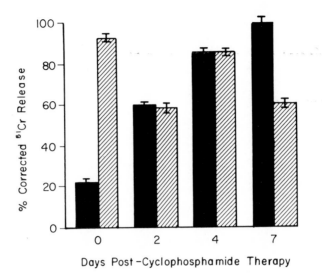

FIG. 6. Cyclophosphamide therapy of MOPC-315 tumor-bearing mice leads to elimination of suppressor cells within 2 days. BALB/c mice bearing 24 mm tumors were injected ip with 15 mg/kg cyclophosphamide and 2, 4, or 7 days later their spleens were excised and single-cell suspensions prepared. Unfractionated (solid bars) or glass wool fractionated (hatched bars) spleen cells were immunized *in vitro* with MOPC-315 tumor cells for 5 days and subsequently tested for their antitumor cytotoxicity in the ^{51}Cr release assay.

hibited some antitumor immunity due to previous immunization than to unimmunized counterparts (Moore and Williams, 1973; Chassoux *et al.*, 1978). Furthermore, CY treatment of tumor bearers that were immunosuppressed [by antithymocyte serum (Radov *et al.*, 1976; Greenberg *et al.*, 1980), X-irradiation (Radov *et al.*, 1976; Lubet and Carlson, 1978), or high doses of drug (Mathe *et al.*, 1977)] has been reported to be less effective than treatment of immunocompetent tumor bearers. Our results illustrate the importance of the timing of CY administration to tumor bearers for successful therapy. CY should be administered at a stage when the cytotoxic potential is well developed and the suppressive activity is developing in order to obtain both reduction of tumor burden and elimination of suppressor cells. Experiments should be performed to determine if these features of CY action are limited to the MOPC-315 tumor system or they can be extended to other tumor systems.

The success of the therapy of animals at early stages of tumor growth by CY administration in conjunction with adoptively transferred immune cells is probably dependent on the ability of the recipient tumor-bearing animals to mount an antitumor response. The need for a recipient antitumor response might be illustrated by the finding of Fefer's group

(Greenberg *et al.*, 1980) in the FBL-3 tumor system. Administration of CY to day 5 tumor bearers reduced the concentration of metastatic tumor cells in the spleen below detectable levels and 5 days passed before metastatic tumor cells were again detectable. When mice were subjected to combined CY and adoptive immunotherapy there was recurrence of metastatic tumor cells in the spleen 15–25 days after therapy. However, the recurrence was transient and metastatic tumor cells were no longer detectable by day 45. The delay in the recurrence of metastatic tumor cells in the spleens of mice subjected to the combined modalities (as compared to recurrence in spleen of mice subjected to CY alone) was attributed to the antitumor activity mediated by the infused immune cells. The later antitumor activity which led to eradication of tumor cells and left 90% of the mice tumor free 150 days posttherapy might have been mediated by recipient antitumor activity. Thus, it appears that the role of adoptively transferred immune cells is to extend the period of time in which the concentration of tumor cells is low allowing the recipient to develop a strong antitumor immunity that can cope with the remaining tumor cells. Repeated injections of immune lymphoid cells with strong antitumor activity might provide the recipient tumor bearer with a longer period of time to develop immunity and/or a smaller tumor burden to handle. Adoptive transfer of immune cells was not needed to aid the effect of CY in the therapy of mice bearing large size MOPC-315 tumors since CY abolished the suppressor elements and the cytotoxic cells regained antitumor activity within 2 days posttherapy (Hengst *et al.*, 1980). This rapid appearance of antitumor activity was possible in the MOPC-315 tumor system, since some of the suppression is at the level of expression of antitumor activity or at late stages of maturation of cytotoxic cells (Mokyr *et al.*, 1979b). However, when suppressor cells inhibit at earlier stages of the development of antitumor immunity even if the chemotherapy eliminates the suppressor activity, it might take too long for an active antitumor immunity to develop, and by that time the tumor burden might be too large for it to handle. In such cases administration of *in vitro* immunized lymphoid cells as an adjunct to chemotherapy might be desirable in order to keep the tumor cells under control long enough for the development of *in vivo* antitumor immunity.

VIII. Summary

The technique of *in vitro* immunization by cocultivation with stimulator tumor cells has been used extensively for the generation of cytotoxic lymphoid cells with the hope of using these cells for immunotherapeutic regimens. The advantages of utilizing *in vitro* immunized lymphoid cells compared to *in vivo* immunized cells include: (1) the level of cell-mediated cytotoxicity produced is significantly higher; (2) antigens which are weakly immunogenic *in vivo* can evoke high levels of cell-mediated cytotoxicity upon *in vitro* immunization; (3) the risks involved in immunizing hosts with malignant cells are eliminated; and (4) a more rapid generation of cytotoxicity occurs. The success of an *in vitro* immunization culture depends on the (1) presence of 1×10^{-5} to 1×10^{-4} M 2-ME, (2) presence of at least 3% macrophages, (3) use of an "appropriate" batch of FCS, (4) appropriate ratio of responder/stimulator cells, and (5) appropriate duration of the process.

In order for *in vitro* immunized lymphoid cells to be effective in adoptive immunotherapy they have to persist in the recipient for several days and implement a potent antitumor response. An ideal source of such lymphoid cells is the tumor-bearer's own cells since they are not only histocompatible but also primed to tumor antigens and upon *in vitro* immunization can mount a secondary type antitumor cytotoxic response.

To facilitate the use of *in vitro* immunized lymphoid cells for adoptive immunotherapy, investigators have searched for means to augment the antitumor cytotoxicity exhibited by the cells. One approach was aimed at altering the composition of responder lymphoid cells by increasing the frequency of (pre-)cytotoxic T lymphocytes and removing suppressor cells. The method used for removal of the suppressor elements depends on their nature. Suppression by T cells may be eliminated by the use of anti-I-J serum, fractionation by velocity sedimentation, adherence to histamine–rabbit serum albumin–Sepharose, or treatment of spleen cell donors with CY. Suppression by macrophages may be eliminated if they are removed by glass adherence or carbonyl iron and magnet or inactivated by silica, carrageenan, trypan blue, or indomethacin. Other methods to potentiate the antitumor cytotoxicity generated upon *in vitro* immunization include the following: (1) administering immunostimulants such as BCG to lymphoid cell donors; (2) adding immunostimulants such as BCG, PEG, Con A, or interleukin 2 to immunization cultures; and (3) heightening the immunogenicity of stimulator tumor cells by chemical or enzymatic modifications.

There is a need for a reliable method to screen immune lymphoid cells for their *in vivo* antitumor potential since their administration into tumor-bearing hosts might not only be without therapeutic effect, but actually have a harmful effect by facilitating tumor growth. The *in vitro* cytotoxicity assays cannot serve this role since in most cases there is no correlation between the cytotoxic activity of lymphoid cells *in vitro* and their ability to transfer local or systemic antitumor immunity. Furthermore, in some cases lymphoid cells capable of mediating strong local antitumor immunity are only marginally effective in conferring systemic antitumor immunity. To confer systemic antitumor immunity, it is not enough to have cells capable of mediating local antitumor immunity; the cells also have to reach the tumor foci. It appears therefore that evaluation of both the migratory patterns of lymphoid cells and their ability to mediate local antitumor immunity will provide valuable information for screening lymphoid cells for their therapeutic potential.

The effectiveness of adoptively transferred, *in vitro*, immunized lymphoid cells for the therapy of tumor bearers is limited by its inability to cope with a large tumor load which is due in part to the limited numbers of cytotoxic cells available. By the establishment of cultures of cytotoxic cells that continuously proliferate *in vitro* in the presence of growth factors, the cytotoxic cells could then be administered repeatedly in large numbers and thereby might increase the potential effectiveness of adoptively transferred cells for immunotherapy. Adoptive immunotherapy might be still more effective as an adjunct to cytostatic therapy. Chemotherapeutic drugs may not only reduce tumor burden but also render the remaining tumor cells more susceptible to immune lysis and/or eliminate suppressor elements while leaving the cytotoxic potential intact. The success of chemoimmunotherapy depends also on the ability of the recipient tumor bearer to mount an antitumor response. It appears, therefore, that the role of adoptively transferred immune cells is to extend the period of time in which the concentration of tumor cells is low, allowing the recipient to develop strong antitumor immunity to cope with the remaining tumor cells.

ACKNOWLEDGMENTS

This work was supported by NIH Grant PHS CA-26480. The authors wish to acknowledge the contributions of James Hengst, Donald Braun, and Donna Przepiorka to the various phases of the research in our laboratory and the invaluable technical assistance of Kathy Siessmann.

REFERENCES

Alexander, P., and Delorme, E. J. (1971). *Isr. J. Med. Sci.* **7**, 239–245.

Alexander, P., Delorme, E. J., and Hall, J. G. (1966). *Lancet* **1**, 1186–1189.

Allison, A. C. (1978). *Immunol. Rev.* **40**, 3–27.

Allison, A. C., Harrington, J. S., and Birbeck, M. (1966). *J. Exp. Med.* **124**, 141–153.

Alter, B. J., Grillot-Courvalin, C., Bach, M. L., Zier, K. S., Sondel, P. M., and Bach, F. H. (1976). *J. Exp. Med.* **143**, 1005–1014.

Baldwin, R. W., and Price, M. R. (1976). *Annu. Rev. Med.* **27**, 151–163.

Basten, A., Sprent, J., and Miller, J. F. A. P. (1972). *Nature (London) New Biol.* **225**, 178–180.

Bean, M. A., Pees, H., Rosen, G., and Oettgen, H. F. (1973). *Natl. Cancer Inst. Monogr.* **37**, 41–48.

Bennett, J. A., Rao, S., and Mitchell, M. S. (1978). *Proc. Natl. Acad. Sci. U.S.A.* **75**, 5142–5144.

Berke, G., Clark, W. R., and Feldman, M. (1971). *Transplantation* **12**, 237–248.

Bernstein, I. D. (1977). *J. Immunol.* **118**, 122–128.

Bernstein, I. D., Wright, P. W., and Cohn, E. (1976). *J. Immunol.* **116**, 1367–1372.

Bonavida, B. (1974). *J. Immunol.* **112**, 926–934.

Bonavida, B. (1977a). *J. Exp. Med.* **145**, 293–301.

Bonavida, B. (1977b). *J. Immunol.* **119**, 1530–1533.

Borberg, H., Oettgen, H. F., Choudy, K., and Beattie, E. J. (1972). *Int. J. Cancer* **10**, 539–547.

Borsos, T., Bast, R. C., Ohanian, S. H., Sereling, M., Zbar, B., and Rapp, H. J. (1976). *Ann. N.Y. Acad. Sci.* **276**, 565–571.

Boyse, E. A., and Cantor, H. (1977). *Hosp. Pract.* **12**, 81–88.

Braun, D. P., Mokyr, M. B., and Dray, S. (1978). *Cancer Res.* **38**, 1626–1632.

Brock, N. (1976). *Cancer Chemother. Rep.* **60**, 301–308.

Brunner, K. T., Maul, J., Rudolf, H., and Chapuis, B. (1970). *Immunology* **18**, 499–516.

Burton, R. C., and Warner, N. L. (1977). *Cancer Immunol. Immunother.* **2**, 91–99.

Burton, R. C., Thompson, J., and Warner, N. L. (1975). *J. Immunol. Methods* **8**, 133–150.

Cerottini, J. C., and Brunner, K. T. (1974). *Adv. Immunol.* **18**, 67–132.

Chassoux, M. D., Gotch, F. M., and MacLennan, J. C. M. (1978). *Br. J. Cancer* **38**, 211–218.

Cheever, M. A., Kempf, R. A., and Fefer, A. (1977). *J. Immunol.* **119**, 714–718.

Cheever, M. A., Greenberg, P. D., and Fefer, A. (1978). *J. Immunol.* **121**, 2220–2227.

Cheever, M. A., Greenberg, P. D., and Fefer, A. (1981a). *J. Immunol.* **126**, 1318–1322.

Cheever, M. A., Greenberg, P. D., and Fefer, A. (1981b). *Cancer Res.* **41**, 2658–2663.

Cohen, A. M., Millar, R. C., and Ketcham, A. S. (1972). *Transplantation* **13**, 57–60.

Cohen, I. R. (1973). *Cell. Immunol.* **8**, 209–220.

Delorme, E. J., and Alexander, P. (1964). *Lancet* **2**, 117–120.

Diamantstein, T., Willinger, E., and Reiman, J. (1979). *J. Exp. Med.* **150**, 1571–1576.

Durkin, H. G., and Thorbecke, G. J. (1972). *Nature (London) New Biol.* **238**, 53–54.

Elgert, K. D., and Farrar, W. L. (1978). *J. Immunol.* **120**, 1345–1353.

Elkins, W. L. (1971). *Prog. Allergy* **15**, 78–187.

Engers, H. D., and MacDonald, H. R. (1976). *Contemp. Top. Immunol.* **5**, 145–180.

Fakhri, O., and Hobbs, J. R. (1972). *Nature (London) New Biol.* **235**, 177–178.

Faraci, R. P. (1974). *Surgery* **76**, 469–471.

Fefer, A. (1970). *Int. J. Cancer* **5**, 327–337.

Fefer, A., Einstein, A. B., and Cheever, M. A. (1976). *Ann. Acad. Sci.* **277**, 492–504.

Feldman, M., Cohen, I. R., and Wekerle, H. (1972). *Transplant. Rev.* **12**, 57–90.

Fernandez-Cruz, E., Halliburton, B., and Feldman, J. D. (1979). *J. Immunol.* **123**, 1772–1777.

Fogel, M., Gorelik, E., Segal, S., and Feldman, M. (1979). *J. Natl. Cancer Inst.* **62**, 585–588.

Folch, H., and Waksman, B. H. (1973). *Cell. Immunol.* **9**, 12–24.

Fortner, G. W., Kuperman, O., and Lucas, Z. J. (1975). *J. Immunol.* **115**, 1269–1276.

Germain, R. N., and Benacerraf, B. (1980). *Springer Sem. Immunopathol.* **3**, 93–127.

Gillette, S., and Bellanti, J. A. (1973). *Cell. Immunol.* **8**, 311–320.

Gillis, S., and Smith, K. A. (1977). *Nature (London)* **268**, 154–156.

Gillis, S., Baker, P. E., Ruscetti, F. W., and Smith, K. A. (1978a). *J. Exp. Med.* **148**, 1093–1098.

Gillis, S., Ferm, M. M., Ou, W., and Smith, K. L. (1978b). *J. Immunol.* **120**, 2027–2032.

Ginsburg, H. (1968). *Immunology* **14**, 621–635.

Glaser, M. (1979). *J. Exp. Med.* **149**, 774–779.

Glaser, M., Lavrin, D. H., and Herberman, R. B. (1976). *J. Immunol.* **116**, 1507–1511.

Gordon, D., Bray, M. A., and Morley, J. (1976). *Nature (London)* **262**, 401–402.

Greenberg, P., Cheever, M., and Fefer, A. (1980). *Cancer Res.* **40**, 4428–4432.

Hamuro, J., Wagner, H., and Rollinghoff, M. (1978). *Cell. Immunol.* **38**, 328–335.

Hardt, C., Pfizenmaier, K., Rollinghoff, M., Klein, J., and Wagner, H. (1980). *J. Exp. Med.* **152**, 1413–1418.

Harris, J. W., MacDonald, H. R., Engers, H. D., Fitch, F. W., and Cerottini, J.-C. (1976). *J. Immunol.* **116**, 1071–1077.

Hawrylko, E. (1977). *J. Natl. Cancer Inst.* **59**, 359–365.

Hawrylko, E., and Macaness, G. B. (1973). *J. Natl. Cancer Inst.* **51**, 1677–1682.

Hengst, J. C. D., Mokyr, M. B., and Dray, S. (1980). *Cancer Res.* **40**, 2135–2141.

Hengst, J. C. D., Mokyr, M. B., and Dray, S. (1981). *Cancer Res.* **41**, 2163–2167.

Herberman, R. B. (1974). *Adv. Cancer Res.* **19**, 207–263.

Hibbs, J. B. (1975). *Transplantation* **19**, 77–81.

Hodes, R. J., and Terry, W. D. (1974). *J. Immunol.* **113**, 39–44.

Howell, S. B., Dean, J. H., Esber, E. C., and Law, L. W. (1974). *Int. J. Cancer* **14**, 662–674.

Humes, J. L., Bonney, R. J., Pelus, L. M., Dahlgren, M. E., Sadowski, S. J., Kuehl, F. A., and Davies, P. (1977). *Nature (London)* **269**, 149–151.

Igarashi, T., Rodrigues, D., and Ting, C.-C. (1979). *J. Immunol.* **122**, 1519–1527.

Jagarlamoddy, S. M., Aust, T. C., Tew, R. N., and McKhann, C. F. (1971). *Proc. Natl. Acad. Sci. U.S.A.* **68**, 1346–1350.

Jeejeebhoy, H. F. (1974). *Int. J. Cancer* **13**, 665–677.

Kedar, E., and Lupu, T. (1978). *J. Immunol. Methods* **21**, 35–50.

Kedar, E., and Weiss, D. W. (1982). *In* "Immunogenicity" (F. Borek, ed.), 2nd ed. (in press).

Kedar, E., Unger, E., and Schwartzbach, M. (1976). *J. Immunol. Methods* **13**, 1–19.

Kedar, E., Nahas, F., Unger, E., and Weiss, D. W. (1978a). *J. Natl. Cancer Inst.* **60**, 1097–1106.

Kedar, E., Raanan, Z., and Schwartzbach, M. (1978b). *Cancer Immunol. Immunother.* **4**, 161–169.

Kedar, E., Schwartzbach, M., Hefetz, S., and Raanan, Z. (1978c). *Cancer Immunol. Immunother.* **4**, 151–160.

Kende, M., Keys, L. D., Gaston, M., and Goldin, A. (1975). *Cancer Res.* **35**, 346–351.

Kirchner, H., Chused, T. M., Herberman, R. B., Holden, H. T., and Lavrin, D. H. (1974). *J. Exp. Med.* **139**, 1432–1487.

Kirchner, H., Muchmoke, A. V., Chused, T. M., Holden, H. T., and Herberman, R. B. (1975). *J. Immunol.* **114**, 206–210.

Klein, G. (1966). *Annu. Rev. Microbiol.* **20**, 223–252.

Klimpel, G. R., and Henney, C. S. (1978). *J. Immunol.* **120**, 563–569.

Kline, I., Gang, M., Tyrer, D. D., Mantel, N., Vendittti, J. J., and Goldin, A. (1968). *Chemotherapy* **13**, 28–41.

Kuperman, O., Fortner, G. W., and Lucas, Z. J. (1975a). *J. Immunol.* **115**, 1277–1281.

Kuperman, O., Fortner, G. W., and Lucas, Z. J. (1975b). *J. Immunol.* **115**, 1282–1287.

Leclerc, J. C., Gomard, E., Plata, F., and Levy, J. P. (1973). *Int. J. Cancer* **11**, 426–432.

Levy, J. G., Maier, T., and Kilburn, D. G. (1979). *J. Immunol.* **122**, 766–771.

Lubet, R. A., and Carlson, D. E. (1977). *Cancer Immunol. Immunother.* **2**, 267–270.

Lubet, R. A., and Carlson, D. E. (1978). *J. Natl. Cancer Inst.* **61**, 896–903.

Mathe, G., Halle-Pannenko, O., and Bourut, C. (1977). *Cancer Immunol. Immunother.* **2**, 139–141.

Mills, G. B., and Paetkau, V. (1980). *J. Immunol.* **125,** 1897–1903.
Mills, G. B., Carlson, G., and Paetkau, V. (1980). *J. Immunol.* **125,** 1904–1909.
Mitchell, M. S., Kirkpatrick, D., Mokyr, M. B., and Gery, I. (1973). *Nature (London) New Biol.* **243,** 216–218.
Mokyr, M. B., and Mitchell, M. S. (1975). *Cell. Immunol.* **15,** 264–273.
Mokyr, M. B., Braun, D. P., Usher, D., Reiter, H., and Dray, S. (1978). *Cancer Immunol. Immunother.* **4,** 143–150.
Mokyr, M. B., Braun, D. P., and Dray, S. (1979a). *Cancer Res.* **29,** 785–792.
Mokyr, M. B., Hengst, J. C. D., Przepiorka, D., and Dray, S. (1979b). *Cancer Res.* **39,** 3928–3934.
Mokyr, M. B., Przepiorka, D., and Dray, S. (1979c). *Proc. Am. Assoc. Cancer. Res.* **20,** 13.
Mokyr, M. B., Bennett, J. A., Braun, D. P., Hengst, J. C. D., Mitchell, M. S., and Dray, S. (1980). *J. Natl. Cancer Inst.* **64,** 339–344.
Moore, M., and Williams, D. E. (1973). *Int. J. Cancer* **11,** 358–368.
Mosier, D. E. (1967). *Science* **158,** 1573–1575.
Nablholz, M., Engers, H. D., Collavo, D., and North, M. (1978). *Curr. Top. Microbiol. Immunol.* **81,** 176–187.
Ogawa, M., Bergsagel, D. E., and McCulloch, E. A. (1973). *Blood* **41,** 7–15.
Okumura, K., Herzenberg, L. A., Murphy, D. B., McDevitt, H. O., and Herzenberg, L. A. (1976). *J. Exp. Med.* **144,** 685–698.
Old, L. J., and Boyse, E. A. (1964). *Annu. Rev. Med.* **15,** 167–186.
Pellis, N. R., Mokyr, M. B., and Kahan, B. D. (1977). *Proc. Am. Assoc. Cancer Res.* **18,** 138.
Pellis, N. R., Mokyr, M. B., Babcock, J. R., and Kahan, B. D. (1978). *Immunol. Commun.* **7,** 431–440.
Pelus, L. M., and Strausser, H. R. (1976). *Int. J. Cancer* **18,** 653–660.
Pelus, L. M., and Strausser, H. R. (1977). *Life Sci.* **20,** 903–913.
Perlman, P., and Holm, G. (1969). *Adv. Immunol.* **11,** 117–193.
Pierce, C. W., Kapp, J. A., Wood, D. W., and Benacerraf, B. (1974). *J. Immunol.* **112,** 1181–1189.
Pilarski, L. (1979). *Eur. J. Immunol.* **9,** 454–460.
Pimm, M. V., and Baldwin, R. W. (1977). *Int. J. Cancer* **20,** 37–43.
Palata, F., Cerottini, J.-C., and Brunner, K. T. (1975). *Eur. J. Immunol.* **5,** 227–233.
Pope, B. L., Whitney, R. B., and Levy, J. G. (1978). *J. Immunol.* **120,** 2033–2040.
Prehn, R. T. (1972). *Science* **176,** 170–171.
Przepiorka, D., Mokyr, M. B., and Dray, S. (1980). *Cancer Res.* **40,** 4565–4570.
Radov, L. A., Haskill, J. S., and Korn, J. H. (1976). *Int. J. Cancer* **17,** 773–779.
Ray, P. K., and Simmons, R. L. (1973). *Proc. Soc. Exp. Biol. Med.* **142,** 217–222.
Rollinghoff, M., and Wagner, H. (1973). *J. Natl. Cancer Inst.* **51,** 1317–1318.
Rosenberg, S. A., and Terry, W. D. (1977). *Adv. Cancer Res.* **25,** 323–388.
Rosenberg, S. A., Schwarz, S., and Spiess, P. J. (1978a). *J. Immunol.* **121,** 1951–1955.
Rosenberg, S. A., Spiess, P. J., and Schwarz, S. (1978b). *J. Immunol.* **121,** 1946–1950.
Rouse, B. T., and Wagner, H. (1973). *Transplantation* **16,** 161–170.
Rouse, B. T., Rollinghoff, M., and Harris, A. W. (1972). *J. Immunol.* **108,** 1352–1361.
Rouse, B. T., Rollinghoff, M., and Warner, N. L. (1973). *Eur. J. Immunol.* **3,** 218–224.
Russell, J. H., Hale, A. H., Ginns, L. C., and Eisen, H. N. (1978). *Proc. Natl. Acad. Sci. U.S.A.* **5,** 441–445.
Ryser, J.-E., Cerottini, J.-C., and Brunner, K. T. (1979). *Eur. J. Immunol.* **9,** 179–184.
Schechter, B., Treves, A. J., and Feldman, M. (1976). *J. Natl. Cancer Inst.* **56,** 975–979.
Schechter, B. Segal, S., and Feldman, M. (1977). *Int. J. Cancer* **20,** 239–246.

Schirrmacher, V., Bosslet, K., Shantz, G., Claver, K., and Hijdsch, D. (1979). *Int. J. Cancer* **23**, 245–252.
Shearer, G. M. (1974). *Eur. J. Immunol.* **4**, 527–533.
Silva, A., Bonavida, B., and Targan, S. (1980). *J. Immunol.* **125**, 479–484.
Sjogren, H. O. (1965). *Prog. Exp. Tumor Res.* **6**, 289–322.
Small, M., and Trainin, A. (1976). *J. Immunol.* **117**, 292–297.
Strausser, J. L., and Rosenberg, S. A. (1978). *J. Immunol.* **121**, 1491–1495.
Sugarbaker, E. V., and Cohen, A. M. (1972). *Surgery* **72**, 155–161.
Tada, T., Taniguchi, M., and David, C. S. (1976). *J. Exp. Med.* **144**, 713–725.
Takasugi, M., and Klein, E. (1970). *Transplantation* **9**, 219–227.
Takei, F., Levy, J. G., and Kilburn, D. G. (1976). *J. Immunol.* **116**, 288–292.
Tarro, G. (1973). *Proc. Natl. Acad. Sci. U.S.A.* **70**, 325–327.
Ting, C-C, Rodrigues, D., and Igarashi, T. (1979). *J. Immunol.* **122**, 1510–1518.
Treves, A. J. (1978). *Immunol. Rev.* **40**, 205–226.
Treves, A. J., Cohen, I. R., and Feldman, M. (1975). *J. Natl. Cancer Inst.* **54**, 777–780.
Treves, A. J., Cohen, I. R., Schechter, B., and Feldman, M. (1976a). *Ann. N.Y. Acad. Sci.* **276**, 165–175.
Treves, A. J., Schechter, B., Cohen, I. R., and Feldman, M. (1976b). *J. Immunol.* **116**, 1059–1064.
Treves, A. J., Honsik, C., Feldman, M., and Kaplan, H. S. (1979). *Cancer Immunol. Immunother.* **6**, 179–184.
Wagner, H., Harris, A., and Feldman, M. (1972). *Cell. Immunol.* **4**, 39–50.
Wagner, H., Rollinghoff, M., and Nossal, J. G. V. (1973). *Transplant. Rev.* **17**, 3–36.
Watson, J. (1979). *J. Exp. Med.* **150**, 1510–1519.
Weiss, D. W., Kuperman, O., Fathallah, N., and Kedar, E. (1976). *Ann. N.Y. Acad. Sci.* **276**, 536–549.
Wing, E. J., and Remington, J. S. (1977). *Cell. Immunol.* **30**, 108–121.
Winn, H. J. (1959). *Natl. Cancer Inst. Monogr.* **2**, 113–138.
Wunderlich, J. R., and Canty, T. G. (1970). *Nature* (*London*) **228**, 62–63.
Yoshinaga, M., Yoshinaga, A., and Waksman, B. H. (1972). *J. Exp. Med.* **136**, 956–961.
Zatz, M. M. (1971). *J. Exp. Med.* **134**, 224–241.
Zatz, M. M., and Lance, E. M. (1970). *Cell. Immunol.* **1**, 3–17.

INDEX

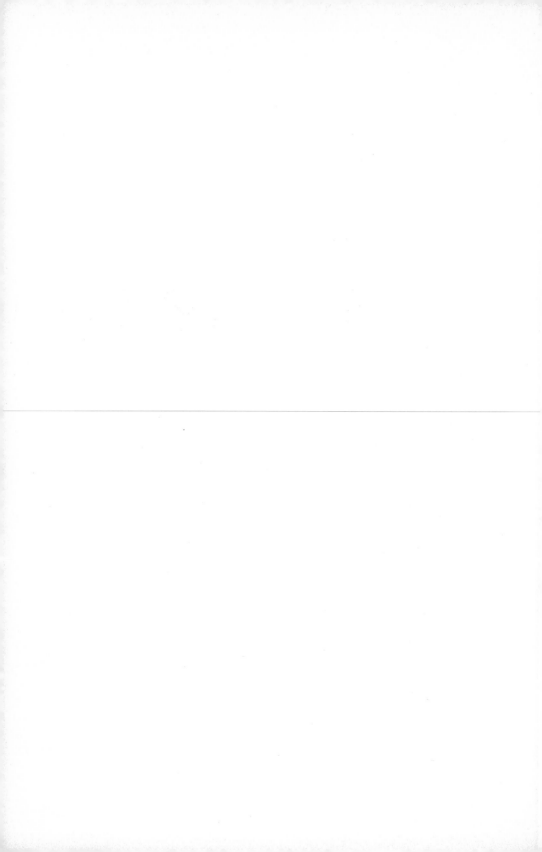